Today's Health Care Issues

Recent Titles in the Across the Aisle Series

Today's Social Issues: Democrats and Republicans
Timothy W. Kneeland

Today's Economic Issues: Democrats and Republicans
Nancy S. Lind, Erik T. Rankin, and Gardenia Harris

Today's Foreign Policy Issues: Democrats and Republicans
Trevor Rubenzer

Today's Environmental Issues: Democrats and Republicans
Teri J. Walker

Today's Health Care Issues

Democrats and Republicans

ROBERT B. HACKEY AND TODD M. OLSZEWSKI

Across the Aisle

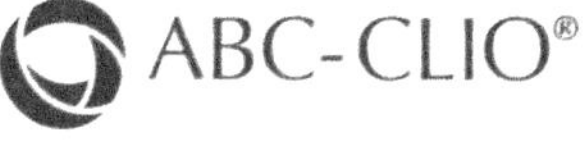

An Imprint of ABC-CLIO, LLC
Santa Barbara, California • Denver, Colorado

Library of Congress Cataloging-in-Publication Data

Names: Hackey, Robert B., author. | Olszewski, Todd M., author.
Title: Today's health care issues : Democrats and Republicans / Robert B. Hackey and Todd M. Olszewski.
Description: Santa Barbara, California : ABC-CLIO, [2021] | Series: Across the aisle | Includes bibliographical references and index.
Identifiers: LCCN 2021000781 (print) | LCCN 2021000782 (ebook) | ISBN 9781440869150 (hardcover) | ISBN 9781440869167 (ebook)
Subjects: LCSH: Medical care—United States. | Medical policy—United States. | Health services administration—United States. | Health—Government policy—United States. | COVID-19 (Disease)—Political aspects—United States.
Classification: LCC RA395.A3 H3314 2021 (print) | LCC RA395.A3 (ebook) | DDC 362.10973—dc23
LC record available at https://lccn.loc.gov/2021000781
LC ebook record available at https://lccn.loc.gov/2021000782

ISBN: 978-1-4408-6915-0 (print)
978-1-4408-6916-7 (ebook)

25 24 23 22 21 1 2 3 4 5

This book is also available as an eBook.

ABC-CLIO
An Imprint of ABC-CLIO, LLC

ABC-CLIO, LLC
147 Castilian Drive
Santa Barbara, California 93117
www.abc-clio.com

This book is printed on acid-free paper ∞
Manufactured in the United States of America

Contents

Introduction

Health policy in the United States is at a crossroads. Will policy makers and the public embrace a larger role for government to address the challenges facing the U.S. health care system? Or will key decisions remain in the hands of providers and other private-sector actors? The 2020 presidential election offered Americans a stark choice about the future direction of U.S. health policy, as health policy issues emerged as a key litmus test for both Democrats and Republicans. During the preceding decade, "divisions in both American society and its politics have widened and hardened" (Seib 2019). These divisions are particularly evident in heated debates over abortion, contraception coverage, the individual health insurance mandate, and Medicaid expansion, among others. The parties' positions on these contested issues, in turn, reflected deep-seated and strongly held beliefs about the proper role of government in American society. While Democrats championed a greater role for government in solving social problems, Republicans prescribed private, market-based policy reforms.

Health policy is not a new battlefield for partisan politics. Democrats and Republicans sparred over national health insurance for most of the 20th century. Current policy debates often evoke a sense of nostalgia: "Democrats talk about public policy as though it were always 1965 and the model of the Great Society welfare state will answer our every concern. And Republicans talk as though it were always 1981 and a repetition of the Reagan Revolution is the cure for what ails us. It is hardly surprising that the public finds the resulting political debates frustrating" (Levin 2017, 15).

President Barack Obama won a historic victory with the passage of the Affordable Care Act (ACA) in 2010, but it came at a high political price. Democrats enacted "Obamacare" without a single Republican vote; ongoing Republican opposition to the ACA led to midterm debacles for Democrats in 2010 and 2014. After regaining control over both houses of Congress in 2014, Republicans worked tirelessly to repeal, replace, or restrict the scope of the ACA. Republican proposals to overturn the ACA sputtered out in 2017, but Republican governors and attorneys general mounted new legal challenges. As James Morone (2014) observed, "There has not been this much conflict over a Congressional act since prohibition." Democrats and Republicans remain locked in a policy stalemate at the federal level. The ACA survived despite repeated attempts to repeal and replace it by Republicans in Congress (and later by the Trump administration). Nevertheless, Republicans succeeded in weakening the law in 2017 by eliminating penalties for individuals who did not purchase health insurance.

Abortion remains a fiercely contested partisan issue nearly five decades after the U.S. Supreme Court's landmark decision in *Roe v. Wade*. The two parties have offered voters diametrically opposing views on this hot-button issue. Donald Trump became the first sitting U.S. president to formally address pro-life supporters when he gave remarks at the annual March for Life in January 2020. All the candidates who sought the 2020 Democratic presidential nomination opposed restrictions on abortion, indicating how pro-life Democrats are now an endangered species (Bailey 2020). Meanwhile, all Republicans in the 2020 House of Representatives held pro-life views, as did all but two Republican senators—thus making pro-choice Republicans an endangered species on the GOP side (Peterson 2019).

Democrats and Republicans continued to wrestle over health policy in a hotly contested electoral environment. Since 2000, both parties have grappled with unstable electoral majorities. Party control of the House, Senate, or White House changed in seven of the nine elections between 2000 and 2016 (Taranto 2018). This trend continued in the 2018 midterm elections when Democrats regained control over the House of Representatives for the first time since 2010. Such intense party competition left control over Congress up for grabs in nearly every election cycle. Under these circumstances, members of the minority party have little incentive to compromise, for victory in the next election could bring a switch in party control and a new governing majority. Consequently, the American political environment has become a "landscape infused with partisanship, polarization, and mutual intolerance. Simmering tensions over politics, economics, and culture have metastasized into an overarching us-versus-them environment" (West 2019, 3).

In such a sharply polarized political environment, the courts emerged as the final arbiter of many controversial health policy questions. In a series of cases beginning in 2012, the U.S. Supreme Court became a pivotal health policy battleground. While the ACA survived two challenges by narrow 5–4 majorities in the cases of *NFIB v. Sebelius* (2012) and *King v. Burwell* (2015), the Roberts Court upheld limits on the ACA's contraception mandate in *Burwell v. Hobby Lobby Stores* (2014).

The Trump administration recognized the significance of the courts as policy makers immediately after taking the reins of the federal government in January 2017 and quickly joined forces with Senate Republicans in an effort to remake the federal judiciary. By the end of his term in office, Donald Trump had nominated—and the Senate confirmed—more than 220 conservative appointees to the federal bench. The confirmation process became a partisan battleground; most judges (77 percent) nominated by President Trump faced a cloture vote in the U.S. Senate, and nearly half (45 percent) were confirmed over the opposition of 25 percent or more senators (Heritage Foundation 2020). However, the Trump administration's success in shepherding nominees through the confirmation process shifted the partisan balance on federal appellate courts and cemented a 6–3 majority on the U.S. Supreme Court with the appointments of Justices Amy Coney Barrett, Neil Gorsuch, and Brett Kavanaugh. By February 2020, Republican presidents had appointed more than half (54 percent) of all active federal appellate judges (Wheeler 2020).

Public opinion polls paint a picture of an electorate where parties are ideologically distinct and deeply polarized. A 2019 poll from the New Center (a bipartisan policy institute) found that two-thirds (65 percent) of Republicans identified with the right, while 27 percent identified with the center on a left-right spectrum. In contrast, 42 percent of Democrats identified with the left and an equal number with the center (Galston 2019). As a result, "one major party has a dominant ideology while the other is divided down the middle" (Galston 2019). Rather than a political realignment, the United States appears to be undergoing a "dealignment" as more Americans describe themselves as political independents (42 percent) than identify with either the Democratic (27 percent) or Republican (27 percent) party (Jones 2019).

While the parties remain locked in a fierce battle for control over Congress and the presidency, the states tell a very different story. At the state level, "America has been experiencing a slow-motion realignment, with broad swaths of the country now off-limits to one party or the other" (Greenblatt 2019). The decline in party competition at the state level has broad implications for health policy, for "in most states, either Democrats or Republicans have held power for years and are unlikely to give it up any time soon" (Greenblatt 2019). The U.S. Supreme Court's decision in the case of *NFIB v. Sebelius*, in particular, underscored the significance of states in shaping health policy, as the justices allowed states to decide whether or not to expand their Medicaid programs, effectively shifting health policy decision-making from Washington, DC, to state capitals. In the wake of the court's decision, a majority of states—most with Republican governors or Republican-controlled legislatures—refused to expand their Medicaid programs. As a result, "Democratic and Republican states are moving in opposite directions on health policy, leaving Americans with starkly divergent options for care depending on where they live" (Armour 2018). California, for example, not only embraced the Affordable Care Act (ACA) but also opted to extend health insurance coverage to undocumented immigrants in 2019. In contrast, Republican state attorneys general continue to fight the ACA in court, and Republican governors and legislatures have enacted new restrictions on abortion providers in recent years.

Markets and Health Care

Should government use its power to regulate the behavior of health providers, payers, and patients, or should it embrace a more laissez-faire approach to encourage competition and innovation? Democrats emphasize the importance of values such as equality and equity in making health policy, while Republicans prioritize choice, efficiency, and personal liberty. In part, this reflects a significant difference in how the parties think about liberty itself. Democrats are more committed to what Isaiah Berlin (2002) described as a "positive" conception of liberty in health care: individuals should be able to realize their potential in life. Poor health limits individuals' ability to work, provide for their families, and achieve their life goals. Thus, Democrats embrace the notion of health care as a social right by supporting policies that expand access to health insurance, reduce health disparities, and prevent illness through public programs. Republicans, in contrast, embrace what Berlin describes as a "negative" concept of liberty. In this view, liberty is the absence of constraint over one's life choices. Thus, while Democrats supported mandates requiring individuals to purchase health insurance or for states to expand their Medicaid programs, Republicans assailed these policies as unwarranted constraints on choice.

Public opinion polls underscore the partisan divide between Democrats and Republicans over government intervention in the marketplace. Seventy-nine percent of Democrats who responded to a 2020 Pew Research poll believed government "should do more to solve problems," but 78 percent of Republicans said government "is doing too many things better left to businesses and individuals" (Pew Research Center 2020). Instead of greater regulation, Republicans favor competitive markets as a way to improve efficiency, drive innovation, and lower costs. Democrats, in contrast, argue that an unregulated business model will adversely affect poor and vulnerable populations while making the rich richer. Most Democrats (78 percent) surveyed in the aforementioned Pew poll agreed that "government regulation of business is necessary to protect the public interest." In contrast, two-thirds (66 percent) of Republicans believed that "government regulation of business usually does more harm than good" (Pew Research Center 2020). Republicans regard free markets and entrepreneurship, rather than publicly funded social programs, as the best vehicles to achieve economic and social progress.

A similar divide appears in congressional voting. In December 2019, House Democrats passed legislation that would permit the Secretary of Health and Human Services to negotiate prices for up to 250 high-cost drugs by a margin of 230 to 192 (Cancryn and Owermohle 2019). While every House Democrat supported the bill, all but two Republican representatives opposed the measure. House Republicans denounced the proposal as a form of creeping socialism and warned that government efforts to set drug prices would stymie innovation and threaten the prospects for developing new cures (Steinhauer 2019). As Sen. Marco Rubio (R-FL) argued, capitalism is an "economic model that allows everyone to rise without pulling anyone down . . . [to] make poor people richer without making rich people poor" (*Washington Post* 2016). Instead of government price setting or expanded regulation, Republicans aim to create "market conditions long proven to bring down prices while improving equality—empowering consumers to seek value, increasing the supply of care, and stimulating competition" (Atlas 2017).

Debates about appropriate levels of government intervention in the marketplace also underscored a deeper divide about public trust in government itself.

Trust in Government

Public trust in government—particularly in the federal government—has fallen precipitously over the past several decades. The Pew Research Center (2019b) reported that the proportion of Americans who "trust the federal government to do what is right just about always or most of the time" declined from 77 percent in 1964 to 17 percent in 2019. Efforts to control costs, increase access to care, or improve the quality of care typically entail an expanded role for government through taxes and regulations that shape the behavior of patients, providers, and payers. As a result, declining public trust in government disproportionately constrains Democrats who seek to address health disparities or control costs by using public funding or regulatory powers. In a 2017 poll, two-thirds (67 percent) of Americans cited "big government" as the principal threat to the country in the future (Fishman and Davis 2017). While Republicans (81 percent) were more likely to view government as a threat than Democrats (51 percent), pervasive skepticism about the role of government creates significant challenges for reformers seeking to remake the U.S. health care system.

Democrats tend to view government as a benevolent problem solver, but Republicans often regard the use of public power as a threat to liberty. The Democratic party's platform, for example, noted that "Democrats have been fighting to secure universal health care for the American people for generations, and we are proud to be the party that passed Medicare, Medicaid, and the Affordable Care Act" (Democratic National Committee 2020). Most candidates seeking the 2020 Democratic presidential nomination supported either a Medicare "buy-in" or some version of "Medicare for All" to provide universal coverage for all Americans. A strong commitment to universal health care is now a core tenet of the Democratic party's social and economic agenda. Republicans, in contrast, remain steadfastly opposed to such an expansion of federal authority in health care and believe that states—not the federal government—should take the lead in health care reform. Seema Verma, the director of the Centers for Medicare and Medicaid Services under President Trump, declared that health care reform must "preserve the right of states to shape your programs in ways that are consistent with the needs of your residents, your cultures and your values. Anything less stifles innovation" (Galewitz 2019).

Taxes and Spending

In recent decades, Democrats and Republicans have responded in different ways to growing inequalities in wealth and income. In one 2020 poll, 61 percent of Democratic and Democratic-leaning voters supported "more assistance to people in need." This view, however, was shared by only 13 percent of Republican voters (Pew Research Center 2020). The survey also found public opinion split along partisan lines on whether upper-income Americans pay enough in taxes. Most Democrats (75 percent) say the rich pay too little in taxes, but this view is shared by less than half of Republicans (45 percent) (Newport 2016). Furthermore, while 80 percent of Democrats polled in a 2016 survey favor increasing taxes on the wealthy to fund redistributive programs, only 22 percent of Republicans support this notion (Newport 2016). By 2020, meanwhile, Pew Research found that 68 percent of Democratic voters described economic inequality as a "very big" problem for the country today, but only 16 percent of Republican voters agreed (Pew Research Center 2020).

Individual Responsibility and Social Determinants of Health

Is health largely determined by personal choices or by social circumstances? Republicans seek to empower individuals to make choices; their perspective emphasizes the importance of "earned success" and hard work (Brooks 2015). Polls underscore Republicans' belief in individual responsibility; in one 2020 poll, 82 percent of Republican voters agreed that "most people who want to get ahead can make it if they're willing to work hard" (Pew Research Center 2020). As a result, Republicans prefer private, rather than public, solutions for most health policy challenges. For example, Republicans responding to the aforementioned 2020 poll overwhelmingly rejected "Medicare for All" proposals that would end private insurance for Americans—78 percent of Republican voters opposed such a plan (Pew Research Center 2020).

For Democrats, health care is a basic human right. In 2020, for example, all Democratic presidential candidates favored some form of universal coverage, even though they often disagreed on the best approach to achieving this goal. As Sen. Elizabeth Warren (D-MA) declared, "Medicare for All is the best way to give every single person in this country a guarantee of high-quality health care. Everybody is covered. Nobody goes broke because of a medical bill" (Warren 2020a). A 2020 Pew Research poll found nearly three-quarters (74 percent) of Democratic voters favored "a single national health insurance program run by the government, sometimes called 'Medicare for all,' that would replace private insurance" (Pew Research Center 2020). Democrats' support for expanded social programs reflects a growing belief that economic opportunity within the United States is often severely limited by socioeconomic factors. The aforementioned poll found that 55 percent of Democratic voters believe that "hard work and determination are no guarantee of success for most people" (Pew Research Center 2020).

The parties' divergent views on personal responsibility for health are particularly evident in the case of Medicaid work requirements and the Trump administration's "public charge" rule. The Trump administration argued work requirements would help "families and individuals attain or retain capability for independence or self-care" (Fadulu 2019). As CMS administrator Seema Verma declared, "We owe our fellow citizens more than just giving them a Medicaid card. We owe a card with care, and more importantly a card with hope. Hope that they can break the chains of generational poverty and no longer need public assistance" (Palosky 2019). In Missouri, legislators proposed a constitutional amendment on the November 2020 ballot to add work requirements for able-bodied Medicaid recipients (Stewart 2020). Democratic governors, in contrast, strongly opposed work requirements as a condition for receiving benefits. After taking office in 2019, Maine's newly elected governor, Janet Mills, withdrew the state's application to institute work requirements for Medicaid beneficiaries that had been filed by her Republican predecessor (Hiltzik 2020).

In August 2019, Ken Cuccinelli, the director of the U.S. Citizenship and Immigration Services for the Trump administration, defended the new public charge rule that allowed federal officials to deny individuals a green card based on their use of public services such as Medicaid: "Through the public charge rule, President Trump's administration is reinforcing the ideals of self-sufficiency and personal responsibility, ensuring that immigrants are able to support themselves and become successful here in America" (Cuccinelli 2019). Democrats expressed outrage at the new requirements. As Sen Mazie Hirono (D-HI) argued, "the true intent of the public charge rule is to create a climate of fear among immigrant families, and sadly its working" (Rodrigo 2019). Democrats raised additional concerns about the impact of the requirement on immigrants' use of health care services—such as testing and treatment for coronavirus—in March 2020. Rep. Raúl M. Grijalva (D-AZ) claimed that "Trump's public charge rule is deterring vulnerable immigrant communities from accessing care in the middle of a public health crisis" (Moreno 2020).

Pandemics and Public Health

The novel coronavirus pandemic presented an unprecedented challenge for the U.S. health care system. Federal, state, and local officials took drastic steps in an effort to "flatten the curve" of new cases to avoid overwhelming overburdened hospitals. Public responses to the pandemic, however, underscored the stark divide between Democratic and Republican perceptions of both the threat and the necessity for a vigorous response. Democrats called for swift and decisive action to protect the health of the public and save lives. The Trump administration, in contrast, downplayed initial media warnings about the pandemic. In his first public statement on the coronavirus in the United States, President Donald Trump reassured the public that "we have it totally under control. It's one person coming in from China, and we have it under control. It's going to be just fine" (Leonhardt 2020). President Trump continued to downplay concerns about the need for significant restrictions on public gatherings or federal preparations to manage the expected surge in hospitalizations for critically ill patients (Edwards 2020). Speaking in late February, the president argued the number of cases were "going down, not up. We're going very substantially down, not up" (Leonhardt 2020). Two days before Gov. Gavin Newsom (D-CA) declared a state of emergency in California to limit the spread of the virus, President Trump told Fox News's Sean Hannity that most coronavirus cases were "very mild" (Leonhardt 2020). Ron Paul—a former Republican senator and presidential candidate—challenged the need for significant public health measures. As he argued, "People should ask themselves whether this coronavirus 'pandemic' could be a big hoax, with the actual danger of the disease massively exaggerated by those who seek to profit—financially or politically—from the ensuing panic" (Remnick 2020).

Democrats called for decisive federal action rather than a piecemeal approach to managing the pandemic. In late February, Senate Minority Leader Chuck Schumer (D-NY) declared, "Congress must act swiftly to confront the threat of this global health crisis." Schumer warned his fellow senators that "time is of the essence" (Schumer 2020). In early March—nearly two weeks before President Trump acknowledged that decisive action was needed to address the coronavirus—House Speaker Nancy Pelosi noted that "Americans urgently need a coordinated, fully-funded, whole-of-government response to keep us safe from the widening coronavirus epidemic" (Pelosi 2020). The pandemic upended the 2020 presidential nominating process, leading Sen. Bernie Sanders (I-VT) and former vice president Joe Biden to hold their final televised debate before an empty auditorium; both candidates canceled rallies and speaking events as the virus spread. Speaking to voters from his home in Delaware, Democratic presidential candidate Joe Biden argued, "This pandemic is a national emergency, akin to fighting a war" (Alter and Villa 2020).

The effectiveness of policy solutions such as social distancing, lockdowns, or other measures to slow the pace of transmission rests upon public acceptance of the need for action. The stark partisan divide in how Democrats and Republicans regarded the coronavirus threat underscores the challenges facing public health officials. A March 2020 Marist College/NPR poll found that 76 percent of Democrats believed that the coronavirus was a "real threat," while less than half of Republicans (40 percent) agreed. In contrast, a majority (54 percent) of Republicans thought warnings about the virus were "blown out of proportion" compared to only 20 percent of Democrats (Allyn and Sprunt 2020). These beliefs, in turn, shaped the personal responses of Democratic and Republican partisans to calls to change personal behaviors. For example, while 59 percent of Democrats reported they sought to avoid large gatherings, 60 percent of Republicans did not. Eating habits also reflected a similar partisan divide; 60 percent of Democrats reported eating in more often, while 63 percent of Republicans reported no changes to their eating and dining habits (Allyn and Sprunt 2020). Partisanship, in short, shaped if, and how, individuals modified their behavior in response to this historic, and indeed unprecedented, public health challenge.

Personal and Moral Decisions

Democrats and Republicans remain sharply divided over the role of government in regulating personal health care decisions. Control over one's body—or over the care provided to family members and loved ones—raises profound moral and religious concerns. These debates also shape the relationships between patients and health providers and between individuals and the state (e.g., public health officials). Many policy arenas that previously enjoyed wide bipartisan support, such as vaccination, are now intensely politicized. For example, Democratic legislators in many states spearheaded efforts to limit personal and religious exemptions to vaccination requirements, but these efforts often met with staunch opposition from Republicans. Public opinion on whether individuals should be free to make personal health care decisions without interference by the state is heavily influenced by party affiliation. Republicans often defend government regulation of personal health care decisions as necessary to preserve moral order. Democrats, in contrast, strongly support the right of individuals to determine what happens to their own bodies. For example, a 2018 Gallup poll found that 80 percent of Democrats believed that doctors should be allowed to end a patient's life at the request of patients or families compared to only 62 percent of Republicans (Brenan 2018).

Abortion underscores the partisan divide on the extent to which government should be able to regulate personal behavior. Since 1995, a majority of Americans have supported the right to abortion in all or most cases; a large majority of the public also opposed overturning the precedent established by *Roe v. Wade* in 1973 (Pew Research Center 2019a). Republicans remain evenly split on whether the Supreme Court should overturn *Roe v. Wade*: 48 percent support reversing the precedent in *Roe*, while 50 percent oppose doing so (Pew Research Center 2019c). In contrast, 87 percent of Democrats oppose any effort to overturn *Roe* (Pew Research Center 2019c). Debates over late-term abortion, meanwhile, have energized both social conservatives and reproductive rights activists. Sen. Mitch McConnell (R-KY) argued that a ban on late-term abortions would "bring our nation's regard for the unborn off this sad and radical fringe" of countries that permit the procedure. Democrats dismissed such appeals as partisan grandstanding and, in the words of Sen. Chuck Schumer (D-NY), "purely an attack on women's health care" (Stolberg 2020).

In recent years, access to care for LGBTQ+ patients also aroused intense passions and sparked heated debates between Democrats and Republicans. Section 1557 of the Affordable Care Act established new protections for LGBTQ+ patients by prohibiting discrimination in health care services or health insurance (Baker

2016). In response, several Republican-led states enacted "freedom of conscience" laws for health providers to "offer legal cover to people of faith who don't want to provide certain goods or services to LBGT people" (Green 2016). Freedom of conscience laws represented a new front in the cultural war between Democrats and Republicans. The new state laws permitted health providers "to opt out of any procedure or choose not to take on any patient if doing so would compromise their conscience" (Green 2016). In 2019, the Trump administration issued new regulations that allowed physicians, nurses, and other health professionals to opt out of "providing, participating in, paying for, or referring for healthcare services that they have personal or religious objections to" (Abutaleb 2019). House Speaker Nancy Pelosi (D-CA) vehemently opposed the new rule, which she argued would grant "an open license to discriminate against Americans who already face serious, systematic discrimination" (Kopp 2019). Republicans legislators dismissed Pelosi's objections and described the rules as an issue of religious freedom, not discrimination. As Rep. Phil Roe (R-TN) declared, "It sickens me to think we would force a health care provider to perform a procedure that violates their conscience or religious beliefs. . . . This is a simple concept—doctors should not be forced to perform abortions, assisted suicides or any other service that would violate their conscience" (Roe 2019).

A Partisan Battlefield

Health care policy making today reflects the deep fault lines separating Democrats and Republicans in contemporary American politics. Partisan polarization in Congress and ideological sorting among voters limit the prospects for bipartisan collaboration to address significant health policy problems. This heightened partisanship is reflected in ongoing struggles over the future of the Affordable Care Act. In addition, Democrats and Republicans learn about health policy issues from different news sources; recent surveys by Gallup found that a majority of Democrats relied upon a "liberal news diet" from sources such as MSNBC, the *New York Times*, or Vox, while a plurality of Republicans turned to a "conservative news diet," such as Fox News, Breitbart, or the *National Review* (Ritter 2020).

The following chapters underscore wide differences in how the United States' two major political parties view the role of government in the health care system in a wide range of policy domains, including children's health insurance, the COVID-19 pandemic, the Affordable Care Act, veterans' health care, and Medicare drug pricing reform. Other chapters highlight significant differences in perspectives between Democrats and Republicans on hotly contested issues such as abortion, assisted suicide, contraception, marijuana, and vaccination. It is our hope that the chapters in this volume enable readers to become better informed and more engaged participants in our national conversation about health care reform over the next decade.

Acknowledgments

Writing this book has been an extraordinary journey. I will always be grateful for Todd Olszewski's willingness to collaborate on this volume—this was a professional challenge unlike any other we have embarked upon. Over the past two years, we assembled a remarkable research team of student coauthors who partnered with us to create what we hope is an accessible, concise analysis of many of our country's most pressing health policy problems. No single volume can provide readers with a comprehensive snapshot of all facets of the U.S. health care system, but we hope that our chapters both inform our readers and inspire them to dig deeper into the problems discussed in the following chapters.

We are particularly grateful for the generous support we received from the Center for Engaged Learning at Providence College. The Center's support enabled us to forge a strong sense of identity for our research team. Funding from the School of Professional Studies at Providence College enabled us to hire two extraordinary student editors and research assistants during the summer of 2019 and also allowed us to hire a professional indexer for this volume. We are deeply indebted to Anne Capozzoli and Theresa Durkee for their careful attention to detail in editing our chapters and their resourcefulness in ferreting out far-flung sources over many months. This project would not have been possible without our talented team of student researchers, each of whom contributed to our volume by coauthoring one or more chapters. We owe a special debt of gratitude to Morgan Bjarno, Olivia Braga, Anne Capozzoli, Emma Collins, Theresa Durkee, Bethany Evans, Nicolette Greco, Alyssa Hartigan, Anxhela Hoti, Delaney Mayette, Amanda McGrath, Shannon McGonagle, Maureen Murphy, Shannon Rowe, Rose Shelley, Keith Vieira Jr., Emily Wall, and Erin Walsh. This book is dedicated to them.

Robert B. Hackey and Maureen Murphy

Further Reading

Abutaleb, Yasmeen. 2019. "U.S. Health Agency Finalizes Conscience and Religious Freedom Rule." Reuters, May 2. Accessed April 10, 2020. https://www.reuters.com/article/us-usa-healthcare-religion/u-s-health-agency-finalizes-conscience-and-religious-freedom-rule-idUSKCN1S81PS.

Allen, Arthur. 2019. "Republicans Reject Democratic Attempts to Tighten Vaccine Laws." Politico, April 16. Accessed January 29, 2020. https://www.politico.com/story/2019/04/16/republican-reject-democrat-vaccines-1361277.

Allyn, Bobby, and Barbara Sprunt. 2020. "Poll: As Coronavirus Spreads, Fewer Americans See Pandemic as a Real Threat." NPR, March 17.

Alter, Charlotte, and Lissandra Villa. 2020. "Welcome to the Coronavirus Campaign." *Time*, March 30.

Armour, Stephanie. 2018. "Red and Blue States Move Further Apart on Health Policy." *Wall Street Journal*, February 28. Accessed January 25, 2020. https://www.wsj.com/articles/red-and-blue-states-move-further-apart-on-health-policy-1519813801.

Atlas, Scott. 2017. "The Health Reform That Hasn't Been Tried." *Wall Street Journal*, October 3. Accessed February 24, 2020. https://www.wsj.com/articles/the-health-reform-that-hasnt-been-tried-1507071808.

Bailey, Sarah Pulliam. 2020. "Why Democrats Who Oppose Abortion Are Finding It Harder to Remain in the Party." *Washington Post*, January 31. Accessed February 1, 2020. https://www.washingtonpost.com/religion/2020/01/31/why-democrats-who-oppose-abortion-rights-are-finding-it-harder-remain-party/.

Baker, Kellan. 2016. "LGBT Protections in Affordable Care Act Section 1557." Health Affairs, *Health Affairs Blog*, June 6. Accessed April 10, 2020. https://www.healthaffairs.org/do/10.1377/hblog20160606.055155/full/.

Berlin, Isaiah. 2002. "Two Concepts of Liberty." In *Liberty: Incorporating Four Essays on Liberty*, edited by Isaiah Berlin and Henry Hardy, 2nd ed., 166–217. London: Oxford University Press.

Brenan, Megan. 2018. "Americans' Strong Support for Euthanasia Persists." Gallup, May 31. Accessed January 25, 2020. https://news.gallup.com/poll/235145/americans-strong-support-euthanasia-persists.aspx.

Brooks, Arthur. 2015. *The Conservative Heart*. New York: Broadside Books/Harper Collins.

Cancryn, Adam, and Sarah Owermohle. 2019. "House Passes Bill Requiring Drug Price Negotiations." Politico, December 12. Accessed February 19, 2020. https://www.politico.com/news/2019/12/12/house-passes-drug-pricing-bill-083792.

Cruz, Ted. 2017. "Sen. Cruz: 'By Reforming the Tax Code, We Can Make the American Dream Achievable Again.'" September 13. Accessed February 4, 2020. https://www.tedcruz.org/press-releases/sen-cruz-reforming-tax-code-can-make-american-dream-achievable/.

Cuccinelli, Ken. 2019. "Press Briefing by USCIS Acting Director Ken Cuccinelli." August 12. Accessed April 12, 2020. https://trumpwhitehouse.archives.gov/briefings-statements/press-briefing-uscis-acting-director-ken-cuccinelli-081219/.

Democratic National Committee. 2020. "Health Care." Accessed April 10, 2020. https://democrats.org/where-we-stand/the-issues/health-care/.

Edwards, Haley Sweetland. 2020. "The Trump Administration Fumbled Its Initial Response to Coronavirus. Is There Enough Time to Fix It?" *Time*, March 19. Accessed April 8, 2020. https://time.com/5805683/trump-administration-coronavirus/.

Fadulu, Lola. 2019. "Why States Want Certain Americans to Work for Medicaid." *The Atlantic Monthly*, April 12. Accessed February 24, 2020. https://www.theatlantic.com/health/archive/2019/04/medicaid-work-requirements-seema-verma-cms/587026/.

Fishman, Noam, and Alyssa Davis. 2017. "Americans Still See Government as Top Threat." Gallup, January 5. Accessed January 30, 2020. https://news.gallup.com/poll/201629/americans-big-government-top-threat.aspx.

Galewitz, Phil. 2019. "Verma Attacks Critics of Medicaid Work Requirement, Pushes for Tighter Eligibility." *Kaiser Health News*, November 12. Accessed January 30, 2020. https://khn.org/news/verma-attacks-critics-of-medicaid-work-requirement-pushes-for-tighter-eligibility/.

Gallup. 2020. "Party Affiliation." Accessed January 25, 2020. https://news.gallup.com/poll/15370/party-affiliation.aspx.

Galston, William. 2019. "Polarized America Still Has a Big Middle." *Wall Street Journal*, December 3. Accessed January 29, 2020. https://www.wsj.com/articles/polarized-america-still-has-a-big-middle-11575417229.

Golshan, Tara. 2019. "Bernie Sanders Defines His Vision for Democratic Socialism in the United States." Vox, June 12. Accessed January 21, 2020. https://www.vox.com/2019/6/12/18663217/bernie-sanders-democratic-socialism-speech-transcript.

Green, Emma. 2016. "When Doctors Refuse to Treat LGBT Patients." *The Atlantic*, April 19. Accessed April 10, 2020. https://www.theatlantic.com/health/archive/2016/04/medical-religious-exemptions-doctors-therapists-mississippi-tennessee/478797/.

Greenblatt, Alan. 2019. "All or Nothing: How State Politics Became a Winner-Take-All World." Governing, January. Accessed February 6, 2020. https://www.governing.com/topics/politics/gov-state-politics-governors-2019.html.

Heritage Foundation. 2020. "Judicial Appointment Tracker." Accessed March 1, 2020. https://www.heritage.org/judicialtracker.

Hiltzik, Michael. 2020. "The Red State Craze for Costly and Useless Medicaid Work Requirements Is Disappearing." *Los Angeles Times*, January 10. Accessed February 24, 2020. https://www.latimes.com/business/story/2020-01-10/red-state-medicaid-work-requirements.

Jones, Jeffrey M. 2019. "Americans Continue to Embrace Political Independence." Gallup, January 7. Accessed January 25, 2020. https://news.gallup.com/poll/245801/americans-continue-embrace-political-independence.aspx.

Jones, Jeffrey M., and Lydia Saad. 2019. "U.S. Support for More Government Inches Up, but Not for Socialism." Gallup, November 18. Accessed January 21, 2020. https://news.gallup.com/poll/268295/support-government-inches-not-socialism.aspx.

Kaplan, Thomas. 2019. "Bernie Sanders Proposes a Wealth Tax: 'I Don't Think That Billionaires Should Exist.'" *New York Times*, September 24. Accessed February 5, 2020. https://www.nytimes.com/2019/09/24/us/politics/bernie-sanders-wealth-tax.html.

Kopp, Emily. 2019. "'Downright Deadly': Pelosi Rips Trump Rule Allowing Providers to Deny Care to LGBTQ, Women." Roll Call, May 3. Accessed April 10, 2020. https://www.rollcall.com/2019/05/03/downright-deadly-pelosi-rips-trump-rule-allowing-providers-to-deny-care-to-lgbtq-women/.

Leonhardt, David. 2020. "A Complete List of Trump's Attempts to Play Down Coronavirus." *New York Times*, March 15. Accessed April 8, 2020. https://www.nytimes.com/2020/03/15/opinion/trump-coronavirus.html.

Levin, Yuval. 2017. *The Fractured Republic*. New York: Basic Books.

Moreau, Julie. 2018. "Texas Judge Who Struck Down ACA to Weigh in on Transgender Health Case." NBC News, December 20. Accessed April 10, 2020. https://www.nbcnews.com/feature/nbc-out/texas-judge-who-struck-down-aca-weigh-transgender-health-case-n950501.

Moreno, J. Edward. 2020. "Dozens of Democrats Raise Concerns over 'Public Charge' Rule and Coronavirus Response." The Hill, March 11. Accessed April 12, 2020. https://thehill.com/homenews/house/486856-democrats-raise-concerns-public-charge-rule-coronavirus-response.

Morone, James A. 2014. *The Devils We Know: Us and Them in America's Raucous Political Culture*. Topeka: University Press of Kansas.

Newport, Frank. 2016. "Americans Still Say Upper-Income Pay Too Little in Taxes." Gallup, April 15. Accessed March 2, 2020. https://news.gallup.com/poll/190775/americans-say-upper-income-pay-little-taxes.aspx.

Newport, Frank. 2019a. "Americans' Long-Standing Interest in Taxing the Rich." Gallup, February 22. Accessed February 24, 2020. https://news.gallup.com/opinion/polling-matters/247052/americans-long-standing-interest-taxing-rich.aspx.

Newport, Frank. 2019b. "The Impact of Increased Political Polarization." Gallup, December 5. Accessed January 25, 2020. https://news.gallup.com/opinion/polling-matters/268982/impact-increased-political-polarization.aspx.

Nichols, John. 2019. "Bernie Sanders: 'We Have to Talk about Democratic Socialism as an Alternative to Unfettered Capitalism.'" *The Nation*, June 12. Accessed March 6, 2020. https://www.thenation.com/article/archive/bernie-sanders-socialism-capitalism-2020/.

Palosky, Craig. 2019. "Poll: On Health Care, Democrats and Democratic-Leaning Independents Trust Sen. Sanders the Most, but Significantly More People Support a Public Option Than Medicare-for-All." Kaiser Family Foundation, November 20. Accessed February 24, 2020. https://www.kff.org/health-reform/press-release/kff-tracking-poll-on-health-care-democrats-and-democratic-leaning-independents-trust-sen-sanders-the-most-but-significantly-more-people-support-a-public-option-than-medicare-for-all/.

Pelosi, Nancy. 2020. "Pelosi Statement on Coronavirus Emergency Response Bill." March 4. Accessed April 8, 2020. https://www.speaker.gov/newsroom/3420.

Peterson, Kristina. 2019. "House Republicans Now Unanimous in Opposing Abortion Rights." *Wall Street Journal*, March 21. Accessed February 1, 2020. https://www.wsj.com/articles/house-republicans-now-unanimous-in-opposing-abortion-rights-11553172954.

Pew Research Center. 2019a. "Public Opinion on Abortion: Views on Abortion, 1995–2019." August 29. Accessed January 25, 2020. https://www.pewforum.org/fact-sheet/public-opinion-on-abortion/.

Pew Research Center. 2019b. "Public Trust in Government: 1958–2019." Accessed January 30, 2020. https://www.people-press.org/2019/04/11/public-trust-in-government-1958-2019/.

Pew Research Center. 2019c. "U.S. Public Continues to Favor Legal Abortion, Oppose Overturning *Roe v. Wade*." August 29. Accessed January 29, 2020. https://www.people-press.org/2019/08/29/u-s-public-continues-to-favor-legal-abortion-oppose-overturning-roe-v-wade/.

Pew Research Center. 2020. "Political Values and Democratic Candidate Support." January 30. Accessed March 1, 2020. https://www.people-press.org/2020/01/30/political-values-and-democratic-candidate-support/.

Remnick, David. 2020. "How the Coronavirus Shattered Trump's Supreme Confidence." *New Yorker*, March 22. Accessed April 11, 2020. https://www.newyorker.com/magazine/2020/03/30/how-the-coronavirus-shattered-trumps-serene-confidence.

Ritter, Zacc. 2020. "Amid Pandemic, News Attention Spikes; Media Favorability Flat." Gallup, April 9. Accessed April 9, 2020. https://news.gallup.com/opinion/gallup/307934/amid-pandemic-news-attention-spikes-media-favorability-flat.aspx.

Rodrigo, Chris Mills. 2019. "Democratic Senators Introduce Bill to Block Trump 'Public Charge' Rule." The Hill, September 17. Accessed April 12, 2020. https://thehill.com/homenews/senate/461735-democratic-sens-introduce-bill-to-block-trump-public-charge-rule.

Roe, Phil. 2019. "Roe Supports HHS Physician Conscience Rule." June 13. Accessed April 10, 2020. https://justfacts.votesmart.org/public-statement/1353105/roe-supports-hhs-physician-conscience-rule.

Schumer, Chuck. 2020. "Schumer Offers Detailed Proposal for $8.5 Billion in Emergency Coronavirus Funding." February 26. Accessed April 8, 2020. https://www.democrats.senate.gov/newsroom/press-releases/schumer-offers-detailed-proposal-for-85-billion-in-emergency-coronavirus-funding.

Seib, Gerald. 2019. "How the U.S. Became a Nation Divided." *Wall Street Journal*, December 17. Accessed March 2, 2020. https://www.wsj.com/articles/how-the-u-s-became-a-nation-divided-11576630802.

Stecula, Dominik. 2019. "Vaccines Should not Become a Partisan Issue." *Philadelphia Inquirer*, July 10. Accessed January 29, 2020. https://www.inquirer.com/opinion/commentary/vaccines-outbreaks-exemption-bills-democrats-republicans-20190710.html.

Steinhauer, Jennifer. 2019. "Democrats Who Flipped Seats in 2018 Have a 2020 Playbook: Focus on Drug Costs." *New York Times*, December 24. Accessed January 21, 2020. https://www.nytimes.com/2019/12/24/us/politics/prescription-drug-costs-democrats.html.

Stewart, Tynan. 2020. "Push for Medicaid Expansion Could Conflict with GOP Work Requirement Efforts." *St. Louis Post-Dispatch*, January 16. Accessed February 24, 2020. https://www.stltoday.com/news/local/govt-and-politics/push-for-medicaid-expansion-could-conflict-with-gop-work-requirement/article_d1f4e305-573f-5721-b966-f5105c9afcb6.html.

Stolberg, Sheryl. 2020. "McConnell, Looking to Energize Social Conservatives, Forces Vote on Abortion." *New York Times*, February 24. Accessed March 1, 2020. https://www.nytimes.com/2020/02/24/us/politics/abortion-bill-votes.html.

Taranto, James. 2018. "Moderate Voters, Polarized Parties." *Wall Street Journal*, January 5. Accessed January 25, 2020. https://www.wsj.com/articles/moderate-voters-polarized-parties-1515193066.

Warren, Elizabeth. 2020a. "Health Care Is a Basic Human Right." Accessed February 24, 2020. https://elizabethwarren.com/plans/health-care.

Warren, Elizabeth. 2020b. "Ultra-Millionaire Tax." Accessed January 21, 2020. https://elizabethwarren.com/plans/ultra-millionaire-tax.

Washington Post. 2016. "Transcript of the New Hampshire GOP Debate, Annotated." February 6. Accessed January 21, 2020.https://www.washingtonpost.com/news/the-fix/wp/2016/02/06/transcript-of-the-feb-6-gop-debate-annotated/.

West, Darrell. 2019. *Divided Politics, Divided Nation*. Washington, DC: Brooking Institution Press.

Wheeler, Russell. 2020. "Judicial Appointments in Trump's First Three Years: Myths and Realities." Brookings Institution, January 28. Accessed February 3, 2020. https://www.brookings.edu/blog/fixgov/2020/01/28/judicial-appointments-in-trumps-first-three-years-myths-and-realities/.

Chronology

1905: The U.S. Supreme Court decides state governments have the right to enact compulsory vaccine mandates in *Jacobson v. Massachusetts*.

1930: President Herbert Hoover (R) reorganizes several veterans' programs—including pension and health care services—into a new independent federal agency called the Veterans' Administration.

1935: President Franklin Roosevelt (D) signs the Social Security Act into law, creating a social insurance program that provides cash benefits to retired individuals over the age of 65 who have worked their entire lives.

1946: President Harry S. Truman (D) becomes the first U.S. president to endorse a national health insurance system.

1952: Dwight D. Eisenhower (R) defeats Adlai Stevenson (D) in the U.S. presidential election.

1953: The Eisenhower administration determines employer contributions to health insurance plans are nontaxable benefits.

1957: Rep. Aime Forand (D-RI) introduces the first Medicare proposal in Congress to provide hospital insurance to the aged.

1965: The U.S. Supreme Court decides in *Griswold v. Connecticut* that married women have the right to contraception.

1965: President Lyndon B. Johnson (D) signs Medicare and Medicaid into law. Medicare is a governmental program that finances health care for the elderly, while Medicaid does so for the poor.

1970: President Richard Nixon (R) signs the Controlled Substances Act, which regulates the manufacture, importation, possession, use, and distribution of certain substances.

1970: The Occupational Safety and Health Act (OSHA) is signed into law and establishes a federal program of standard setting and enforcement activities to ensure healthy and safe workplaces.

1971: Sen. Edward M. Kennedy (D-MA) holds hearings across the nation on a Canadian-style single-payer health insurance system and introduces legislation in Congress.

1971: The U.S. Supreme Court decides in *Graham v. Richardson* that state restrictions on legal immigrants' eligibility for public benefits violates the U.S. Constitution's equal protection clause.

1971: President Richard Nixon (R) declares "a war on drugs" after a report of a heroin epidemic among U.S. soldiers in Vietnam.

1971: President Nixon issues nationwide wage and price controls to counter inflation.

1972: The Social Security Amendments establish professional standards review organizations (PSROs) to monitor the quality of services provided to Medicare beneficiaries and the medical necessity for the services.

1973: The U.S. Supreme Court's decision in *Roe v. Wade* affirms a woman's right to abortion without interference during the first trimester. The court rules that states may, at their discretion, regulate the abortion procedure during the second trimester to protect maternal health and, if they choose, proscribe it during the third trimester to protect the "potentiality of human life" once the fetus has reached viability.

1973: The Health Maintenance Organization Act amends the Public Health Service Act to "provide assistance and encouragement for the establishment and expansion of health maintenance organizations."

1974: The Employee Retirement Income Security Act (ERISA) provides the regulation of almost all pension and benefit plans for employees, including pensions, medical or hospital benefits, disability, and death benefits.

1976: Connecticut and Minnesota become the first states to create high-risk pools for individuals who have been denied health insurance coverage by insurers in the health insurance market.

1978: Alain Enthoven, a health economist at Stanford University, proposes a "consumer choice health plan."

1980: Congress approves work requirements for food assistance programs.

1980: The U.S. Supreme Court upholds the constitutionality of the Hyde Amendment, prohibiting federal funding for abortion services in the case of *Harris v. McRae*.

1980: Ronald Reagan (R) defeats incumbent Jimmy Carter (D) in the U.S. presidential election.

1983: The Social Security Amendments introduces a new prospective payment system (PPS) for Medicare that includes provisions to reimburse hospitals for inpatient services on predetermined rates per discharge using diagnosis-related groups (DRGs).

1984: The Deficit Reduction Act expands Medicaid coverage of children up to the age of 5 born to families eligible for federal cash welfare payments.

1984: The Drug Price Competition and Patent Term Restoration Act provides brand-name pharmaceutical manufacturers with patent term extensions, significantly increasing manufacturers' opportunities for earning profits during the longer effective patent life of their affected products.

1985: The Terminally Ill Act is enacted, allowing adults to determine decisions regarding life-sustaining treatments.

1986: The Emergency Medical Treatment and Active Labor Act (EMTALA) guarantees that any individual who goes into an emergency room cannot be turned away regardless of insurance status or ability to pay.

1986: The Anti-Drug Abuse Act is enacted under the Reagan administration; it increases penalties for drug possession, creates minimum sentences for drug-related offenses, and increases funds for drug enforcement measures.

1990: Congress institutes work requirements for housing assistance.

1990: The U.S. Supreme Court decides in *Cruzan v. Director, Missouri Department of Health* that competent Americans have a constitutional right to refuse treatment.

1990: The Omnibus Budget Reconciliation Act of 1990 (OBRA 90) is enacted to reduce the federal budget.

1992: The Centers for Disease Control and Prevention (CDC) launches the National Center on Injury Prevention and Control to conduct public health research on gun violence.

1992: Bill Clinton (D) defeats incumbent George H. W. Bush (R) in the U.S. presidential election.

1993: President Bill Clinton (D) creates a task force, headed by First Lady Hillary Clinton, that is charged with developing a national health reform plan.

1993: Congressional Republicans, including Sen. John Chafee (R-RI), endorse an individual health insurance mandate as an alternative to the Clinton administration's proposed Health Security Act.

1993: President Bill Clinton (D) signs the Brady Bill, which requires individuals to submit to a background check before purchasing a gun.

1994: Oregon becomes the first state to allow terminally ill patients to end their own lives.

1994: Republicans regain majority control of the House of Representatives.

1994: The Clinton administration's proposed Health Security Act fails to pass Congress.

1995: Forty states implement work requirements through state waivers.

1996: The Health Insurance Portability and Accountability Act (HIPAA) grants citizens the right to retain their health coverage when they have lost or changed jobs.

1996: The Personal Responsibility and Work Opportunity Act (PRWORA) is enacted, requiring individuals to work to receive welfare assistance.

1996: California passes Proposition 215 and becomes the first state to legalize medical marijuana.

1996: Congress passes the Dickey Amendment, which prohibits the CDC from using its funding to advocate for or promote gun control.

1997: The U.S. Supreme Court rules the U.S. Constitution does not enshrine a right to die; Oregonians vote to keep their physician-assisted death act in place.

1997: The U.S. Supreme Court issues rulings on two cases pertaining to assisted suicide: *Washington v. Glucksberg* and *Vacco v. Quill*. *Washington v. Glucksberg* challenges Washington State's ban on physician-assisted suicide in its Natural Death Act (*Compassion in Dying v. State of Washington* 1994).

1997: The Department of Health and Human Services (HHS) defines short-term, limited-duration insurance (STLDI) plans as policies with a term of less than one year.

1997: President Bill Clinton (D) signs the Balanced Budget Act. This law creates the Children's Health Insurance Plan (CHIP) to provide health coverage to uninsured children whose families do not qualify for Medicaid.

1997: The Food and Drug Administration Modernization and Accountability Act directs the secretary of HHS to identify new drugs as a "fast track products" and to facilitate development and expedite review if the new drugs are intended for serious conditions and demonstrate the potential to address unmet medical needs for those conditions.

1998: The U.S. House of Representatives votes 310–93 to oppose subsequent state efforts to legalize medical marijuana.

2000: George W. Bush (R) defeats Al Gore (D) in the U.S. presidential election.

2001: The Best Pharmaceuticals for Children Act amends the Public Health Service Act to develop an annual list of approved drugs for which (1) there is a referral, an approved or pending new drug application, or no patent or market exclusivity protection and (2) additional pediatric safety and effectiveness studies are needed.

2003: The Medicare Modernization Act (MMA) is signed into law, establishing a voluntary prescription drug benefit program known as Medicare Part D.

2005: The U.S. Supreme Court decides in *Gonzales v. Raich* that Congress can criminalize marijuana use.

2005: The Patient Navigator Outreach and Chronic Disease Prevention Act authorizes a demonstration grant program to provide patient navigator services to reduce barriers and improve health care outcomes.

2006: Massachusetts incorporates a health insurance exchange and an individual health insurance mandate into its landmark health reform bill.

2006: Democrats regain a majority in both houses of Congress.

2008: The U.S. Supreme Court decides in *District of Columbia v. Heller* that the Second Amendment guarantees an individual the right to own a firearm for self-defense.

2008: Barack Obama (D) defeats John McCain (R) in the U.S. presidential election.

2009: The uninsurance rate in Massachusetts drops from 10.4 percent in 2006 to 4.4 percent.

2009: President Barack Obama (D) signs the Children's Health Insurance Reauthorization Act (CHIPRA).

2010: The Patient Protection and Affordable Care Act of 2010 (ACA, also known as Obamacare), a major health reform law that expands health insurance coverage to millions of uninsured Americans, is passed by a Democrat-led Congress and signed into law by President Barack Obama (D).

2010: Twenty-six states file suits against the ACA in federal court, arguing Congress exceeded its authority by threatening noncompliant states with the loss of all Medicaid funding.

2010: States can expand eligibility for Medicaid under the ACA, but a majority of Republican-led states opt against expanding their Medicaid programs.

2010: Republicans regain a majority in the House of Representatives.

2012: The U.S. Supreme Court decides the ACA's individual mandate is constitutional but mandatory Medicaid expansion is unduly coercive in the case of *National Federation of Independent Business v. Sebelius*. States have discretion over whether or not to expand Medicaid.

2012: President Barack Obama (D) defeats Mitt Romney (R) to win reelection.

2012: President Barack Obama (D) signs the Deferred Action for Childhood Arrivals (DACA) program, which protects children who have been brought into the country illegally from being deported for two years.

2013: The ACA reforms the individual and small group health insurance markets by limiting the ability of insurers to use individuals' health status to set premiums.

2013: The first ACA open enrollment period begins on October 1, but the newly created health insurance marketplaces are beset by technical problems.

2013: Vermont policy makers legalize assisted death by enacting Act 39, or the Vermont Patient Choice and Control at the End-of-Life Act, as a less restrictive adaptation of Oregon's law.

2013: The ACA's new health insurance marketplaces enroll their first subscribers.

2013: President Barack Obama (D) apologizes to the nation for the administration's problem-plagued rollout of the ACA.

2014: The Veterans Choice Program (VCP) allows veterans who face a delay of more than 30 days for an appointment or procedure to receive care outside of the VA.

2014: The ACA's individual mandate takes effect and requires individuals to maintain "minimum essential coverage" or pay a tax penalty.

2014: The U.S. Supreme Court decides in *Burwell v. Hobby Lobby* that some for-profit employers with religious objections can refuse to cover contraceptives in their health insurance plans.

2014: Medicaid expansion is implemented.

2014: President Barack Obama (D) signs the Veterans Access, Choice, and Accountability (VACA) Act, which provides veterans with improved health care and more options when it comes to receiving health care.

2014: Republicans regain majority control of the Senate.

2015: The U.S. Supreme Court decides in *King v. Burwell* that individuals who reside in states that have not established health insurance exchanges still qualify for federal subsidies, saving the ACA once again.

2015: The Centers for Medicare and Medicaid Services (CMS) declares that requiring employment for Medicaid may not be a condition of eligibility because Medicaid is a health coverage program.

2015: Gov. Jerry Brown (D-CA) signs S.B. 277, removing personal belief as a lawful reason for seeking an exemption from the state's vaccination requirements.

2015: Gov. Jerry Brown (D-CA) signs the California End of Life Option Act, which allows adults to request medical assistance in dying from their physician if they are suffering from a terminal illness.

2016: The Obama administration issues new regulations limiting the maximum term of short-term health insurance plans to 90 days and bans the guaranteed renewal of such policies.

2016: Donald Trump (R) defeats Hillary Clinton (D) in the U.S. presidential election.

2016: The New Mexico State Supreme Court issues a unanimous ruling that medical aid in dying is not a constitutional right.

2016: Several of the nation's largest insurers—Aetna, Anthem, Humana, and United Health Group—report mounting losses on ACA marketplace plans.

2016: Colorado voters approve Proposition 106, the End-of-Life Option Act.

2017: President Donald Trump (R) ends Cost-Sharing Reduction (CSR) payments to insurance companies.

2017: The American Health Care Act (AHCA) passes the House by a slim margin (217–213) but fails to pass the Senate. Two other GOP-led bills to repeal and replace the ACA also fail to pass Congress.

2017: President Donald Trump (R) repeals the ACA's individual mandate penalty by signing the Tax Cuts and Jobs Act (TCJA), which reset the penalty for not having health insurance to $0.

2018: The Centers for Medicare and Medicaid Services (CMS) endorses the ability of states to impose work requirements for Medicaid recipients.

2018: President Donald Trump (R) signs a six-year extension of the CHIP program.

2018: Arkansas becomes the first state to implement work requirements for Medicaid recipients.

2018: President Donald Trump (R) signs the VA Maintaining Internal Systems and Strengthening Integrated Outside Networks (MISSION) Act into law, which allows veterans to have more provider options when choosing a health care plan.

2018: The Trump administration finalizes a rule allowing individuals to extend the term of short-term, limited-duration health insurance plans for up to one year, with the possibility of renewal for up to three years.

2018: Gov. Gavin Newsom (D-CA) signs S.B. 910, which prohibits short-term, limited-duration health insurance policies within the state.

2018: Judge Reed O'Connor rules that after the passage of the TCJA repealed the penalty for not purchasing health insurance, the individual health insurance mandate can no longer be upheld under Congress' tax power in the case of *Texas v. United States*. This decision, which would have invalidated the ACA, is stayed pending appeal.

2019: An outbreak of 425 cases of measles prompts New York state legislators to introduce bills eliminating all nonmedical exemptions to state vaccine mandates.

2019: U.S. Citizenship and Immigration Services revokes and then reinstates a policy enabling immigrants to avoid deportation while undergoing lifesaving medical treatment.

2019: Chinese officials report a cluster of pneumonia cases caused by SARS-CoV-2, later known as COVID-19.

2019: U.S. District Court Judge James Boasberg sets aside the Trump administration's approved work requirement waivers in Arkansas, Kentucky, and New Hampshire.

2019: The Fifth Circuit Court of Appeals upholds Justice O'Connor's ruling in *Texas v. United States* in a 2–1 decision.

2019: The Trump administration issues new rules to implement the VA MISSION Act, allowing veterans to seek care from private-sector providers if they live 30 or more minutes away from a VA facility or if the wait time exceeds 20 days for an appointment.

2020: COVID-19 appears in the United States. The nation records 19.6 million cases and more than 340,000 deaths by year's end.

2020: Joseph Biden (D) defeats President Donald Trump (R) to win the presidency.

2020: The U.S. Supreme Court hears oral arguments about the constitutionality of the ACA's individual mandate in the case of *California v. Texas*.

Children's Health Insurance

At a Glance

Congress created the Children's Health Insurance Program (CHIP) as part of the Balanced Budget Act of 1997 (Pub. L. 105-33). The Balanced Budget Act passed with strong bipartisan support in both the House (346–85) and Senate (85–15). President Clinton signed it into law on August 5, 1997. CHIP offered federal matching funds for states to expand access to health coverage for children from low-income families who did not qualify for Medicaid. All 50 states and the District of Columbia had created CHIP programs by 2000. States had the option of extending Medicaid eligibility, creating a combined CHIP/Medicaid program, or establishing a new freestanding program for children. Most (42) states opted to create independent or partnership programs rather than using CHIP funds to expand Medicaid to cover higher-income children (Hayes and Catalanotto 2017). Each state received a federal block grant that covered 65 percent to 81 percent of the cost of insuring eligible children. Before the passage of CHIP in 1997, over 10 million children in the United States were uninsured; by 2017, fewer than 4 million children lacked health insurance coverage. In 2018, more than 9.4 million children received comprehensive health insurance coverage through this joint federal-state program.

Over the past two decades, the goals of CHIP have enjoyed strong bipartisan support, but ongoing debates about funding have often sparked intense partisan conflicts. Unlike Medicaid, CHIP is funded through a capped block grant that must be reauthorized by Congress. In 2007, President George W. Bush vetoed two CHIP reauthorization bills that included funding for expectant mothers. Bush argued that adults should not be eligible for CHIP; he criticized the proposal as a thinly veiled attempt to expand the federal government's role in financing health care. This standoff over the future of CHIP was resolved after the 2008 presidential election. Soon after taking office in February 2009, President Barack Obama signed the Children's Health Insurance Reauthorization Act (CHIPRA), which funded the program through 2013 and also extended coverage to pregnant women. However, the yearlong impasse over reauthorizing CHIP exposed a growing partisan rift over funding children's health insurance.

The most recent standoff over CHIP funding began in 2017. In 2015, Congress passed the Medicare Access and CHIP Reauthorization Act (MACRA), which funded CHIP through September 30, 2017, without making any substantive changes to the program (Burak 2015). By 2017, the debate over reauthorizing CHIP had become enmeshed with several other high-profile issues, including Republican efforts to repeal and replace the Affordable Care Act (ACA), competing proposals for immigration reform, a sweeping tax reform bill, and a shutdown of the federal government. With no guarantees of continued federal funding, several states prepared notices of cancellation for program beneficiaries. After a monthslong standoff, President Donald Trump signed a six-year extension of the program in January 2018. Although CHIP funding is now secure through 2023, this most recent debate underscored the difficulty of finding bipartisan solutions in Washington today, even when beneficiaries are widely acknowledged as deserving of public aid.

According to Many Democrats . . .

- CHIP funding should cover as many children as possible.
- Pregnant women depend on CHIP for health care coverage. Investing in coverage for expectant mothers is an investment in healthy pregnancies and healthy children.
- Republicans held CHIP reauthorization hostage to their efforts to cut taxes for wealthy Americans and their efforts to repeal and replace the Affordable Care Act.

According to Many Republicans . . .

- CHIP should focus on covering poor children, not middle-income families, and should not replace private health insurance for families who can afford it.
- Expectant mothers should not be covered by CHIP. Expanding the program beyond its target population of children is inconsistent with the program's original purpose.
- Democrats "played games" with CHIP by withholding their support in an effort to force a vote on immigration reform.

Overview

Proposals to expand access to health insurance for nonindigent children first appeared in the 1970s. The Carter administration's proposed Child Health Assessment Program (CHAP) sought to expand Medicaid eligibility to 700,000 poor children under the age of 6 (CQ Almanac 1977). As Joseph Califano, Carter's secretary of Health, Education, and Welfare, explained, CHAP would "identify the poorest children in our society, have them examined by doctors, [and] have them treated on an out-patient basis" (CQ Almanac 1977). However, CHAP never received a vote in Congress.

The prospects for any "stand-alone" health care legislation for children faded after the election of Ronald Reagan in 1980 (Smith 2011). The Reagan administration increased defense spending and slashed taxes, resulting in large peacetime budget deficits. The administration also sought to rein in rising spending on welfare programs, including Medicaid. Since state eligibility rules for welfare varied widely, many poor women and children did not qualify for Medicaid benefits. Nevertheless, Congress took tentative steps to expand health insurance for children and pregnant women during the Reagan administration. The Tax Equity and Fiscal Responsibility Act of 1982 (Pub. L. 97-248) gave states the option to cover disabled children under the age of 18 who lived at home, regardless of their family income. These "Katie Beckett waivers"—named for a young girl in Iowa with complex medical needs—marked a significant departure from traditional Medicaid eligibility criteria (Catalyst Center 2016). Two years later, the 1984 Deficit Reduction Act (Pub. L. 98-639) mandated coverage of children up to age of 5 born to families eligible for federal cash welfare payments. However, Congress declined to expand health insurance coverage to nonindigent children.

Despite the Reagan administration's efforts to curtail social welfare spending, congressional Democrats used the budget reconciliation process to incrementally expand access to Medicaid for children and pregnant women. Rep. Henry Waxman (D-CA), the chair of the House Ways and Means Subcommittee on Health and Environment, led Democratic efforts to expand health insurance coverage for poor women and children. From 1984 to 1990, Rep. Waxman helped to pass 24 new Medicaid initiatives. Thomas Scully, the administrator for the Centers for Medicare and Medicaid Services under President George W. Bush, quipped that "fifty percent of the social safety net was created by Henry Waxman when no one was looking" (U.S. House of Representatives, Committee on Energy and Commerce 2014). Rep. Waxman "would first offer the states an attractive option and then, a year or two later, mandate it for all states. By securing broad acceptance of optional expansion, and then waiting for a majority of states to take up that option before making it mandatory, he was able to minimize political resistance" (Rose 2013, 125). For example, the Omnibus Budget Reconciliation Act of 1989 (OBRA 89) mandated coverage for pregnant women and children under the age of 6 in families whose income was at or below 133 percent of the federal poverty line (FPL). A year later, the Omnibus Budget Reconciliation Act of 1990 (OBRA 90) mandated coverage of children ages 6 through 18 in families with incomes at or below 100 percent of the FPL (Kaiser Family Foundation 2008).

By the early 1990s, national health care reform had returned to the forefront of the policy agenda. During the 1992 presidential campaign, Democrats and Republicans proposed options for comprehensive health care reform. As the national policy conversation shifted toward universal coverage for all Americans, the need for a separate children's health insurance program receded. With the election of

Bill Clinton in 1992, many observers argued that universal health insurance was an idea "whose time has come" (Hackey 1993).

Republicans, however, steadfastly opposed the Clinton administration's health care reform agenda. Conservative critics of national health insurance used the specter of "big government" to undermine public support for universal coverage. Conservative critics attacked President Clinton's proposed Health Security Act (H.R. 3600) as a thinly veiled blueprint for "socialized medicine" (Skocpol 1996). With dozens of competing reform bills in Congress in 1993 and 1994, Democrats failed to forge a working majority to enact a comprehensive health care reform plan. The two-year push for health care reform died a quiet death in the summer of 1994 after enduring months of withering attacks by Republicans, who claimed that the bill represented a "government takeover" of the health care system (Skocpol 1996).

President Clinton argued that his comprehensive health care reform plan—the Health Security Act—offered "the promise of a new era of security for every American" (Clinton 1993). The president believed that the resulting plan "builds on the existing private sector system. It responds to market forces" while still guaranteeing comprehensive coverage for all. Under Clinton's plan, all children would be insured—not through their parents' employment or eligibility gained through Medicaid, but through their own coverage that could not be taken away.

Republicans charged that universal coverage would raise taxes, erode the quality of patient care, and lead to rationing. Over time, these charges resonated with the American public. Public opinion polls revealed a steady erosion of support for the Clinton plan. When President Clinton announced his plan in September 1993, 59 percent of Americans favored it. By April 1994, support had fallen to 43 percent, and only 33 percent of Americans believed that the president's health care reform proposal would be good for the country (Blendon, Brodie, and Benson 1995). Opposition to health care reform was a cornerstone of Republicans' strategy for the 1994 midterm elections. Their assault on health reform paid off handsomely, as Republicans regained control of the House of Representatives for the first time in 40 years.

In the wake of defeat, Democrats did not abandon the pursuit of health care reform. Instead, reformers focused on smaller, incremental changes to improve access to health care. During the mid-1990s, advocacy groups pressed Congress to consider an updated version of the Carter administration's Children's Health Assurance Program. Beginning in 1994, the Children's Health Fund organized children's health care providers and advocacy groups to lobby for targeted insurance programs for children who did not qualify for Medicaid (Children's Health Fund). After hosting a national symposium in 1995, the Children's Health Fund sponsored the Kids First, Kids Now campaign to raise public awareness about children's health issues through a series of conferences. Harvard economist David Cutler described the new approach as the "Titanic strategy" because "it meant saving women and children first" (Cutler and Gruber 2001).

Children's health insurance had strong bipartisan appeal for both practical and political reasons. As a practical matter, many children did not qualify for employer-sponsored health insurance coverage, even if one or more of their parents worked. Furthermore, expanding coverage to children was comparatively inexpensive relative to adults with chronic illnesses or other uninsured groups. As a political matter, children represented a "deserving" target for reformers that had demonstrated need; reformers often framed the call for expanded coverage in moral terms.

Children's health insurance brought together odd bedfellows, including liberal Democrats such as Sen. Edward Kennedy (D-MA) and conservative Republicans such as Sen. Orrin Hatch (R-UT). This "legislative odd couple" announced a plan to insure over 10 million uninsured children at a Children's Defense Fund conference in March 1997 (Pear 1997). Hatch framed the issue as a moral question, noting that "children are being terribly hurt and perhaps scarred for the rest of their lives" because of a lack of access to timely health care (Pear 1997). As Sen. Kennedy noted in his testimony before the Senate Finance Committee that year, "The largest growth in the uninsured in this country today are children. Their numbers are increasing. That is a recent phenomenon" (U.S. Senate, Committee on Finance 1997). The passage of the Balanced Budget Act (Pub. L. 105-33) provided $40 billion in federal matching funds to states over a 10-year period for a new Children's Health Insurance Program financed by increasing the federal excise tax on cigarettes. Sen. Kennedy defended the use of tobacco taxes, despite Republican opposition to tax increases. "We should make sure the sons and daughters of working families get a healthy start," Kennedy declared. "The best way to fund this is a tax on tobacco, which causes five million premature deaths a year and weighs down our whole health system" (Clymer 1997).

The new Children's Health Insurance Program (CHIP) championed by Kennedy and Hatch had broad appeal for states, which could tailor the program to provide coverage and services in ways that reflected their unique circumstances and characteristics (Institute of Medicine 1998). Sen. Kennedy described the new law as "the most far-reaching step that Congress has ever taken to help the nation's children, and the most far-reaching advance in health care since the enactment of Medicare and Medicaid a generation ago" (Kaiser Family Foundation 2008). CHIP enrollment increased tenfold from 1998 to 2006. In its first full year, CHIP covered 660,351 low-income children; by 2006, enrollment in the program exceeded 6.7 million children. Between 1997 and 2012, the uninsured rate among children fell by 50 percent, from 14 percent to 7 percent (Paradise 2014). Beginning in 2000, many states expanded outreach programs and simplified enrollment procedures for families to help children enroll (and stay enrolled) in coverage (Kaiser Family Foundation 2008). The expansion of CHIP produced tangible improvements in children's health, as avoidable hospitalizations and child mortality declined during the program's first decade. Children's access to—and utilization of—preventive services, dental care, and primary care also improved after enrolling in CHIP (Paradise 2014). In addition, CHIP also reduced racial and ethnic disparities in access to care.

A decade after it was first enacted, Congress took up the reauthorization of CHIP in 2007. Public opinion surveys revealed that Democrats overwhelmingly supported the reauthorization and expansion of CHIP—more than 80 percent of self-identified Democrats favored expansion compared to 54 percent of Republicans (NPR, Kaiser Family Foundation, and the Harvard School of Public Health 2007). The first attempt to pass the Children's Health Insurance Program Reauthorization Act of 2007 (H.R. 976) passed the House by a margin of 265 to 159 and sailed through the Senate with a vote of 68–31. However, President George W. Bush vetoed the reauthorization bill, arguing that it strayed beyond the program's initial purpose of prioritizing low-income children by expanding coverage to include expectant mothers.

Bush's veto was highly unpopular with the public; nearly two-thirds opposed this action (NPR, Kaiser Family Foundation, and the Harvard School of Public Health 2007). Congress passed a revised version of CHIPRA (H.R. 3963) by a margin of 64 to 30 in the Senate and 265 to 142 in the House. President Bush remained unpersuaded and vetoed a second reauthorization bill in December 2007. After an unsuccessful attempt by the House to override the president's veto, Congress passed, and President Bush ultimately signed into law, a short-term extension bill (S. 2499) that maintained already established funding levels for the program. The standoff over reauthorizing CHIP became a proxy fight over "the role of government in organizing and overseeing the health care marketplace" (Rosenbaum 2008, 870).

The election of Barack Obama in 2008 marked a fundamental shift in the politics of CHIP reauthorization. Within weeks of taking office, President Barack Obama signed the Children's Health Insurance Program Reauthorization Act (CHIPRA) into law; the bill passed the House on a 290–135 vote and sailed through the Senate by a margin of 66 to 32. CHIPRA reauthorized the program through 2013, eliminated the five-year waiting period that barred legal immigrants from participating in Medicaid, and expanded coverage to include pregnant women. Two years later, President Obama's signature domestic policy achievement—the Affordable Care Act (ACA)—passed Congress without a single Republican vote. The ACA extended CHIP funding through September 30, 2015, but also required states to enroll children between the ages of 6 and 19 in families with incomes between 100 percent and 138 percent of the FPL into Medicaid by January 1, 2014. This policy change was designed to streamline coverage for low-income families; parents and children could now share one insurance plan with a unified network of doctors and hospitals. This change affected more than 1.5 million children and reduced CHIP enrollment by 30 percent in 2014. The ACA, however, substantially increased federal funding for CHIP by increasing the matching rate by 23 percentage points; after the passage of the ACA, federal funding accounted for more than 93 percent of total CHIP expenditures. In 2015, CHIP was once again due for reauthorization. In contrast to previous clashes over CHIP reauthorization in 2007 and 2009, the Medicare Access and CHIP Reauthorization Act (MACRA) passed with a strong bipartisan majority in both the House and the Senate. MACRA funded CHIP through September 30, 2017.

As the funding deadline drew near, more than 130 children's health organizations—including the American Academy of Pediatrics, the Children's Hospital Association, the Children's Defense Fund, and the March of Dimes—urged legislators to take immediate action to reauthorize the program for an additional five years. However, Congress failed to reach agreement on a reauthorization bill. On September 30, 2017, federal funding for CHIP expired, and several states began preparations to freeze enrollment and mailed notices to beneficiaries that warned them of a potential gap in coverage (Quinn 2017). The debate became enmeshed with several contentious issues in Congress, including Republican efforts to "repeal and replace" the Affordable Care Act and Democrats' desire to help "Dreamers" affected by the end of the Deferred Action for Childhood Arrival program (DACA). In December 2017, Republicans proposed to link the CHIP reauthorization to a continuing resolution to keep the government open. Democrats balked, arguing that any funding measure needed to address the plight of the "Dreamers." With both sides at an impasse, federal funding for CHIP lapsed for nearly four months.

CHIP Needs Stable, Long-Term Financing

In December 2017, Sen. Orrin Hatch (R-UT), one of the original sponsors of CHIP, defended Republicans' commitment to reauthorize CHIP and urged his colleagues to support a stable, long-term approach to financing the program.

> There have been a number of claims from our friends on the other side and some of their allies in the media that Republicans have ignored the CHIP program; that we don't intend to reauthorize it; or that we supposedly placed a higher priority on tax cuts for the rich than on providing health insurance for needy children. Those claims are absolutely ridiculous, and they know it. It gets a little old sometimes—some of the stupid politics that are being played by the other side.
>
> I come at this issue from two angles. I am both the original author of CHIP, and I currently chair the committee with jurisdiction over the program. Nobody should doubt my commitment to continuing the CHIP program. For two decades now, I have been a supporter of CHIP, and I worked with Members of both parties to keep it moving forward and functioning properly—even in times when my Democratic colleagues have pursued a more divisive approach with the program. That commitment continues to this day.
>
> On October 4, the Senate Finance Committee unanimously reported a bipartisan bill that would reauthorize CHIP for 5 years. In my view, a long-term reauthorization is essential so that States, including my home State of Utah, can plan well into the future and the families who benefit from CHIP can be sure that coverage for their needy children won't just disappear.

Source

Congressional Record, vol. 163, no. 209 (Thursday, December 21, 2017): S8213–S8214. Accessed January 22, 2021. https://www.congress.gov/congressional-record/2017/12/21/senate-section/article/S8213-1.

Republican leaders refused to bring CHIP to the floor as a freestanding issue and instead incorporated the reauthorization into a larger short-term spending bill (Cunningham 2018). By linking CHIP funding to the larger spending bill, Republicans hoped to persuade Democrats to vote for the overall funding package, thereby averting a federal government shutdown. As a result, CHIP reauthorization became enmeshed with larger debates about enacting protections for Dreamers, an ongoing budget impasse, and lingering partisan discord over the passage of the Tax Cuts and Jobs Act in December 2017. The continuing standoff over CHIP funding even emerged as a topic on late-night talk shows. Television personality Jimmy Kimmel made an emotional plea for Congress to act. Holding his son Billy (who survived open heart surgery as a newborn), Kimmel told the audience that "CHIP—[it] has become a bargaining chip. It's on the back burner while they work out the new tax plans. Parents of children with cancer, diabetes and heart problems are about to get letters saying their coverage could be cut off next month. Merry Christmas, right?" (Weiss 2018).

In an effort to break the legislative logjam over CHIP reauthorization, Sens. Orrin Hatch (R-UT) and Ron Wyden (D-OR) proposed legislation—the Keeping Kids' Insurance Dependable and Secure (KIDS) Act (S.1827)—that preserved the enhanced funding authorized during the Obama administration for two years before tapering it off over the final three years. However, S. 1827 failed to pass the Senate and the House. On November 3, 2017, the House passed the Championing Healthy Kids Act (H.R. 3922) to fund CHIP until 2022, but the bill died in the Senate. In January 2018, President Donald Trump signed a continuing appropriations bill (Pub. L. 115-120) that extended funding for CHIP through 2023. Sen. Hatch expressed relief over the six-year extension, which was nearly identical to the bill he had cosponsored with Sen. Ron Wyden in 2017. "For this moment, let us not overlook the success we've achieved this week. A six-year CHIP extension gives security and certainty to millions of American families and allows states to plan their budgets for several years into the future" (Hatch 2018). Although the passage of the reauthorization bill was a relief for supporters, many Democrats were dissatisfied with new limitations included in the bill, which allowed states to adopt more restrictive eligibility standards with respect to children in families whose income exceeds 300 percent of the poverty line. Following the lead of Hatch and Wyden's original proposal, the reauthorization bill continued the 23 percent enhanced the federal match through FY 2020, but returned to the standard CHIP matching rate beginning in FY 2021 (Kaiser Family Foundation 2017.

Throughout the most recent standoff in late 2017 and early 2018, the public strongly supported reauthorization of CHIP. In September 2017, three out of four respondents to the Kaiser Health Tracking Poll described "reauthorizing funding for the State Children's Health Insurance Program, which provides health care coverage for uninsured children," as either an "extremely important" or "very important" priority for Congress (Kirzinger, DiJulio, Hamel, Wu, and Brodie 2017). This issue garnered more support than stabilizing the ACA marketplaces, reforming the tax code, or repealing and replacing the ACA. Notably, support for CHIP was bipartisan; 89 percent of Democrats felt it was "extremely important" or "very important" to reauthorize CHIP compared to 62 percent of Republicans and 72 percent of Independents (Kirzinger, DiJulio, Hamel, Wu, and Brodie 2017). By November 2017, 62 percent of Americans viewed the reauthorization of CHIP as a "top priority." Public support for CHIP outpaced federal funding for hurricane relief, addressing the prescription painkiller epidemic, tax reform, and legislation to protect "Dreamers" (Kirzinger, DiJulio, Muñana, and Brodie 2017). The partisan divide on CHIP—first evident in 2007—is significant. Democrats are more likely to support CHIP funding than Republicans. By January 2018, 84 percent of Democrats supported renewing funding for CHIP compared to only 48 percent of Republicans (Kirzinger, Wu, and Brodie 2018).

The creation of CHIP underscored the possibilities of bipartisan policy making on health care reform. In 1997, Sen. Orrin Hatch declared that "this is not a Democrat/Republican issue; this is a bipartisan debate on an issue that literally needs to be solved" (U.S. Senate, Committee on Finance 1997). Writing in the *New York Times* in 2015, former senators Hillary Clinton (a Democrat) and Bill Frist (a Republican) underscored the need for swift bipartisan action to reauthorize CHIP: "As parents, grandparents, and former legislators, we believe that partisan politics should never stand between our kids and quality health care" (Clinton and Frist 2015). Yet, time and again, CHIP has been buffeted by broader political tensions and hostilities. Indeed, "CHIP is a good way to measure the health of our government, revealing that it struggles to pass uncontroversial legislation on time that exists to help children, possibly the last group of citizens who can muster universal sympathy and support" (Chang 2017).

Over the past two decades, funding CHIP has been a flashpoint for the parties' views on the proper role of government in the U.S. health care system and the larger economy. Recurring struggles over reauthorizing CHIP illustrate the contentious and polarized state of American politics in the 21st century. The most recent standoff ended in January 2018 when Congress finally enacted a six-year extension of the program that reauthorized federal funding for CHIP through 2023. After a 114-day lapse in funding threatened access to care for millions of children, H.R. 1892 passed by a margin of 245 to 182 in the House and 71 to 28 in the Senate and was signed into law by President Trump on February 9, 2018, as Pub. L. 115-123 (Congress.gov 2018). After its passage, the director of Families USA—a health care advocacy group—noted that "this action ends months of anxiety and worry for the hard-working families who rely on CHIP for life-saving health care" (Hellman 2018).

Democrats on Children's Health Insurance

Democrats embrace an expansive view of CHIP's role in the American health care system. The Democratic party platform includes a long-standing commitment to universal health insurance; CHIP represents an incremental yet important step in this direction. From the program's first years, Democrats strongly encouraged outreach and education efforts to sign up eligible families for coverage. Beginning in 2007, Democrats in Congress—later joined by President Barack Obama—viewed CHIP as an effective tool to decrease the number of uninsured children. As a result, Democrats favored an approach to CHIP funding that sought to maximize enrollment and expand eligibility. As Rep. Tom Perriello (D-VA) argued during the debate over reauthorizing CHIP in 2009, this is "morally the right thing to do by our children. . . . At a time when the cost of health care is crushing America's families . . . this is an important lifeline" (CNN 2009).

Democrats enthusiastically supported the reauthorization of CHIP in 2009. They viewed CHIP as part of a larger strategy to expand access to health care for all Americans. As President Barack Obama observed, "Since it was created more than ten years ago, the Children's Health Insurance Program has been a lifeline for millions of kids whose parents work full time, and don't qualify for Medicaid, but through no fault of their own don't have—and can't afford—private insurance" (Obama 2009). Rep. Henry A. Waxman (D-CA), who had previously championed

CHIP Needs Immediate, Bipartisan Reauthorization

In December 2017, the minority leader of the U.S. House of Representatives, Nancy Pelosi (D-CA), spoke at the Democratic Women's Working Group, where she called on House Republicans to join Democrats in supporting the reauthorization of CHIP.

> The health and well-being of our children is a primary responsibility for those of us in Congress—for me, personally, my motivation for me to be in politics is the one in five [children] who live in poverty in our country, go to sleep hungry at night in America, the greatest country that has ever existed in the history of the world. That we should be addressing their health issues is without question, and even if you are oblivious to the concerns—and it's amazing how much patience people have for other peoples' suffering—the threshold is so high for other peoples' suffering. But nonetheless, this issue should have been done by September 30 when the reauthorization ended. The Republicans—because they wanted to pay for it in a strange way—we could not come to an agreement on it. . . . For example, the Walden bill, which they continue to put forth, is a bill that says . . . 5-year reauthorization of CHIP must be paid for . . . at the same time that the Republicans have given a nearly one and a half trillion dollar tax break, permanently, unpaid-for, to corporate America. So where is their value system? Corporations are people, okay, so corporate people get more attention than little children to that ratio of difference—that's intolerable, that's unconscionable.

Source

Pelosi, Nancy. 2017. "Pelosi Remarks at Democratic Women's Working Group Press Conference Calling for Immediate, Bipartisan CHIP Reauthorization." Press Release, December 20, 2017. Accessed January 22, 2021. https://pelosi.house.gov/news/press-releases/pelosi-remarks-at-democratic-women-s-working-group-press-conference-calling-for.

congressional efforts to expand Medicaid eligibility, also celebrated the passage of CHIPRA. "While this bill is short of our ultimate goal of health reform," Waxman argued "it is a down payment, and is an essential start." As President Obama declared at the signing ceremony for CHIPRA in 2009, "This bill is only a first step. The way I see it, providing coverage to 11 million children through CHIP is a down payment on my commitment to cover every single American" (Obama 2009). As Sen. Tammy Baldwin (D-WI) argued, "Achieving health care for all is the reason I got into politics." As a result, Democrats oppose proposals that set restrictions on enrollment for legal immigrants, middle-income families, and pregnant women, preferring to cast a wide net to increase enrollment among eligible families.

Since 2007, Democrats have fought to include—and then maintain—coverage for expectant mothers in the CHIP program. Democrats argued that investing in coverage for pregnant women would provide newborn babies with a healthier start; better prenatal care would improve health outcomes and also save money. In 2017, more than 370,000 pregnant women received health insurance coverage through CHIP. As Sen. Debbie Stabenow (D-MI) declared, "When a mom can go and get prenatal care and a baby is born healthy, we all benefit by that" (Terkel 2017). Stabenow noted, "Providing maternity care as part of basic health care actually saves tremendously in health care costs—rather than a complicated pregnancy [and] health problems for babies" (Terkel 2017).

Preserving access to coverage for expectant mothers took on a new sense of urgency for Democrats in 2017, as Republicans introduced several bills to repeal and replace the Affordable Care Act. Several Republican bills proposed to eliminate the "minimum essential coverage" requirement of the ACA, which required insurers to include coverage for maternity benefits. Colorado Lt. Gov. Donna Lynne compared the standoff over CHIP reauthorization to "a little hostage taking with kids and pregnant women in the middle." Lynne worried about "the cost to the people and the magnitude of the anxiety it is producing. Imagine if you're a pregnant woman and you're going to lose your insurance?" (Weiss 2018).

During the 2017–2018 debate over reauthorizing CHIP, Democrats charged that Republicans held poor children hostage to their efforts to cut taxes for wealthy Americans and their efforts to repeal and replace the ACA. House Minority Leader Nancy Pelosi (D-CA) dismissed Republicans' decision to incorporate CHIP reauthorization within the short-term spending bill before Congress as a political ploy. Pelosi scoffed, "This is like giving you a bowl of doggy doo, put[ting] a cherry on top and call[ing] it a chocolate sundae" (Cunningham 2018). In particular, Democrats strongly objected to Republican proposals to pay for the reauthorization bill by increasing Medicare premiums for high-income seniors and cutting funds for prevention and public health to support community health centers (Dickson 2017). As Sen. Bob Casey (D-PA) wrote in 2017, "Senate Republicans took up a partisan tax bill to cut the corporate tax rate, which creates a $1.4 trillion hole in the federal budget, all while claiming that we don't have the money for CHIP" (Casey 2017). At a news conference before Christmas in 2017, Democratic legislators holding lumps of coal demanded that Republicans bring a "clean" vote on CHIP funding for a vote before the holiday recess. Rep. Jackie Speier (D-CA) described the continuing stalemate over CHIP as "the ultimate bad Christmas carol story. This may be the most shameful day in the history of Congress." Speier said, "What we're doing here today is basically saying, 'Wealthy Americans, big fat Christmas present for you; Tiny Tim, we're taking your crutch away from you and all the other kids in this country, and we're putting a lump of coal into your Christmas stocking'" (Chuck 2017).

Republicans on Children's Health Insurance

Republicans supported the creation of CHIP in 1997, but over time, they expressed growing concerns about the expanding reach of the program. Republicans in Congress continue to favor a limited role for the program—focused on children, not adults—rather than expanding eligibility to include mothers. In addition, Republicans argue that CHIP should not replace private health insurance for families who can afford it. During the debate about reauthorizing CHIP in 2007, President George W. Bush and most congressional Republicans argued that CHIP should focus on covering poor children who did not qualify for Medicaid.

Republicans believe that efforts to expand CHIP to higher-income families or undocumented individuals are inconsistent with the program's primary purpose. During the floor debate over reauthorizing SCHIP in 2007, Rep. Nathan Deal (R-GA) argued, "We should put the poorest children at the front of the line. This means we should require states to enroll 90 percent of their SCHIP and Medicaid eligible children under 200 percent of the poverty line before they start enrolling children at higher income levels." As Rep. Wally Herger (R-CA) noted during the congressional debate over CHIP reauthorization in 2007, "All of us support SCHIP, and we all want to reauthorize it, but we need to put low-income kids first. This bill would expand the program to families making more than $60,000 a year. That is not low income. It is a majority of the households in America. There is a better way. Reauthorize SCHIP and keep it focused on truly needy children" (U.S. Congress 2007). Many Republicans charged that the proposed expansion to SCHIP fundamentally redefined the program's mission and the intent of original legislation. Rep. Kenny Hulshof (R-MO) declared, "The Federal Government should not be, in my humble opinion, in the business of paying for states who want to cover childless adults that are grandfathered in this bill. And on behalf of my constituents in Missouri, should I ask them to reach into their pockets then and to pay for a family of four in New Jersey making $70,000 or a family of four in New York making $80,000?" (U.S. Congress 2007).

In December 2007, President George W. Bush vetoed H.R. 3963, the Children's Health Insurance Program Reauthorization Act of 2007. The crux of the president's opposition lay in his belief that the proposed reauthorization and expansion represented a fundamental change in the nature of the program. This was not a new concern for Republicans in Congress. A fear of "crowding out"—in which people drop private plans for less expensive (or free) public coverage—led Republicans to oppose expanded eligibility for middle- and upper-income families. During the initial debate over SCHIP in 1997, Sen. William Roth (R-DE) noted that "the greatest challenge facing the various child health proposals before us is to reach more children without eroding the present system which provides health care coverage for seven out of eight children. Two-thirds of all children gain access to health care through the private sector. Thus, we need to proceed carefully to make certain that we do not displace the private sector role in providing health insurance for children" (U.S. Senate, Committee on Finance 1997).

A decade later, President Bush reaffirmed this point: "Ultimately, our Nation's goal should be to move children who have no health insurance to private coverage—not to move children who already have private health insurance to government coverage. The legislation would still shift SCHIP away from its original purpose by covering adults. It would still include coverage of many individuals with incomes higher than the median income in the United States. It would still result in government health care for approximately 2 million children who already have private health care coverage" (Bush 2007). Republicans believe that federal policy to support children's health insurance should encourage private insurance, not replace private insurance for families who can afford to purchase their own coverage. Public coverage, when necessary, serves as a backstop for families unable to obtain private coverage. Rep. Marsha Blackburn (R-TN) supported President Bush's veto of the reauthorization bill in 2007, warning, "It would remove people from private insurance and put them over on the government rolls" (U.S. Congress 2007).

For Republicans, the reauthorization of CHIP raised fundamental questions about the role of government in the health care system. As the *Wall Street Journal* editorialized in 2007, "SCHIP expansion has become the consensus Democratic strategy for quietly growing the government's share of health spending." The editors warned that "what the Senate, and the country need is a bigger debate over whether Americans really want this stealthy, slow-motion socialism" (*Wall Street Journal* 2007). During the floor debate in the House of Representatives over overriding President Bush's first veto of the CHIP reauthorization bill in October 2007, Rep. Steve King (R-IA) attacked the reauthorization bill as "socialized medicine." He parodied the usual acronym, arguing that "SCHIP stands for Socialized, Clinton-style Hillarycare for Illegals and their Parents" (Congress.gov 2007). King declared, "This is the cornerstone of socialized medicine. It's put in place. That's what this debate is about: make people dependent so they don't have individual responsibility and you can have more people dependent upon your votes on the floor of this Congress and less vitality in America" (Congress.gov 2007). As a result, Republicans argued that expectant mothers should not be covered by CHIP. Expanding the program beyond its target population of children is inconsistent with the program's original purpose.

Republicans charged Democrats "played games" with CHIP in a heavy-handed effort to force a vote on immigration reform and other policy priorities. In January 2018, House Republicans tweeted, "Children's lives are at stake. It's time for our friends across the aisle to stop playing games with CHIP funding." Minority Leader Nancy Pelosi (D-CA) lent credence to Republicans' charges in her public remarks about the short-term funding bill before Congress in December 2017. Pelosi described the temporary spending measure as "a waste of time" and declared that the members of the House "will not leave here (for the holidays) without a . . . fix" to the problem of illegal immigrants who had arrived in the United States as children and are sometimes referred to as "Dreamers" (Reuters 2017). Pelosi complained that the spending bill "has nothing about (the) opioid epidemic. There's nothing about veterans' funding, nothing about CHIP—CHIP—children's health insurance, community health centers, nothing about, well, the DREAM Act, among other things" (Reuters 2017).

Republicans charged Democrats with obstruction. House Republican Conference Chair Cathy McMorris Rodgers (R-WA) expressed frustration that "nearly all of the Democrats, unfortunately in the House, have voted against CHIP three times now. They've pushed us to this critical deadline when the government funding runs out on Friday. And now they're threatening to hold this up over DACA" (House Republicans 2018). As Rep. Greg Walden (R-OR) argued, "It was the Democrats on the Energy and Commerce Committee that repeatedly moved to delay consideration of bipartisan legislation to extend these vital programs in the first place. And ultimately the majority of Democrats voted against funding CHIP and community health centers on the House Floor at every turn, while Republican majorities carried every vote to passage" (Walden 2018).

Robert B. Hackey and Rose Shelley

Further Reading

Blendon, Robert, Mollyann Brodie, and John Benson. 1995. "What Happened to Public Support for the Clinton Health Plan?" *Health Affairs* (Summer): 7–23. Accessed October 10, 2020. https://www.healthaffairs.org/doi/full/10.1377/hlthaff.14.2.7.

Burak, Elisabeth. 2015. "What, Exactly, Is in That CHIP Extension?" Georgetown University Health Policy Institute, May 27. Accessed February 7, 2019. https://ccf.georgetown.edu/2015/05/27/exactly-chip-extension/.

Bush, George W. 2007. "Message to the House of Representatives." White House, Office of the Press Secretary, December 12. Accessed January 2, 2019. https://georgewbush-whitehouse.archives.gov/news/releases/2007/12/20071212-10.html.

Casey, Bob. 2017. "Millions Depend on the Children's Health Insurance Program. Save It Before It Is Too Late." *USA Today*, December 20. Accessed January 28, 2019. https://www.usatoday.com/story/opinion/2017/12/20/millions-children-depend-chip-republicans-would-rather-cut-corporate-taxes-than-fun/962144001/.

Catalyst Center. 2016. "The TEFRA Medicaid State Plan Option and Katie Beckett Waiver for Children—Making It Possible to Care for Children with Significant Disabilities at Home." Accessed November 20, 2018. https://cahpp.org/wp-content/uploads/2016/07/TEFRA.pdf.

Chang, Clio. 2017. "The GOP's Struggles to Re-Authorize CHIP Is a Devastating Indictment." *New Republic*, September 28. Accessed February 7, 2019. https://newrepublic.com/article/145084/gops-struggles-re-authorize-chip-devastating-indictment.

Children's Health Fund. 2018. "Advocacy Milestones." Accessed November 21, 2018. https://www.childrenshealthfund.org/advocacy-milestones/.

Chuck, Elizabeth. 2017. "Democrats Demand Republicans Reauthorize CHIP Kids' Health Plan before Christmas." NBC News, December 20. Accessed February 7, 2019. https://www.nbcnews.com/politics/congress/democrats-demand-republicans-re-authorize-chip-christmas-n831496.

Clinton, Hillary Rodham, and Bill Frist. 2015. "Save the Children's Insurance." *New York Times*, February 13. Accessed February 27, 2021. https://www.nytimes.com/2015/02/13/opinion/hillary-clinton-and-bill-frist-on-health-care-for-americas-kids.html.

Clinton, William J. 1993. "Remarks on Presenting Proposed Health Care Reform Legislation to the Congress." In *Public Papers of the Presidents of the United States: William J. Clinton*, vol. 2, 1830–1834. Washington, DC: U.S. Government Publishing Office. October 27. Accessed October 10, 2020. https://www.govinfo.gov/content/pkg/PPP-1993-book2/html/PPP-1993-book2-doc-pg1830-2.htm.

Clymer, Adam. 1997. "Expanding Children's Health Care." *New York Times*, February 28. Accessed November 20, 2018. https://www.nytimes.com/1997/02/28/us/expanding-children-s-health-care.html.

CNN. 2009. "Obama Signs Children's Health Initiative into Law." Accessed November 21, 2018. http://www.cnn.com/2009/POLITICS/02/04/schip.vote/index.html.

Congress.gov. 2007. "The State Children's Health Insurance Program." *Congressional Record – House of Representatives*, October 17. Accessed February 27, 2021. https://www.congress.gov/110/crec/2007/10/17/CREC-2007-10-17-pt1-PgH11720-3.pdf.

Congress.gov. 2018. *Bipartisan Budget Act of 2018*. H.R.1892. 115th Congress (2017–2018). Accessed October 10, 2020. https://www.congress.gov/bill/115th-congress/house-bill/1892/actions?q=%7B%22search%22%3A%5B%22Bipartisan+Budget+Act+of+2018%22%5D%7D&r=2&s=2.

CQ Almanac. 1977. "Child Health Program." Accessed November 23, 2018. https://library.cqpress.com/cqalmanac/document.php?id=cqal77-1203337.

Cunningham, Paige. 2018. "The Health 202: Here's How Children's Health Became a Bargaining CHIP in Government Shutdown Talks." *Washington Post*, January 19. Accessed February 14, 2014. https://www.washingtonpost.com/news/powerpost/paloma/the-health-202/2018/01/19/the-health-202-here-s-how-children-s-health-became-a-bargaining-chip-in-government-shutdown-talks/5a60e36c30fb0469e88401f7/.

Cutler, David, and Jonathan Gruber. 2001. "Health Care in the Clinton Era: Once Bitten, Twice Shy." Cambridge, MA: Kennedy School of Government. Accessed November 23, 2018. https://sites.hks.harvard.edu/m-rcbg/Conferences/economic_policy/CUTLER-GRUBER.pdf.

Dickson, Virgil. 2017. "House, Senate Committees Pass CHIP Bill Proposals." *Modern Healthcare*, October 4. Accessed February 27, 2021. https://www.modernhealthcare.com/article/20171004/NEWS/171009974/house-senate-committees-pass-chip-bill-proposals.

Hackey, Robert. 1993. "The Illogic of Health Care Reform: Policy Dilemmas for the 1990s." *Polity* 26, no. 2: 233–258.

Hatch, Orrin. 2018. "Hatch: Longest CHIP Extension Ever Provides Certainty for Families and States." Accessed January 28, 2019. https://www.finance.senate.gov/chairmans-news/hatch-longest-chip-extension-ever-provides-certainty-for-families-and-states.

Hayes, Heather, and Anna Catalanotto. 2017. "Primer: The Children's Health Insurance Program (CHIP)." American Action Forum, July 17. Accessed February 27, 2021.

https://www.americanactionforum.org/research/primer-childrens-health-insurance-program-chip/.

Hellman, Jessie. 2018. "Congress Funds Children's Health Program after Four-Month Delay." The Hill, January 22. Accessed October 10, 2020. https://thehill.com/policy/healthcare/370195-congress-funds-childrens-health-program-after-four-month-delay.

House Republicans. 2018. "Why Won't the Democrats Vote for CHIP Funding." January 17. Accessed January 29, 2019. https://www.gop.gov/roundups/democrats-are-blocking-chip-funding/.

Institute of Medicine. 1998. *Systems of Accountability: Implementing Children" Health Insurance Programs.* Washington, DC: The National Academies Press. https://doi.org/10.17226/6317.

Kaiser Family Foundation. 2008. "Medicaid: A Timeline of Key Developments." Accessed November 20, 2018. https://kaiserfamilyfoundation.files.wordpress.com/2008/04/5-02-13-medicaid-timeline.pdf.

Kaiser Family Foundation. 2017. "Extending Federal Funding for CHIP: What Is at Stake?" November 2. Accessed February 27, 2021. https://www.kff.org/medicaid/fact-sheet/extending-federal-funding-for-chip-what-is-at-stake/.

Kenney, Genevieve, and Justin Yee. 2007. "SCHIP at a Crossroads: Experiences to Date and Challenges Ahead." *Health Affairs* 26, no. 2: 356–369. Accessed January 28, 2019. https://doi.org/10.1377/hlthaff.26.2.356.

Kirzinger, Ashley, Bianca DiJulio, Liz Hamel, Bryan Wu, and Mollyann Brodie. 2017. "Kaiser Health Tracking Poll—September 2017: What's Next for Health Care?" September 22. Accessed February 7, 2019. https://www.kff.org/health-reform/poll-finding/kaiser-health-tracking-poll-september-2017-whats-next-for-health-care/.

Kirzinger, Ashley, Bianca DiJulio, Cailey Muñana, and Mollyann Brodie. 2017. "Kaiser Health Tracking Poll—November 2017: The Role of Health Care in the Republican Tax Plan." November 15. Accessed February 7, 2019. https://www.kff.org/health-reform/poll-finding/kaiser-health-tracking-poll-november-2017-the-role-of-health-care-in-the-republican-tax-plan/.

Kirzinger, Ashley, Bryan Wu, and Mollyann Brodie. 2018. "Kaiser Health Tracking Poll—January 2018: The Public's Priorities and Next Steps for the Affordable Care Act." January 26. Accessed February 7, 2019. https://www.kff.org/health-reform/poll-finding/kaiser-health-tracking-poll-january-2018-publics-priorities-next-steps-affordable-care-act/.

National Public Radio (NPR), Kaiser Family Foundation, and the Harvard School of Public Health. 2007. Public Views on SCHIP Reauthorization—Survey Highlights. Accessed February 7, 2019. https://kaiserfamilyfoundation.files.wordpress.com/2013/01/7703.pdf.

Obama, Barack. 2009. "Remarks by President Barack Obama on Children's Health Insurance Program Bill Signing." White House, Office of the Press Secretary, February 4. Accessed January 28, 2019. https://obamawhitehouse.archives.gov/the-press-office/remarks-president-barack-obama-childrenrsquos-health-insurance-program-bill-signing.

Paradise, Julie. 2014. "The Impact of the Children's Health Insurance Program (CHIP): What Does the Research Tell Us?" July 17. Accessed November 21, 2018. https://www.kff.org/report-section/the-impact-of-the-childrens-health-insurance-program-chip-issue-brief/.

Pear, Robert. 1997. "Hatch Joins Kennedy to Back a Health Program" *New York Times*, March 14. Accessed November 21, 2018. https://www.nytimes.com/1997/03/14/us/hatch-joins-kennedy-to-back-a-health-program.html.

Pear, Robert. 2009. "Obama Signs Children's Health Insurance Bill." *New York Times*, February 5. Accessed January 28, 2019. https://www.nytimes.com/2009/02/05/us/politics/05health.html.

Quinn, Maddie. 2017. "Congress Lets CHIP Expire, and States Scramble." Governing, September 29. Accessed January 2, 2019. http://www.governing.com/topics/health-human-services/gov-congress-chip-states-childrens-health-insurance-program.html.

Reuters. 2017. "Pelosi Says Democrats Will Not Back Short-Term Funding Bill on Thursday." December 7. Accessed February 7, 2019. https://www.reuters.com/article/us-usa-tax-house-democrats/pelosi-says-democrats-will-not-back-short-term-funding-bill-on-thursday-idUSKBN1E12DU.

Rose, Shanna. 2013. *Financing Medicaid: Federalism and the Growth of America's Health Care Safety Net*. Ann Arbor: University of Michigan Press, 2013.

Rosenbaum, Sara. 2008. "The Proxy War: SCHIP and the Government's Role in Health Care Reform." *New England Journal of Medicine* 358, no. 9: 869–872. Accessed February 14, 2019. https://www.nejm.org/doi/full/10.1056/NEJMp0800623.

Skocpol, Theda. 1996. *Boomerang: Clinton's Health Security Effort and the Turn Against Government in U.S. Politics*. New York: W.W. Norton.

Smith, David G. 2011. *The Children's Health Insurance Program: Past and Future*. New York: Transaction Books. Accessed January 28, 2019. https://books.google.com/books?isbn=135148513X.

Terkel, Amanda. 2017. "Trump Plan to Eliminate Universal Maternity Coverage Would Put a High Price on Being a Woman." *Huffington Post*, March 18. Accessed February 14, 2019. https://www.huffingtonpost.com/entry/trump-maternity-coverage_us_58c84f0ce4b022994fa2dd41.

U.S. Congress. House. 2007. "Children's Health Insurance Program Reauthorization Act of 2007—Veto Message from the President of the United States." *Congressional Record* (October 18): H11735–11754. Washington, DC: Government Printing Office. Accessed January 10, 2019. https://www.congress.gov/crec/2007/10/18/CREC-2007-10-18-pt1-PgH11735.pdf.

U.S. House of Representatives, Committee on Energy and Commerce—Minority Staff. 2014. "Rep. Henry A. Waxman's Record of Accomplishment." Accessed November 20, 2018. https://www.eenews.net/assets/2016/06/24/document_gw_10.pdf.

U.S. Senate, Committee on Finance. 1997. "Increasing Children's Access to Health Care." Hearing before the Committee on Finance, United States Senate. 105th Congress (April 30). S. Hrg.: 105–459.

Walden, Greg. 2018. "Walden Sets the Record Straight on Community Health Center Funding." January 26. Accessed January 29, 2019. https://republicans-energycommerce.house.gov/news/in-the-news/walden-sets-record-straight-community-health-center-funding/.

Wall Street Journal. 2007. "SCHIP Ahoy." July 17: A16.

Weiss, Brennan. 2018. "Over 2 Million Children and Pregnant Women Are on the Brink of Losing Health Insurance." *Business Insider*, January 3. Accessed February 14, 2019. https://www.businessinsider.com/chip-funding-1-million-children-pregnant-women-losing-health-care-2017-11.

COVID-19 Pandemic

At a Glance

In December 2019, Chinese officials reported a cluster of pneumonia cases caused by SARS-CoV-2, a novel strain of coronavirus (COVID-19). By late January 2020, the United States had recorded its first documented coronavirus case in Washington State. Within weeks, more cases appeared around the country, and in March, New York City became the epicenter of a national outbreak of the disease. Intense partisanship quickly punctuated the growing national emergency. The first weeks of the pandemic spurred accusations from Democrats that Republicans were downplaying the seriousness of the pandemic and accusations from Republicans that Democrats were fearmongering. Democrats and Republicans differed in how they defined and first responded to the epidemic, how they perceived state and federal measures to protect public health and mitigate viral transmission, and how they planned to reopen state economies and return to normalcy.

Democrats responded to the pandemic by emphasizing that governments had a responsibility to implement public health measures that would protect and preserve the ability of individuals to remain healthy and economically secure. For Democrats, COVID-19 represented a public health emergency that demanded decisive federal action, and they heavily criticized the response of Republican President Donald Trump and his administration as inadequate and incompetent. Moreover, Democrats insisted that the pandemic reinforced the social contract that governments—local, state, and federal—have with their citizens. Democrats widely supported federal aid to state and local governments and called for federal spending to support Americans in need as a result of the pandemic through a combination of sick pay, family leave, unemployment benefits, and other social assistance programs. Democrats also called for increased state authority to set regulations, typically a Republican emphasis.

Republicans responded to the pandemic by emphasizing conservative conceptions of liberty, individual freedom, and limited government. For Republicans, the prospect of government overreach was great, and some regarded statewide stay-at-home and masking orders as threats to individual freedom. GOP lawmakers, officials, and media figures also emphasized that actions taken by state and federal governments to combat COVID-19 had to be measured against their economic impact and their implications for civil liberties. While the pandemic necessitated federal action, Republicans were wary of significant increases in federal spending that, according to them, would encourage state dependency on the federal government. Republicans advocated for financial support for industries harmed by the pandemic and called for liability protections for employers to necessitate economic reopening.

According to Many Democrats . . .

- By downplaying the severity of the pandemic, President Trump and his fellow Republicans unnecessarily jeopardized the nation's health and safety.
- State governments require financial and logistical support from the federal government.
- State governments have the responsibility to mandate social distancing and stay-at-home orders, even if their prolonged practice may impose severe economic impacts on local, state, and national economies.

According to Many Republicans . . .

- Democrats and the media capitalized on public fear in a partisan attempt to damage President Trump.
- Citizens should exercise their personal responsibility for social distancing rather than be forced to do so by government mandate.
- Virus mitigation measures are important, but only if their impacts do not curtail the individual liberties of American citizens or the fundamental well-being of the American economy.

Overview

COVID-19 became a national public health crisis in the United States during the first months of 2020. Following the nation's first documented case in January, all 50 states reported at least one COVID-19 fatality by mid-April. State and federal officials struggled to contain the spread of the virus and engaged in tense political debates about how to manage the pandemic and its aftermath. As one political pollster observed, "It is very clear that partisanship has infected our views of the coronavirus" (McCormick 2020). Over the course of the first half of 2020, the COVID-19 pandemic magnified long-standing differences between the two political parties with respect to attitudes about civil liberties and personal responsibility, emergency powers, public health, and economic policy.

The first COVID-19 hot spots in the United States were major metropolitan areas in coastal states with Democratic leadership. On January 29, 2020, President

Donald Trump announced the formation of the White House Coronavirus Task Force, led first by U.S. Health and Human Services Secretary Alex Azar and then by Vice President Mike Pence. Six weeks later, Trump declared a state of emergency. On March 19, Gavin Newsom (D-CA) became the first governor to announce and implement a mandatory statewide stay-at-home order. Within four days of California's announcement, 9 states—8 of which were led by Democratic governors—had announced their own stay-at-home orders. Within one week, 19 states, 12 led by Democrats, had announced statewide orders. By April 3, 41 states and Washington, DC, had announced stay-at-home orders. One month after California's announcement, the 6 states that had yet to implement statewide stay-at-home orders were all led by Republican governors. By late April, data indicated that while states with Democratic governors had more COVID-19 cases and deaths than states with Republican governors, the number of cases was increasing more quickly in states with Republican governors than those with Democratic governors (Altman 2020).

During March and April 2020, governors and state health agencies announced public health directives that included limitations on public gatherings, social distancing guidelines, stay-at-home orders, the closure of nonessential businesses, and the wearing of face coverings in public spaces. Partisan tensions reflected differences of opinion regarding how restrictive these virus mitigation measures should be. Democratic mayors in Republican-led states sought to institute local measures that were more restrictive than statewide measures; Republican officials in Democratic-led states sought to ease or even ignore statewide measures. In some states, Democratic mayors issued executive orders at the municipal level before Republican governors did so at the state level.

For example, after Mississippi's Gov. Tate Reeves (R) closed schools but issued no other social distancing directives in March 2020, Tupelo Mayor Jason Shelton (D) established limits on public gatherings in the city and restricted its restaurants to only carryout, curbside service, and delivery (Pittman 2020). After Reeves issued a subsequent executive order that allowed restaurants to limit indoor dining capacity to 10 people, Shelton and other mayors argued that the less restrictive statewide orders superseded their more stringent measures (Vance 2020). In Florida, the Democratic mayors of Miami Beach and Fort Lauderdale closed beaches after Gov. Ron DeSantis (R) elected not to do so in mid-March 2020 (NBC Miami 2020). DeSantis defended his decision by emphasizing local control. He explained, "We want [mayors] to have the freedom to [keep beaches open], but we also want them to have the freedom to do more if they see fit" (Willis 2020). In March, Gov. Doug Ducey (R) of Arizona signed an executive order prohibiting city and county governments from closing any essential businesses or declaring stay-at-home orders (Ducey 2020). At times, the opposite pattern was observed with Republican officials in Democratic-led states. In May, the Republican president of the Narragansett, Rhode Island, town council filed (but quickly withdrew) a resolution that directed town police to not enforce penalties if any establishments violated Gov. Gina Raimondo's (D) coronavirus executive orders (Milkovits 2020).

Some Republican governors broke with their colleagues by implementing restrictive measures early or by criticizing the Trump administration's response to COVID-19. For example, Gov. Mike DeWine of Ohio was one of the first Republican governors to regulate activities to prevent or limit the rate of disease spread. DeWine's first COVID-related action in early March came before the state had any documented cases, and Ohio was among the first states to close public schools and issue a statewide stay-at-home order (Witte and Zezima 2020). Similarly, Maryland's Gov. Larry Hogan (R) issued his first COVID-related press release in late January and mobilized state public health officials before the state had any confirmed COVID cases (Office of Governor Larry Hogan 2020). In April, Hogan criticized the Trump administration's handling of the pandemic. After Trump speculated about injecting disinfectants into COVID patients at an April coronavirus task force briefing—a suggestion that deeply alarmed health care professionals and researchers across the country—Hogan remarked, "It's critical that the president of the United States, when people are really scared and in the middle of this worldwide pandemic, in these press conferences that we really get the facts out there, and unfortunately some of the messaging has not been great" (Quinn 2020). Amid a nationwide testing shortage, Hogan also obtained a bulk shipment of a half million COVID test kits from South Korea in late April, sparking Trump's ire. As Trump argued, "the governor of Maryland didn't really understand" the state's COVID-19 testing capacity after the governor had questioned whether enough COVID-19 tests were available to ensure the reopening of the state's economy (Rupar 2020). Hogan responded by defending his decision to obtain test kits from South Korea: "This is exactly what the president has told us to do. Just yesterday, he was saying the governors are responsible for this" (Swalec 2020). By May, Hogan had one of the highest approval ratings among governors nationwide from either party (WJZ 2020).

Public officials also debated who was deserving of relief during the pandemic—individual taxpayers, small businesses, large corporations, or state governments—and to what extent. In March 2020, Democrats and Republicans proposed direct relief payments to individual taxpayers, but in different ways and to different degrees. Some Democrats, including Reps. Tulsi Gabbard (HI) and Alexandria Ocasio-Cortez (NY), advocated for emergency universal basic income, while others, including Reps. Ro Khanna (CA) and Tim Ryan (OH) proposed emergency tax credits. Sen. Mitt Romney (R-UT) favored a onetime cash payment of $1,000, while Sen. Tom Cotton (R-AR) favored monthly payments (Romney 2020). Sen. Bernie Sanders (I-VT), a longtime proponent of Medicare for All, also proposed that Medicare cover all health care expenses during the pandemic (Marans 2020). Ultimately, the Coronavirus Aid, Relief, and Economic Security (CARES) Act unanimously passed the Republican-led Senate on March 25, 2020, and the

Democratic-led House by voice vote the next day. President Trump signed the economic relief package on March 27, 2020. The bill included cash payments to qualifying individuals, unemployment assistance, small business emergency grants and loans, and funding for hospitals and health agencies.

Partisanship became even more pronounced during subsequent economic stimulus debates. In late April, Senate Majority Leader Mitch McConnell (R-KY) suggested that states should declare bankruptcy rather than obtain federal bailout funds. Both Democrats and Republicans criticized the proposal. As Sen. Pat Roberts (R-KS) explained, "There has to be some assistance to state and local governments. . . . This should not be a partisan issue" (Andrews and Wise 2020). Yet, Sen. Rand Paul (R-KY) warned, "We can't continue on this course. No amount of bailout dollars will stimulate an economy that is being strangled by quarantine" (Andrews and Wise 2020). Rep. Alexandria Ocasio-Cortez was the only Democrat who voted against the additional relief plan for small businesses and hospitals. As she argued, "If you had urgency, you would legislate like rent was due on May 1 and make sure we include rent and mortgage relief for our constituents" (Da Silva 2020). As former Vice President Joe Biden and Sen. Elizabeth Warren (D-MA) suggested in early May 2020, "Even the most ideological conservatives have been forced to acknowledge that government is an essential part of the COVID-19 solution. Government delivers best when its actions are fair, transparent and accountable" (Biden and Warren 2020).

In mid-May 2020, the Democratic-led House passed the $3 trillion HEROES Act, which extended unemployment benefits, provided hazard pay for essential workers, increased Supplemental Nutritional Assistance Program (SNAP) benefits, and included funding for state and local governments. Republicans dismissed the legislation as a "liberal wish list" that would never be approved by the Republican-led Senate (Collins 2020).

Democrats and Republicans debated how long social distancing and nonessential business closures would and should remain in force. At one coronavirus task force press briefing in April 2020, President Trump asserted that he could reopen the country regardless of any state or local stay-at-home orders in place. As he argued, "When somebody is the President of the United States, the authority is total" (White 2020). Gov. Andrew Cuomo (D) of New York contradicted Trump: "We would have a constitutional challenge between the state and the federal government, and that would go into the courts, and that would be the worst possible thing he could do at this moment" (Forgey and Oprysko 2020).

As statewide stay-at-home orders remained in place across the country through mid-April, conservative activists held a series of protests at statehouses, challenging Democratic and Republican governors who had issued the orders (Behrmann 2020). Protestors in Minnesota, for example, posted on Facebook, "Our freedoms and economy are under full blown attack by a radical anti-American Governor!" (Liberate Minnesota 2020). Another protest group, Reopen Virginia, argued that "the government mandating healthy citizens to stay home, forcing businesses and churches to close is called tyranny" (WWBT/WHSV 2020). President Trump encouraged these efforts, declaring on Twitter that such states should be "liberated." In response, governors across the country expressed concern that Trump's tweets conflicted with the administration's own guidelines for reopening and would encourage Americans to ignore stay-at-home orders. As Washington's Gov. Jay Inslee (D) argued, "It is dangerous because it can inspire people to ignore things that actually can save their lives." Gov. Gretchen Whitmer (D) of Michigan defended her state's stay-at-home order: "It's working. We are seeing the curve start to flatten. And that means we're saving lives" (Cummings 2020).

In several regions across the country, state governors joined together to announce a series of multistate partnerships to reopen regional economies. In mid-April, the Democratic governors of California, Oregon, and Washington announced a "shared approach for reopening our economies" (Office of Governor Gavin Newsom 2020). That same day, the governors of Connecticut, Delaware, Massachusetts, New Jersey, New York, Pennsylvania, and Rhode Island—six Democrats and one Republican—announced a Northeast regional coalition. Seven Midwestern governors—five Democrats and two Republicans—also established an economic reopening partnership for Illinois, Indiana, Kentucky, Michigan, Minnesota, Ohio, and Wisconsin. Reports indicated that the Republican governors of Iowa, Missouri, North Dakota, and South Dakota declined to participate (Klayman 2020).

Across the country, Republicans filed lawsuits against Democratic governors or sought to introduce alternate recovery plans, concerned that prolonged shutdowns would prolong economic hardship. In Michigan, House Republicans issued Michigan's Comeback Roadmap, which called for reopening less impacted areas rather than maintaining Gov. Whitmer's statewide restrictions (Michigan House Republicans 2020). In Illinois, 11 downstate counties unveiled a plan for regional reopening sooner than allowed under Gov. J. B. Pritzker's (D) Restore Illinois plan. As Peoria Mayor Jim Ardis (R) stated in mid-May 2020, "If the governor comes out and says no, our plan is to move forward" (Register-Mail 2020). All these partisan battles reflected a stark divide in the populace at large. In one April poll, 81 percent of Democrats and Democratic leaners indicated that their greatest concern was that governments would ease restrictions too quickly, while 46 percent of Republicans and Republican leaners feared that restrictions would not be lifted quickly enough (Pew Research Center 2020a). In another poll, 31 percent of Republicans indicated a readiness to return "immediately" to normal activities compared to 11 percent of Democrats (Saad 2020).

Despite partisan differences on reopening, public polls indicated that many Democratic and Republican governors viewed as prioritizing public health and safety over economic considerations received bipartisan support for their handling of the pandemic. In New Jersey, 92 percent of Democrats and 57 percent of Republicans approved of Gov. Phil Murphy's (D) handling (Quinnipiac University Poll

2020). In New Hampshire, public polls indicated even stronger bipartisan support for Gov. Chris Sununu (R): 86 percent of Democrats and 93 percent of Republicans approved of his pandemic response by late April. In fact, 91 percent of Democrats strongly supported Sununu's stay-at-home order versus 45 percent of Republicans (University of New Hampshire Survey Center 2020). In Massachusetts, 80 percent of Democrats and 91 percent of Republicans approved of Gov. Charlie Baker's (R) handling (*Boston Globe* 2020). However, some Republican governors who sought to reopen their states more quickly faced opposition from both sides of the aisle. One May poll found that the Republican governors of Florida, Georgia, and Texas, all of whom sought to reopen their states on a faster schedule, had the three lowest approval ratings among 12 states surveyed (Clement and Balz 2020).

President Trump's approval ratings during the COVID-19 pandemic illustrated the deepening political divide between Democrats and Republicans. In one *Wall Street Journal* poll from March 2020, 81 percent of Republicans approved of Trump's handling of the pandemic, while 84 percent of Democrats disapproved (McCormick 2020). In a University of New Hampshire poll, 97 percent of Democrats disapproved of Trump's handling, while 88 percent of Republicans approved (McKinley, Azem, and Smith 2020). In the midst of an upcoming presidential election, another poll recorded a 15-point favorability drop for Trump in battleground states between March and April 2020 (PPRI 2020). Elsewhere, moderate Republicans in competitive districts voiced concern that Trump's handling of the pandemic would jeopardize their own election chances (Edmonson and Ruiz 2020). One group of Republicans opposed to Trump's reelection, the Lincoln Project, launched television advertisements that reimagined President Ronald Reagan's 1984 reelection campaign ad to "[put] the blame for the government's failures in responding to covid-19 right where it belongs—on Trump," as George Conway explained (Conway 2020). Trump's approval ratings continued to decline throughout the summer, and by mid-July, 60 percent of ABC News poll respondents disapproved of Trump's handling of the pandemic (Langer 2020). Trump's own COVID-19 diagnosis in October 2020 did not shift public opinion in his favor: in one Reuters poll, 65 percent of respondents agreed that if "President Trump had taken coronavirus/COVID-19 more seriously, he probably would not have been infected" (Reuters 2020).

Democrats and Republicans not only disagreed about how politicians were managing the pandemic but also about the scope and severity of the pandemic more generally. This disparity reinforced the fact that Democrats and Republicans learn about health policy issues from different news sources. Gallup surveys highlighted how many Republicans relied on a "conservative news diet" of sources such as Fox News and One America News, while many Democrats relied on a "liberal news diet" of sources that included MSNBC and the *New York Times* (Ritter 2020). In one late March poll, 76 percent of Republicans responded that national media was "overreacting" compared to 21 percent of Democrats (CBS News 2020). In April,

64 percent of Democrats indicated that "the worst is yet to come" compared to 27 percent of Republicans (Kirzinger et al. 2020). By early May, 63 percent of Democrats indicated that they believed that the actual number of COVID-19 deaths was higher than the reported number. Meanwhile, 40 percent of Republicans assumed that the actual number was less than the reported number (Talev 2020).

Other polls suggested that although Americans favored having the federal government in charge of handling the pandemic, they expressed greater trust in their local and state governments (Galston 2020). In one Pew poll from March 2020, 66 percent of Democrats and 73 percent of Republicans agreed that their local officials were doing a "good" or "excellent" job of handling the COVID-19 pandemic (Pew Research Center 2020b).

During the first months of the pandemic, however, the relationships among state governors and the federal government were particularly strained by frustrations regarding states' access to the federal stockpile of personal protective equipment (PPE) and ventilators and by questions about who would fund and administer COVID-19 testing sites across the country. The conservative Heritage Foundation posited that "success will depend on strong federal-state cooperation—and even more so on the capacity and competence of governors and state public health authorities to fashion policies appropriate to the conditions on the ground" (Moffit and Badger 2020). In March, Senior Advisor to the President Jared Kushner responded to public criticism from governors by arguing that the federal stockpile was "not supposed to be states' stockpiles that they then use" (Ordoñez 2020). Kushner also emphasized ceding the federal government's responsibility for the pandemic response to the private sector. He argued, "The federal government is not designed to solve all our problems; a lot of the muscle is in the private sector and there's also a lot of smart people" (Abutaleb, Parker, and Dawsey 2020).

In April, federal funding for testing sites transitioned to the states. One Health and Human Services spokesperson justified the shift by saying, "The transition will ensure each state has the flexibility and autonomy to manage and operate testing sites within the needs of their specific community and to prioritize resources where they are needed the most" (Brady 2020). Democratic governors, on the other hand, argued that this shift and the lack of a national testing strategy signaled the shirking of federal responsibility. As New York's Gov. Andrew Cuomo (D) declared, "Don't give [the states] this massive undertaking that has never been done before and then not give them any resources to do it" (Shabad 2020). Gov. Ned Lamont (D) of Connecticut also criticized the administration's stance, stating, "Obviously, if the Feds would take the lead on [testing], it would be a lot more effective" (CNN 2020).

Democrats and Republicans responded differently to calls to change personal behaviors during the COVID-19 pandemic. For example, in March 2020, 59 percent of Democrats reported they sought to avoid large gatherings, while 60 percent of Republicans did not (Allyn and Sprunt 2020). In one study of geolocation and debit card usage, residents in Democratic counties were more likely to comply with stay-at-home orders than residents in Republican counties. Moreover, compliance rose when a governor's political affiliation aligned with the political makeup of a given county (Painter and Qiu 2020). Mask wearing became an ideologically charged gesture, particularly among public officeholders. As two political correspondents observed, "The mask has become the ultimate symbol of this new cultural and political divide" (Lizza and Lippman 2020).

At an early April 2020 Coronavirus Task Force press conference, President Trump announced new Centers for Disease Control and Prevention (CDC) guidelines for mask wearing but also acknowledged that "this is voluntary. I don't think I'm going to be doing it" (Bennett 2020). While many Democratic legislators wore face coverings in public, some members of the Trump administration and Republican legislators forewent doing so, despite repeated declarations from public health officials in the administration that mask wearing was the most effective practice that citizens could adopt to protect themselves and others when out in public. U.S. House Rules Committee Chairman Jim McGovern (D-MA) criticized Republican colleagues for not wearing masks during committee hearings in late April: "While we all want to show how fearless we are, we should be mindful of the people that are surrounding us" (Nelson 2020). By mid-June, Speaker Nancy Pelosi (D-CA) required all members of the House to wear masks at all hearings (Axelrod 2020).

Although public polls suggested that the percentage of Americans who wore face masks outside the home had increased in early April, partisan differences remained: 75 percent of Democrats reported wearing masks compared to 58 percent of Republicans (Brenan 2020). By May, Democrats were more likely than Republicans to report that social distancing measures were helping slow the spread of COVID-19 "a lot" (Funk, Kennedy, and Johnson 2020). As the pandemic surged through red states in June and July, prominent Republicans began encouraging Americans to wear masks to slow the spread of COVID-19. In late June, Senate Majority Leader Mitch McConnell (R-KY) said, "We must have no stigma, none, about wearing masks when we leave our homes and come near other people" (Phillips 2020). After weeks of public statements minimizing the importance of wearing masks, in late July, President Trump tweeted a photo of himself wearing a face mask for the first time and wrote, "Many people say that it is Patriotic to wear a face mask when you can't socially distance" (Trump 2020b).

Democrats on COVID-19

Democratic responses to COVID-19 embodied liberal conceptions of civil rights, social responsibility, and the role of government in solving social problems. For Democrats, COVID-19 represented a public health emergency that demanded decisive federal, state, and local action. Moreover, Democrats insisted that the pandemic reinforced the social contract that governments have with their citizens.

Early on, Democrats argued that the Trump administration had unnecessarily jeopardized the nation's health and safety by destabilizing the federal pandemic preparedness apparatus. In mid-February 2020, 27 Democratic senators sent a letter to the White House inquiring why the position of head of global health security on the National Security Council had remained vacant since 2018 (Warren et al. 2020). As Joe Biden later tweeted, "The Obama-Biden Administration set up the White House National Security Council Directorate for Global Health Security and Biodefense to prepare for future pandemics like COVID-19. Donald Trump eliminated it—and now we're paying the price" (Biden 2020). When Trump remarked that "nobody ever expected a thing like this" at a town hall in March 2020, former Obama administration officials publicly argued otherwise (Trump 2020a).

Virus terminology became politically contested as Democrats drew attention to rising anti-Asian sentiment associated with the pandemic. Even after the World Health Organization (WHO) warned against employing geographic signifiers when referring to COVID-19, some conservative politicians referred to the virus as the "Chinese virus" or the "Wuhan virus," in part to blame the Chinese government for its presumed lack of transparency about the disease outbreak. Democrats argued that identifying COVID-19 by geographic terms was racist and xenophobic. Rep. Ted Lieu (D-CA) tweeted, "Calling COVID-19 the Wuhan Virus is an example of

Coronavirus Requires Federal Leadership

In a July 15, 2020, press release, Rep. Maxine Waters (D-CA) issued a strong rebuke of President Donald Trump's management of the COVID-19 pandemic.

> Instead of a real president, the American people are left to suffer through the repeated failures of an impeached criminal who lacks the knowledge, experience, or common human decency to provide the leadership that our country needs to survive this public health nightmare. Donald Trump is too much of a coward to use his authority to fully invoke the Defense Production Act (DPA) in order to meet the PPE and medical device needs of our healthcare industry and communities. He's too insecure to respect the life-saving guidance of Dr. Anthony Fauci, our top infectious disease expert whose approval and trustworthiness ratings are greater than his in the eyes of the American people. He's too untrustworthy to allow hospitals and the Centers for Disease Control (CDC) to maintain autonomy in recording COVID-19 cases and patient information, and instead wants them to send the data to his administration cronies. He's too ignorant to wear a mask, and he's too incompetent, dangerous, and too much of an international disgrace to serve in office of the presidency for another day.

Source

Maxine Waters. 2020. "Rep. Maxine Waters: This President Is Failing & People Are Dying." July 15. Accessed March 13, 2021. https://waters.house.gov/media-center/press-releases/rep-maxine-waters-president-failing-americans-are-dying.

the myopia that allowed it to spread in the US. The virus is not constrained by country or race" (Lieu 2020). In one March *Economist*/YouGov poll, 73 percent of Democratic primary voters agreed with the proposition that individuals who referred to COVID-19 as the "Chinese virus," "Kung flu," or "Wuhan virus" were racist (YouGov 2020). In mid-May, Sens. Kamala Harris (D-CA), Tammy Duckworth (D-IL), and Mazie Hirono (D-HI) introduced a resolution condemning anti-Asian rhetoric and discrimination related to the pandemic (S. Res. 580 2020).

Democrats emphasized that state governments had a responsibility to mandate social distancing and stay-at-home orders and argued that such measures were imperative. Days after he implemented a statewide stay-at-home order in March 2020, Gov. Gavin Newsom (D) of California remarked, "There's a social contract here. People, I think, recognize the need to do more and to meet this moment" (Drezner 2020). In contrast to Republican governors who insisted on voluntary social distancing to preserve individual liberty, Gov. Kate Brown (D) of Oregon argued for the need for greater government restrictions to save lives: "I started by asking Oregonians to stay home and practice social distancing. Then I urged the public to follow these recommendations. Instead, thousands crowded the beaches of our coastal communities, our trails, our parks, and our city streets, potentially spreading COVID-19 and endangering the lives of others across the state. Now, I'm ordering it. To save lives and protect our community" (KATU 2020). In April, after conservative groups protested Michigan's Gov. Gretchen Whitmer's (D) stay-at-home order, Michigan State Attorney General Dana Nessel emphasized that "if people all around our state do not have their lives cut short and instead go on to rebuild their future in the aftermath of this terrible time, then Governor Whitmer will have done her job" (Nichols and Demas 2020).

Democratic governors also argued that they required substantive financial and logistical support from the federal government. The pandemic had significantly impacted supply chains for foodstuffs, household products, and medical supplies, such as surgical masks, N95 respirators, and other PPE. As Gov. Andrew Cuomo (D-NY) asserted, "State and local governments alone simply do not have the capacity or resources to do what is necessary" without federal assistance (Cuomo 2020). When that federal assistance failed to arrive, state governments were forced to compete on the open market for medical supplies. The situation prompted Gov. J. B. Pritzker (D) of Illinois to lament, "It's a Wild West out there. And, indeed, we are overpaying" (Knutson 2020).

Democratic governors suggested that the federal government had actively impeded their purchase efforts following reports of federal seizures of state supply orders. As the Trump administration invoked the Defense Production Act to acquire medical supplies ahead of states and hospitals, Kentucky's Gov. Andy Beshear (D) remarked, "It's very hard to buy things when the federal government is there and anytime they want to buy it, they get it first" (Van Velzer 2020). In response to this challenge, Rep. Anthony Brown (D-MD) and Sen. Elizabeth Warren (D-MA) sponsored bills to centralize the purchasing and distribution of medical supplies. Warren argued, "We can't confront a national crisis with bidding wars and massive price increases—we need a national strategy" (Caygle 2020). Lacking a national strategy, a group of Northeast and mid-Atlantic governors agreed to develop a regional supply chain. Gov. John Carney (D) of Delaware emphasized, "We'll be better positioned to continue tackling this crisis working together with the states around us" (Office of Governor Andrew Cuomo 2020).

Democratic governors in states significantly impacted by COVID-19 also sought to deescalate partisan tensions by calling for national unity. As Gov. Cuomo offered during one press briefing, "Forget the politics. We have a national crisis. We are at war. There is no politics. There is no red and blue. It's red, white and blue. So let's get over it and, again, lead by example" (Allassan 2020). In response to public protests against her executive actions, Gov. Whitmer of Michigan remarked, "We must remember that the enemy is not one another, it is the coronavirus, a threat unconstrained by state lines or party registration" (Whitmer 2020). By late June, the United States set multiple daily records for confirmed COVID-19 cases, spurring Democrats to call for a federal mandate on wearing masks. As negotiations for additional COVID-19 relief bills remained deadlocked leading up to the 2020 presidential election, Democrats repeatedly emphasized that economic recovery would not happen without an effective and coordinated pandemic response. As the Democratic party's 2020 platform put it, "Solving the public health crisis posed by the pandemic is the surest way to get the economy back on track" (Democratic National Committee 2020).

Republicans on COVID-19

Republican responses to COVID-19 have reflected conservative conceptions of civil liberties, individual freedom, and limited government. For Republicans, the prospect of government overreach in the name of public health was great, whether restricting freedom of religion or freedom of public assembly. Any actions taken by state and federal governments had to be measured against their economic impact and their imposition on individual civil liberties.

Throughout January and February 2020, members of the Trump administration argued that initial media coverage about the pandemic was excessive and melodramatic. On February 25, then Trump campaign spokeswoman Kayleigh McEnany said, "We will not see diseases like the coronavirus come here" (Kaczynski, Steck, and McDermott 2020). The administration also claimed that Democrats sought to stoke public fear about COVID-19 in a partisan attempt to damage President Trump. As White House Chief of Staff Mick Mulvaney intimated at the Conservative Political Action Conference (CPAC), "They think this is going to be what brings down the president. That's what this is all about" (Behrmann and Fritze 2020). On February 29, the day before the announcement of the first COVID-19 death in the

United States, Trump said during a rally in South Carolina, "The Democrats are politicizing the coronavirus. . . . This is their new hoax" (Cook and Choi 2020).

The Trump administration's strategy of minimizing the likely severity and duration of the pandemic was reflected in conservative media. In late March, one poll found that only 33 percent of Republicans perceived the spread of COVID-19 as a "crisis" (CBS News 2020). By April, some Republicans suggested that the media had overhyped the pandemic because COVID-related deaths had not reached the original projections at that point. As former U.S. Secretary of Education William Bennett and Seth Leibsohn posited, "A panic and hysteria over a pandemic that does not look to be what so many frightened us into thinking has radically degraded this country" (Bennett and Leibsohn 2020). As the number of COVID-19 deaths exceeded 100,000 by the end of May, some prominent Republicans distanced themselves from Trump's efforts to minimize the scope

Ingenuity Will Reopen America

On March 25, 2020, Sen. Tom Cotton (R-AR) emphasized industrial ingenuity on the path toward reopening the American economy.

> America must, indeed, reopen. When we do, these decisions must be based on local conditions, not an arbitrary nationwide timeline. Our Governors and mayors understand their local conditions. They can make gradual, rolling, calibrated decisions in a way that is responsible when the tools to effectively fight this virus are ready and available.
>
> What I have outlined may seem like a daunting and even impossible challenge, but our Nation has overcome far greater challenges before. Already, America is rising to take on the China virus. The giant of American industry is awakening and retooling our factories to join this fight just as we did during World War II. Never bet against America's workers and American ingenuity. All across this country, Americans are springing into action. We know the vital role our doctors and nurses will play in the coming months alongside our first responders, our factory workers, our farmers, our grocers, and on down the list.
>
> Ask yourself now how you can help. Can you keep your distance from those who are most at risk, realizing that the China virus preys on our most earnest desires for society and companionship? Can you offer your charity to a friend in need? Can you pick up groceries for your elderly neighbor? Can you keep your workers on payroll and benefits for just a little longer until our legislation kicks in? Can you postpone your tenant's rent for a month? Can you pray for the deliverance of our Nation and the world?

Source

Congressional Record, vol. 166, no. 59 (March 25, 2020): S2033. Washington, DC: Government Printing Office. Accessed May 24, 2020. https://www.congress.gov/116/crec/2020/03/25/CREC-2020-03-25-pt1-PgS2022-4.pdf.

and severity of the pandemic. Public opinion polls indicated that Maryland's Gov. Larry Hogan—one of Trump's most vocal Republican critics—was the most popular governor in the nation with an 85 percent approval rating (Blake 2020). In one June interview, Hogan suggested that Trump should prepare for the pandemic's second wave by "listen[ing] to the scientists, look[ing] at the science, and mak[ing] the decisions based on that" (Kroll 2020). Reporters from other news outlets documented how programming on Fox News, the conservative news outlet favored by Trump, evolved from initially downplaying the pandemic to declaring it a public health crisis and de-emphasizing controversial positions on mask wearing (Nazaryan 2020).

Republicans insisted that steps taken to combat COVID-19 also had to be judged by whether they threatened civil liberties or took too heavy an economic toll. As President Trump tweeted, "We cannot let the cure be worse than the problem itself" (Trump 2020b). Some Republicans compared COVID-19 to other public health risks and warned against what they perceived as disproportionate policy responses. As Sen. Ron Johnson (R-WI) suggested, "We don't shut down our economy because tens of thousands of people die on the highways. It's a risk we accept so we can move about. We don't shut down our economies because tens of thousands of people die from the common flu" (Gilbert 2020). Some Republican officials and allies in conservative media criticized public health officials who called for significant curtailments in social and economic activity to reduce disease transmission. Drs. Anthony Fauci and Deborah Birx, prominent members of the White House Coronavirus Task Force, were particular targets of this type of criticism. Reps. Andy Biggs (R-AZ) and Ken Buck (R-CO), for example, dismissed Fauci and Birx as "the dynamic duo of economic destruction" who were preventing the reopening of state economies (Biggs and Buck 2020).

Republican governors encouraged citizens to exercise their personal responsibility to practice social distancing rather than be forced to do so by government mandate. Gov. Kristi Noem (R) of South Dakota justified not issuing a statewide stay-at-home order by stating that citizens should be able to decide "to exercise their right to work, to worship and to play. Or to even stay at home" (Witte 2020). Similarly, Nebraska's Gov. Pete Ricketts (R) touted his voluntary social distancing order as "about [you] making that decision, not the heavy hand of government taking away your freedoms" (Ollstein, Goldberg, and McCaskill 2020). Some Republican governors intimated that stay-at-home orders were akin to communism or socialism. When Gov. Tate Reeves (R) of Mississippi first rejected issuing a statewide order, he remarked, "Mississippi's never going to be China. Mississippi's never going to be North Korea" (Judin 2020). Other Republican governors proudly characterized their stances as ones that reflected their states' individual needs. When Alabama's Gov. Kay Ivey (R) declined to issue a statewide order in late March, she remarked, "Y'all, we are not Louisiana, we are not New York state, we are not California" (Bump 2020). Eight days later, Ivey ordered the closing of nonessential businesses and issued a statewide stay-at-home order as cases continued to rise in the state (Fulmore 2020).

Republican governors were particularly hesitant to impose size limits on public gatherings in churches and other spaces, characterizing such mandates as threats to religious freedom. Gov. Greg Abbott (R) of Texas and Gov. Ron DeSantis (R) of Florida included religious exemptions in their statewide orders, for example. As DeSantis suggested, "I don't think government has the authority to close churches, and I'm certainly not going to do that" (Garza 2020). In Kansas, the state's Legislative Coordinating Council voted along party lines to revoke Gov. Laura Kelly's (D) order that limited religious gatherings in the state to 10 people. As Kansas State Senate President Susan Wagle (R) indicated, "I think they were just very upset with the fact that the government was going to tell them that they couldn't practice their religion" (Shorman, Leiker, and Stavola 2020). After Greenville, Mississippi, issued fines to church congregants who attended religious services held in a parking lot, U.S. Attorney General William Barr issued a statement in defense of religious liberty. Barr asserted, "The United States Department of Justice will continue to ensure that religious freedom remains protected if any state or local government, in their response to COVID-19, singles out, targets, or discriminates against any house of worship for special restrictions" (U.S. Department of Justice, Office of Public Affairs 2020).

In part, Republicans interpreted viral mitigation measures as a worrisome turn from limited government. In April 2020, Attorney General Barr indicated that the Justice Department would consider legal action against governors if strict measures continued. As he explained, "These are very, very burdensome impingements on liberty. And we adopted them, we have to remember, for the limited purpose of slowing down the spread, that is bending the curve. We didn't adopt them as the comprehensive way of dealing with this disease" (Strohm 2020). As former Senator Phil Gramm (R-TX) argued, "Democrats hold a strong advantage in their efforts to define post-pandemic America. . . . The role of government in post-coronavirus America will be significantly expanded" (Gramm and Solon 2020).

Around the country, Republicans initiated legal challenges to statewide shutdown orders, insisting that governors that issued such orders were exceeding their emergency powers. In May 2020, Rhode Island conservatives announced their intention to sue Gov. Gina Raimondo (D), arguing that "the Governor cannot use the pandemic as an excuse to suspend constitutional rights" (Flanders, Fabisch, and MacAdams 2020). That same month, Wisconsin Republicans brought a lawsuit to strike down Gov. Tony Evers's (D) statewide shutdown order. The conservative majority of the Wisconsin State Supreme Court issued a ruling that upheld school closures but lifted all restrictions on businesses and public gatherings. Following the ruling, Wisconsin State Assembly Speaker Robin Vos (R) declared, "As a Republican, I believe in local control," and dismissed the need for a new statewide plan (Beck and Marley 2020).

As lawsuits rescinded some statewide orders and governors across the country began implementing phased reopening plans in May and June 2020, how to best mitigate risk via mask wearing and social distancing remained a politically sensitive topic. As Rep. Dan Crenshaw (R-TX) argued in a *Wall Street Journal* editorial, "Just because you don't want to confront risk doesn't mean others should be prevented from doing so" (Crenshaw 2020). By July 2020, partisan debates on reopening shifted to determining whether and how schools would reopen in the fall. By the end of that month, the United States surpassed 4 million cases and 150,000 deaths from COVID-19 (COVID Tracking Project 2020).

Todd M. Olszewski

Further Reading

Abutaleb, Yasmeen, Ashley Parker, and Josh Dawsey. 2020. "Kushner Coronavirus Team Sparks Confusion, Plaudits Inside White House Response Efforts." *Washington Post*, March 18. Accessed July 11, 2020. https://www.washingtonpost.com/politics/kushner-coronavirus-team-sparks-confusion-plaudits-inside-white-house-response-efforts/2020/03/18/02038a16-6874-11ea-9923-57073adce27c_story.html.

Agiesta, Jennifer. 2020. "CNN Poll: Americans Divided over Government Handling of Coronavirus Outbreak." CNN, March 30. Accessed July 10, 2020. https://www.cnn.com/2020/03/30/politics/cnn-poll-americans-coronavirus-government-approval/index.html.

Allassan, Fadel. 2020. "Cuomo: Engaging in Politics during Coronavirus Crisis Is 'Anti-American.'" Axios, March 30. Accessed July 11, 2020. https://www.axios.com/andrew-cuomo-trump-politics-coronavirus-new-york-a3612adc-2dac-48c9-b2c6-c2d5c476a220.html.

Allyn, Bobby, and Barbara Sprunt. 2020. "Poll: As Coronavirus Spreads, Fewer Americans See Pandemic as a Real Threat." NPR, March 17. Accessed July 11, 2020. https://www.npr.org/2020/03/17/816501871/poll-as-coronavirus-spreads-fewer-americans-see-pandemic-as-a-real-threat.

Altman, Drew. 2020. "Reopening Is a Risk for Republican Governors." Axios, May 4. Accessed July 17, 2020. https://www.axios.com/coronavirus-reopening-republican-governors-cases-deaths-c0233fd4-8f92-448e-a11c-ec5bded1def1.html.

Andrews, Natalie, and Lindsay Wise. 2020. "Lawmakers Set to Take Gloves Off in Next Coronavirus Aid Fight." *Wall Street Journal*, April 23. Accessed July 9, 2020. https://www.wsj.com/articles/lawmakers-set-to-take-gloves-off-in-next-coronavirus-aid-fight-11587655822?mod=hp_lead_pos4.

Axelrod, Tal. 2020. "Pelosi Asks House Chairs to Enforce Mandatory Mask-Wearing during Hearings." The Hill, June 16. Accessed July 20, 2020. https://thehill.com/homenews/house/503100-pelosi-requests-committee-chairs-require-members-to-wear-masks-during.

Beck, Molly, and Patrick Marley. 2020. "Top GOP Lawmakers Now Want to Leave Virus Plan in the Hands of Local Officials." *Milwaukee Journal Sentinel*, May 14. Accessed July 13, 2020. https://www.jsonline.com/story/news/politics/2020/05/14/tony-evers-gop-lawmakers-meet-after-supreme-court-ruling-on-coronavirus-orders/5189390002/.

Behrmann, Savannah. 2020. "Protests Draw Thousands over State Stay-at-Home Orders during Coronavirus Pandemic." *USA Today*, April 15. Accessed July 13, 2020. https://

www.usatoday.com/story/news/politics/2020/04/15/coronavirus-multiple-states-see-protests-over-stay-home-rules/5142499002/.

Behrmann, Savannah, and John Fritze. 2020. "Mick Mulvaney Says Media Covering Coronavirus because They Think It Will 'Bring Down' Trump." *USA Today*, February 28. Accessed July 6, 2020. https://www.usatoday.com/story/news/politics/2020/02/28/mick-mulvaney-says-media-hopes-coronavirus-bring-down-trump/4907058002/.

Bennett, Brian. 2020. "President Trump Say Americans Should Cover Their Mouths in Public—But He Won't." *Time*, April 3. Accessed March 11, 2021. https://time.com/5815615/trump-coronavirus-mixed-messaging/.

Bennett, William, and Seth Leibsohn. 2020. "Coronavirus Lessons: Fact and Reason vs. Paranoia and Fear." Real Clear Politics, April 15. Accessed July 9, 2020. https://www.realclearpolitics.com/articles/2020/04/15/coronavirus_lessons_fact_and_reason_vs_paranoia_and_fear_.html.

Biden, Joe (@JoeBiden). 2020. "The Obama-Biden Administration set up the White House National Security Council Directorate for Global Health Security and Biodefense to Prepare for Future Pandemics Like COVID-19. Donald Trump Eliminated It—And Now We're Paying the Price." Twitter, March 19, 2020. Accessed February 18, 2021. https://twitter.com/JoeBiden/status/1240646710021537792.

Biden, Joe, and Elizabeth Warren. 2020. "Biden, Warren: There's No Oversight of Coronavirus Relief—Because That's What Trump Wants." *Miami Herald*, May 3. Accessed July 11, 2020. https://www.miamiherald.com/article242350451.html.

Biggs, Andy, and Ken Buck. 2020. "The Fauci-Birx Doctrine of Destruction." *Washington Examiner*, April 27. Accessed July 11, 2020. https://www.washingtonexaminer.com/opinion/op-eds/the-fauci-birx-doctrine-of-destruction

Blake, Aaron. 2020. "49 of 50 Governors Have Better Coronavirus Poll Numbers Than Trump." *Washington Post*, May 19. Accessed October 31, 2020. https://www.washingtonpost.com/politics/2020/05/19/49-50-governors-have-better-coronavirus-numbers-than-trump/.

Boston Globe. 2020. "Read the Full Results of the Suffolk/Globe Poll about the Coronavirus Response." *Boston Globe*, March 30. Accessed July 16, 2020. https://www.bostonglobe.com/2020/03/29/metro/read-full-results-suffolkglobe-poll-about-coronavirus-response/.

Brady, Jeff. 2020. "Federal Support Ends for Coronavirus Testing Sites as Pandemic Peak Nears." NPR, April 8. Accessed July 12, 2020. https://www.npr.org/sections/coronavirus-live-updates/2020/04/08/829955099/federal-support-for-coronavirus-testing-sites-end-as-peak-nears.

Brenan, Megan. 2020. "Americans' Reported Use of Face Masks Surges in Past Week." Gallup, April 17. Accessed July 8, 2020. https://news.gallup.com/poll/308678/americans-reported-face-masks-surges-past-week.aspx.

Bump, Philip. 2020. "Alabama Governor Won't Issue Stay-at-Home Order because 'We Are Not California.' By Population, It's Worse." *Washington Post*, March 27. Accessed July 11, 2020. https://www.washingtonpost.com/politics/2020/03/27/alabama-governor-wont-order-shelter-in-place-because-we-are-not-california-by-population-its-worse/.

Caygle, Heather. 2020. "Democrats Push for Federal Control during Medical Supply Shortage." Politico, May 1. Accessed July 13, 2020. https://www.politico.com/news/2020/05/01/democrats-supply-chain-226968.

CBS News. 2020. "CBS News Poll. March 21–23, 2020." March 23. Accessed July 11, 2020. https://drive.google.com/file/d/1TofJVeuCbZN8cRGBN97kWGqhO6tlQ7VA/view.

Clement, Scott, and Dan Balz. 2020. "Many Governors Win Bipartisan Support for Handling of Pandemic, but Some Republicans Face Blowback over Reopening Efforts." *Washington Post*, May 12. Accessed July 9, 2020. https://www.washingtonpost.com/politics/many-governors-win-bipartisan-support-for-handling-of-pandemic-but-some-republicans-face-blowback-over-reopening-efforts/2020/05/11/8e98500e-93d2-11ea-9f5e-56d8239bf9ad_story.html.

CNN. 2020. "Transcripts. Cuomo Prime Time." CNN, April 13. Accessed October 31, 2020. http://transcripts.cnn.com/TRANSCRIPTS/2004/13/CPT.01.html.

Collins, Doug. 2020. "Collins Statement on Pelosi's Liberal Wish List." May 15. Accessed July 12, 2020. https://dougcollins.house.gov/media-center/press-releases/collins-statement-pelosi-s-liberal-wish-list.

Conway, George, III. 2020. "George Conway: Trump Went Ballistic at Me on Twitter. Here's Why He Reacts with Such Rage." *Washington Post*, May 6. Accessed July 14, 2020. https://www.washingtonpost.com/opinions/2020/05/06/george-conway-trump-lashed-out-me-twitter-its-because-he-knows-truth/.

Cook, Nancy, and Matthew Choi. 2020. "Trump Rallies His Base to Treat Coronavirus as a 'Hoax.'" Politico, February 28. Accessed July 7, 2020. https://www.politico.com/news/2020/02/28/trump-south-carolina-rally-coronavirus-118269.

COVID Tracking Project. 2020. "US Historical Data." Accessed July 29, 2020. https://covidtracking.com/data/us-daily.

Crenshaw, Dan. 2020. "Why Does Reopening Polarize Us?" *Wall Street Journal*, May 18. Accessed July 15, 2020. https://www.wsj.com/articles/why-does-reopening-polarize-us-11589842995.

Cummings, William. 2020. "Governors Slam Trump's Call to 'Liberate' States Where Protestors Object to Coronavirus Restrictions." *USA Today*, April 19. Accessed October 31, 2020. https://www.usatoday.com/story/news/politics/2020/04/19/governors-decry-trump-call-liberate-states-coronavirus-restrictions/5162196002/.

Cuomo, Andrew. 2020. "Andrew Cuomo to President Trump: Mobilize the Military to Help Fight Coronavirus." *New York Times*, March 15. Accessed July 8, 2020. https://www.nytimes.com/2020/03/15/opinion/andrew-cuomo-coronavirus-trump.html.

Da Silva, Chantal. 2020. "Alexandria Ocasio-Cortez Explains Why She Voted against Coronavirus Relief Package." *Newsweek*, April 24. Accessed July 12, 2020. https://www.newsweek.com/alexandria-ocasio-cortez-explains-why-she-voted-against-coronavirus-relief-package-1499998.

Democratic National Committee. 2020. *2020 Democratic Party Platform*. Accessed October 31, 2020. https://www.demconvention.com/wp-content/uploads/2020/08/2020-07-31-Democratic-Party-Platform-For-Distribution.pdf.

Drezner, Daniel. 2020. "So How Is Society's Response to the Coronavirus Going?" *Washington Post*, March 23. Accessed July 12, 2020. https://www.washingtonpost.com/outlook/2020/03/23/so-how-is-societys-response-coronavirus-going/.

Ducey, Douglas. 2020. "Executive Order 2020-12. Prohibiting the Closure of Essential Services." March 23. Accessed July 10, 2020. https://azgovernor.gov/sites/default/files/eo_2021_0.pdf.

Edmonson, Catie, and Rebecca Ruiz. 2020. "Fearing Political Peril, Republicans Edge Away from Trump on Pandemic Response." *New York Times*, May 2. Accessed July 14, 2020.

https://www.nytimes.com/2020/05/02/us/politics/coronavirus-trump-republicans.html.

Flanders, Robert, Matthew Fabisch, and Richard MacAdams. 2020. "Limits on Emergency Executive Powers in Rhode Island." Rhode Island Center for Freedom & Prosperity, May 13. Accessed July 12, 2020. http://rifreedom.org/wp-content/uploads/FlandersCenter-EmergencyPowers-final.pdf.

Forgey, Quint, and Caitlin Oprysko. 2020. "Governors Defy Trump, Who Cries 'Mutiny.'" Politico, April 14. Accessed July 13, 2020. https://www.politico.com/news/2020/04/14/cuomo-new-york-reopen-trump-185313.

Fulmore, Miranda. 2020. "Gov. Ivey Issues Statewide Stay-at-Home Order Effective April 4." WBHM, April 3. Accessed July 8, 2020. https://wbhm.org/feature/2020/gov-ivey-issues-statewide-stay-home-order-effective-april-4/.

Funk, Cary, Brian Kennedy, and Courtney Johnson. 2020. "Trust in Medical Scientists Has Grown in U.S., but Mainly among Democrats." Pew Research Center, May 21. Accessed July 9, 2020. https://www.pewresearch.org/science/2020/05/21/trust-in-medical-scientists-has-grown-in-u-s-but-mainly-among-democrats/.

Galston, William. 2020. "Polling Shows Americans See COVID-19 as a Crisis, Don't Think US Is Overreacting." Brookings Institute, March 30. Accessed July 11, 2020. https://www.brookings.edu/blog/fixgov/2020/03/30/polling-shows-americans-see-covid-19-as-a-crisis-dont-think-u-s-is-overreacting/.

Garza, Lisa Maria. 2020. "Despite Coronavirus Concerns, Worshippers Gather at Orlando Church under Statewide Exemption." *Orlando Sentinel*, April 5. Accessed July 9, 2020. https://www.orlandosentinel.com/coronavirus/os-ne-coronavirus-orlando-church-open-20200405-eu3rpyapr5cjtoh4zcnlvtzhxu-story.html.

Gilbert, Craig. 2020. "Sen. Ron Johnson Is Telling People to Keep Coronavirus in Perspective." *Milwaukee Journal Sentinel*, March 18. Accessed July 20, 2020. https://www.jsonline.com/story/news/politics/analysis/2020/03/18/coronavirus-sen-ron-johnson-says-keep-outbreak-perspective/5074145002/.

Gramm, Phil, and Michael Solon. 2020. "More 'Stimulus' Would Crush the Recovery." *Wall Street Journal*, April 14. Accessed March 11, 2021. https://www.wsj.com/articles/more-stimulus-would-crush-the-recovery-11586882680.

Jayapal, Pramila. 2020. "Jayapal to Vote No on Heroes Act." May 15. Accessed July 12, 2020. https://jayapal.house.gov/2020/05/15/jayapal-to-vote-no-on-heroes-act-as-legislation-fails-to-protect-the-paychecks-of-workers-guarantee-families-affordable-health-care-provide-sufficient-relief-to-all-businesses-and-safeguard-pensions/.

Judin, Nick. 2020. "Governor Rejects State Lockdown for COVID-19: 'Mississippi's Never Going to Be China.'" *Jackson Free Press*, March 23. Accessed July 10, 2020. https://www.jacksonfreepress.com/news/2020/mar/23/governor-rejects-state-lockdown-covid-19-mississip/.

Kaczynski, Andrew, Em Steck, and Nathan McDermott. 2020. "'Nothing to Worry About' and "It's Being Contained': How Trump Officials Downplayed the Coronavirus." CNN, April 18. Accessed July 10, 2020. https://amp.cnn.com/cnn/2020/04/18/politics/kfile-trump-officials-coronavirus/index.html.

KATU. 2020. "Gov. Brown Issues 'Stay at Home' Order, Closes Many Non-Essential Businesses." KATU, March 23. Accessed July 9, 2020. https://katu.com/news/local/oregon-gov-brown-likely-to-order-stay-at-home-order-monday-amid-coronavirus-outbreak.

Kirzinger, Ashley, Liz Hamel, Cailey Muñana, Audrey Kearney, and Mollyanne Brodie. 2020. "KFF Health Tracking Poll—Late April 2020: Coronavirus, Social Distancing, and Contact Tracing." Kaiser Family Foundation, April 24. Accessed July 11, 2020. https://www.kff.org/global-health-policy/issue-brief/kff-health-tracking-poll-late-april-2020/.

Klayman, Ben. 2020. "U.S. Midwest Governors to Coordinate Reopening Economies Battered by Coronavirus." Reuters, April 16. Accessed July 10, 2020. https://mobile.reuters.com/article/amp/idUSKBN21Y2ZB.

Knutson, Jacob. 2020. "Illinois Governor: States Are 'Competing against Each Other' for Medical Supplies." Axios, March 22. Accessed July 7, 2020. https://www.axios.com/illinois-gov-states-competing-medical-supplies-822678c5-4301-4c4c-a5a5-887da539b63f.html.

Kroll, Andy. 2020. "Republican Larry Hogan, America's Most Popular Governor, Has Some Advice for Trump." *Rolling Stone*, June 11. Accessed October 31, 2020. https://www.rollingstone.com/politics/politics-features/larry-hogan-maryland-governor-coronavirus-trump-white-house-covid-republican-party-1013038/.

Langer, Gary. 2020. "64% Distrust Trump on Coronavirus Pandemic; Approval Declines as Cases Grow: Poll." ABC News, July 17. Accessed October 31, 2020. https://abcnews.go.com/Politics/64-distrust-trump-coronavirus-pandemic-approval-declines-cases/story?id=71779279.

Liberate Minnesota. 2020. "Minnesota Citizens Now Is the Time to Demand Governor Walz and Our State Legislators End This Lock Down!" Facebook, April 17, 2020. Accessed February 18, 2021. https://www.facebook.com/events/1201743216823346/.

Lieu, Ted (@tedlieu). 2020. "Dear @DrPaulGosar: I Will Pray for You, Your Staff & the Person Hospitalized. Also, Calling #COVID-19 the Wuhan Virus Is an Example of the Myopia That Allowed It to Spread in the US. The Virus Is Not Constrained by Country or Race. Be Just as Stupid to Call it the Milan Virus." Twitter, March 8, 2020. https://twitter.com/tedlieu/status/1236832456793186304.

Lizza, Ryan, and Daniel Lippman. 2020. "Wearing a Mask Is for Smug Liberals. Refusing to Is for Reckless Republicans." Politico, May 1. Accessed July 13, 2020. https://www.politico.com/news/2020/05/01/masks-politics-coronavirus-227765.

Marans, Daniel. 2020. "Bernie Sanders Proposes $2 Trillion Coronavirus Relief Effort." *Huffington Post*, March 17. Accessed July 12, 2020. https://www.huffpost.com/entry/bernie-sanders-coronavirus-relief-plan-income-support-medicare-expansion_n_5e717a39c5b6eab7793e670d.

McCormick, John. 2020. "Americans Fear Worst Is Yet to Come from Coronavirus, WSJ/NBC Poll Finds." *Wall Street Journal*, March 15. Accessed July 10, 2020. https://www.wsj.com/articles/americans-fear-worst-is-yet-to-come-from-coronavirus-wsj-nbc-poll-finds-11584277201.

McKinley, Sean, Zachary Azem, and Andrew Smith. 2020. "COVID-19 Response: Bipartisan Approval of Sununu's Handling, Majority Disapprove of Trump's." University of New Hampshire Survey Center, March 27. Accessed July 13, 2020. https://scholars.unh.edu/cgi/viewcontent.cgi?article=1579&context=survey_center_polls.

Michigan House Republicans. 2020. "Michigan's Comeback Roadmap." April 20. Accessed July 13, 2020. http://gophouse.org/michigans-comeback-roadmap/.

Milkovits, Amanda. 2020. "Narragansett Council President's Call to Defy R.I. Governor's COVID Orders Fizzles." *Boston Globe*, May 18. Accessed July 10, 2020. https://azgovernor.gov/sites/default/files/eo_2021_0.pdf.

Moffit, Robert, and Doug Badger. 2020. "Defeating COVID-19—What Policymakers Can Do to Change the Conditions on the Ground." Heritage Foundation, April 9. Accessed July 14, 2020. https://www.heritage.org/sites/default/files/2020-04/BG3485.pdf.

Nazaryan, Alexander. 2020. "As Coronavirus Surges, Fox New Shifts Its Message on Masks." Yahoo! News, July 2. Accessed October 31, 2020. https://news.yahoo.com/as-coronavirus-surges-fox-news-shifts-its-message-on-masks-200834996.html.

NBC Miami. 2020. "Restrictions Placed on Bars, Restaurants and Beaches to Help Stop COVID-19 Spread." March 15. Accessed July 10, 2020. https://www.nbcmiami.com/news/local/miami-beach-to-close-and-clear-beaches-to-stop-the-spread-of-covid-19/2205741/.

Nelson, Steven. 2020. "House Republicans Anger Democrats by Refusing to Wear Protective Masks." *New York Post*, April 23. Accessed July 20, 2020. https://nypost.com/2020/04/23/republicans-refuse-to-wear-coronavirus-masks-angering-democrats/.

Nichols, Anna Liz, and Susan J. Demas. 2020. "Whitmer Stay Home Order Protest Turns into Trump Celebration with Confederate Flags and Guns." Michigan Advance, April 15. Accessed July 8, 2020. https://www.michiganadvance.com/2020/04/15/whitmer-stay-home-order-protest-turns-into-trump-celebration-with-confederate-flags-and-guns/.

Office of Governor Andrew Cuomo. 2020. "Amid Ongoing COVID-19 Pandemic, Governor Cuomo, Governor Murphy, Governor Lamont, Governor Wolf, Governor Carney, Governor Raimondo & Governor Baker Announce Joint Multi-State Agreement to Develop Regional Supply Claim for PPE and Medical Equipment." May 3. Accessed July 8, 2020. https://www.governor.ny.gov/news/amid-ongoing-covid-19-pandemic-governor-cuomo-governor-murphy-governor-lamont-governor-wolf.

Office of Governor Gavin Newsom. 2020. "California, Oregon & Washington Announce Western States Pact." April 13. Accessed July 12, 2020. https://www.gov.ca.gov/2020/04/13/california-oregon-washington-announce-western-states-pact/.

Office of Governor Larry Hogan. 2020. "Governor Hogan Provides Update on Maryland's Response to Novel Coronavirus." January 29. Accessed July 29, 2020. https://governor.maryland.gov/2020/01/29/governor-hogan-provides-update-on-marylands-response-to-novel-coronavirus/.

Ollstein, Alice Miranda, Dan Goldberg, and Nolan McCaskill. 2020. "Hot Spots Erupt in Farm Belt States Where Governors Insist Lockdowns Aren't Needed." Politico, April 15. Accessed July 11, 2020. https://www.politico.com/news/2020/04/15/coronavirus-hot-spots-farm-belt-189272.

Ordoñez, Franco. 2020. "Jared Kushner's Role in Coronavirus Response Draws Scrutiny, Criticism." NPR, April 4. Accessed July 9, 2020. https://www.npr.org/2020/04/04/826922646/jared-kushners-role-in-coronavirus-response-draws-scrutiny-criticism.

Painter, Marcus, and Tian Qiu. 2020. "Political Beliefs Affect Compliance with COVID-19 Social Distancing Orders." SSRN, April 6. Accessed July 12, 2020. https://papers.ssrn.com/sol3/papers.cfm?abstract_id=3569098.

Pew Research Center. 2020a. "Most Americans Say Trump Was Too Slow in Initial Response to Coronavirus Threat." April 16. Accessed July 13, 2020. https://www.pewresearch.org/politics/2020/04/16/most-americans-say-trump-was-too-slow-in-initial-response-to-coronavirus-threat/.

Pew Research Center. 2020b. "Worries about Coronavirus Surge, as Most Americans Expect a Recession—Or Worse." March 26. Accessed July 10, 2020. https://www.pewresearch

.org/politics/2020/03/26/worries-about-coronavirus-surge-as-most-americans-expect-a-recession-or-worse/.

Phillips, Morgan. 2020. "McConnell Makes Appeal for Wearing Masks: 'It Is about Protecting Everyone We Encounter.'" Fox News, June 29. Accessed July 29, 2020. https://www.foxnews.com/politics/mcconnell-face-masks-protecting-everyone.

Pittman, Ashton. 2020. "With No State Mandate, Mississippi Mayors Using Patchwork of COVID-19 Safety Options." *Mississippi Free Press*, March 21. Accessed July 10, 2020. https://www.mississippifreepress.org/1912/with-no-state-mandate-mississippi-mayors-using-patchwork-of-covid-19-safety-options/.

PPRI. 2020. "President Trump's Favorability Ratings Recede from March's Peak." PPRI, April 30. Accessed July 14, 2020. https://www.prri.org/research/president-trumps-favorability-ratings-recede-from-archs-peak/.

Quinn, Melissa. 2020. "Maryland Governor Says Trump's 'Mixed Messages' on Disinfectants Led to Confusion in His State." CBS News, April 26. Accessed July 29, 2020. https://www.cbsnews.com/news/coronavirus-maryland-governor-larry-hogan-trumps-mixed-messages-disinfectants-confusion/.

Quinnipiac University Poll. 2020. "NY/NJ/CT Poll: Majority Say Take Months Not Weeks to Reopen, Quinnipiac University Poll Finds; More Than 6 in 10 Know Someone Who Has Had Coronavirus." May 6. Accessed July 14, 2020. https://poll.qu.edu/connecticut/release-detail?ReleaseID=3660.

Register-Mail. 2020. "Peoria Pushes Plan to Reopen Faster." May 13. Accessed July 9, 2020. https://www.galesburg.com/news/20200513/peoria-pushes-plan-to-reopen-faster.

Reuters. 2020. "Reuters/Ipsos: President Trump Diagnosed with COVID-19." October 4. Accessed October 31, 2020. https://www.ipsos.com/sites/default/files/ct/news/documents/2020-10/topline_with_write_up_reuters_trump_covid_diagnosis_10_04_2020.pdf.

Ritter, Zacc. 2020. "Amid Pandemic, News Attention Spikes; Media Favorability Flat." Gallup, April 9. Accessed July 15, 2020. https://news.gallup.com/opinion/gallup/307934/amid-pandemic-news-attention-spikes-media-favorability-flat.aspx.

Romney, Mitt. 2020. "Romney Calls for Urgent Action on Additional Coronavirus Response Measures." March 16. Accessed July 11, 2020. https://www.romney.senate.gov/romney-calls-urgent-action-additional-coronavirus-response-measures.

Rupar, Aaron. 2020. "Trump Attacks a Republican Governor for Following His Coronavirus Testing Advice." Vox, April 20. Accessed July 29, 2020. https://www.vox.com/2020/4/20/21228817/trump-larry-hogan-coronavirus-testing-kits.

Saad, Lydia. 2020. "Americans Remain Risk Averse about Getting Back to Normal." Gallup, April 14. Accessed July 13, 2020. https://news.gallup.com/poll/308264/americans-remain-risk-averse-getting-back-normal.aspx.

Shabad, Rebecca. 2020. "Trump and Gov. Cuomo Clash over Coronavirus Response after President Tells Him to Stop 'Complaining.'" NBC News, April 17. Accessed October 31, 2020. https://www.nbcnews.com/politics/politics-news/cuomo-trump-clash-over-coronavirus-response-after-president-says-stop-n1186396.

Shorman, Jonathan, Amy Renee Leiker, and Michael Stavola. 2020. "War over Easter: Kansas Lawmakers Revoke Gov. Kelly's Order Limiting Church Gatherings." *Wichita Eagle*, April 8. Accessed July 10, 2020. https://www.kansas.com/news/politics-government/article241861126.html.

Skahill, Patrick. 2020. "Lamont Orders Residents 'Stay Safe, Stay Home'; Jobless Claims in Connecticut Skyrocket." WNPR, March 20. Accessed July 9, 2020. https://www.wnpr

.org/post/lamont-orders-residents-stay-safe-stay-home-jobless-claims-connecticut-skyrocket.

Strohm, Chris. 2020. "Barr Threatens Legal Action against Governors over Lockdowns." Bloomberg, April 21. Accessed July 11, 2020. https://www.bloomberg.com/news/articles/2020-04-21/barr-says-doj-may-act-against-governors-with-strict-virus-limits.

Swalec, Andrea. 2020. "Maryland Governor Defends Coronavirus Test Kit Deal after Trump Criticism." NBC Washington, April 21. Accessed July 29, 2020. https://www.nbcwashington.com/news/local/maryland-governor-defends-coronavirus-test-kit-deal-after-trump-criticism/2280441/.

Talev, Margaret. 2020. "Axios-Ipsos Coronavirus Index, Week 8: Second-Guessing the Death Toll." Axios, May 5. Accessed July 10, 2020. https://www.axios.com/axios-ipsos-coronavirus-week-8-5a1947d5-9850-4e58-9583-9b617e6fdc1b.html.

Trump, Donald. 2020a. "Remarks in a Question-and-Answer Session at a Fox News Virtual Town Hall on the Coronavirus Pandemic." Online by Gerhard Peters and John T. Woolley, the American Presidency Project. Accessed March 11, 2021. https://www.presidency.ucsb.edu/node/341628.

Trump, Donald (@realDonaldTrump). 2020b. "We are United in Our Effort to Defeat the Invisible China Virus, and Many People Say That It Is Patriotic to Wear a Face Mask When You Can't Socially Distance. There Is Nobody More Patriotic Than Me, Your Favorite President!" Twitter, July 20, 2020. https://twitter.com/realDonaldTrump/status/1285299379746811915.

Trump, Donald (@realDonaldTrump). 2020c. "WE CANNOT LET THE CURE BE WORSE THAN THE PROBLEM ITSELF. AT THE END OF THE 15 DAY PERIOD, WE WILL MAKE A DECISION AS TO WHICH WAY WE WANT TO GO!" Twitter, March 22, 2020. https://twitter.com/realDonaldTrump/status/1241935285916782593.

University of New Hampshire Survey Center. 2020. "Granite Staters Approve of Sununu's Handling of Coronavirus, Stay at Home Order 4/22/2020." April 22. Accessed February 18, 2021. https://scholars.unh.edu/survey_center_polls/582/.

U.S. Department of Justice, Office of Public Affairs. 2020. "Attorney General William P. Barr Issues Statement on Religious Practice and Social Distancing; Department of Justice Files Statement of Interest in Mississippi Church Case." April 14. Accessed July 15, 2020. https://www.justice.gov/opa/pr/attorney-general-william-p-barr-issues-statement-religious-practice-and-social-distancing-0.

Van Velzer, Ryan. 2020. "Federal Government Outbids Kentucky for Medical Equipment amid Shortage. WFPL, April 4. Accessed July 13, 2020. https://wfpl.org/federal-government-outbids-kentucky-for-medical-equipment-amid-shortage/amp.

Vance, Taylor. 2020. "Tupelo Mayor Issues New COVID-19 Order Complying with Governor's Latest Mandate." *Daily Journal*, March 25. Accessed July 10, 2020. https://www.djournal.com/news/local/tupelo-mayor-issues-new-covid-19-order-complying-with-governors-latest-mandate/article_8f93f353-d4ad-50b9-a5fb-5e29b8bba0c3.html.

Warren, Elizabeth, et al. 2020. Letter to Robert O'Brien. Washington, DC, February 13, 2020. Accessed July 11, 2020. https://www.schatz.senate.gov/imo/media/doc/021320%20NSC%20Novel%20Coronavirus%20Letter%20final%20pdf.pdf.

White, Jeremy. 2020. "Trump Claims 'Total Authority' over State Decisions." Politico, April 13. Accessed March 11, 2021. https://www.politico.com/states/california/story/2020/04/13/trump-claims-total-authority-over-state-decisions-1275506.

Whitmer, Gretchen. 2020. "I Have Made Gut-Wrenching Choices to Keep People Safe." *New York Times*, April 21. Accessed July 8, 2020. https://www.nytimes.com/2020/04/21/opinion/gretchen-whitmer-coronavirus-michigan.html.

Willis, Andrew. 2020. "Coronavirus in Florida: Beaches Not Ordered to Close amid Pandemic." WFLA, March 17. Accessed July 11, 2020. https://www.wfla.com/community/health/coronavirus/florida-beaches-not-ordered-to-close-amid-coronavirus-pandemic/.

Witte, Griff. 2020. "South Dakota's Governor Resisted Ordering People to Stay Home. Now It Has One of the Nation's Largest Coronavirus Hot Spots." *Washington Post*, April 13. Accessed July 10, 2020. https://www.washingtonpost.com/national/south-dakotas-governor-resisted-ordering-people-to-stay-home-now-it-has-one-of-the-nations-largest-coronavirus-hot-spots/2020/04/13/5cff90fe-7daf-11ea-a3ee-13e1ae0a3571_story.html.

Witte, Griff, and Katie Zezima. 2020. "Ohio Gov. Mike DeWine's Coronavirus Response Has Become a National Guide to the Crisis." *Washington Post*, March 16. Accessed July 29, 2020. https://www.washingtonpost.com/national/coronavirus-ohio-dewine-outbreak/2020/03/16/9bde6b1e-67b2-11ea-9923-57073adce27c_story.html.

WJZ. 2020. "Hogan's Approval Rating up 8 Percent amid Coronavirus Pandemic; Trump's Approval Rating in Maryland Drops to 40 Percent." CBS Baltimore, May 26. Accessed July 29, 2020. https://baltimore.cbslocal.com/2020/05/26/may-gonzales-poll-hogan-trump-approval/.

WWBT/WHSV. 2020. "Police Temporarily Bar Entry to Capitol Square amid 'Reopen Virginia' Protest." WHSV, April 16. Accessed July 13, 2020. https://www.whsv.com/content/news/Protesters-gather-at-Virginia-Capitol-to-demand-end-to-states-closures-569694311.html.

YouGov. 2020. "The Economist/YouGov Poll. March 22–24, 2020." March 24, 2020. Accessed July 20, 2020. https://docs.cdn.yougov.com/bfiid7tfh3/econTabReport.pdf.

Guns and Public Health

At a Glance

Although the Second Amendment to the U.S. Constitution grants Americans the right to bear arms, Democrats and Republicans continue to debate how to interpret its language. In particular, the two parties disagree over the extent to which the right to bear arms exists, to whom, and how. While considerable debate centers on the constitutionality of restricting gun ownership, government-sponsored research on firearms-related violence and gun safety also garners partisan attention. Congress first included the Dickey Amendment in the 1996 omnibus spending bill, which prohibited the Centers for Disease Control and Prevention (CDC) from using its funding to advocate or promote gun control. Policy makers have renewed the provision in subsequent spending bills. Although the provision did not explicitly prohibit government-funded gun safety research, government health agencies essentially ceased funding and conducting research into firearms-related violence in the United States. In turn, this lack of data spurred ongoing partisan debates about the causes and scope of gun violence and the effectiveness of public health policies intended to reduce firearms-related deaths.

The resulting ambiguity of statistical data on firearms violence has heightened partisan differences. Democrats cite recent mass shootings as evidence that an epidemic of gun violence requires policy action. Democrats also argue that evidence-based data can and should inform legislative efforts to minimize gun violence. Gun safety technology should be encouraged, mental health treatment and reporting should be strengthened, and physicians should be able to counsel patients about household gun safety practices.

Republicans, on the other hand, insist that mass shootings, while tragic, should not be politicized. Moreover, they assert that any legislative efforts to address gun violence must not impose upon the rights of law-abiding gun owners. Republicans argue that any government-funded research on gun violence and gun safety will be used to partisan ends in service of a Democratic effort to institute strict gun control measures. Instead, Republicans maintain that mental illness is at the root of much gun violence in the United States, so improving mental health care should be the legislative priority.

According to Many Democrats . . .

- Gun violence is a public health emergency, and mass shootings require political action.
- The federal government should fund evidence-based public health research on firearms-related violence and gun safety.
- It is important to reduce the number of guns and to implement reasonable reform measures, such as gun safety technology and comprehensive background checks that include mental health reporting.

According to Many Republicans . . .

- Lawmakers must preserve Second Amendment rights and refrain from politicizing mass shootings.
- Government-funded research is tantamount to public advocacy for gun control.
- Mental illness causes gun violence, so reinforcing criminal law enforcement measures and improving mental health care services should be the priority—rather than imposing onerous restrictions on law-abiding gun owners.

Overview

The United States has a long-standing tradition of gun ownership. According to one survey conducted between 2016 and 2018, 30 percent of Americans own a gun, and 43 percent report living with someone who does (Saad 2019). Another poll conducted in 2017 found that 48 percent of Americans reported having grown up in a household with a gun (Gramlich and Schaeffer 2019). Although a significant proportion of Americans either grew up or continue to live in gun households, recent surveys point to a decades-long decline in gun ownership that dates to the late 1970s (Smith and Son 2015).

Gun owners offer different reasons for why they own firearms that range from protection to sport to gun collecting; 67 percent report protection and 38 percent indicate hunting as the major reasons for their gun ownership (Parker et al. 2017). Gun ownership is also particularly concentrated: 66 percent of gun owners report owning more than one gun, and 29 percent report owning more than five (Parker et al. 2017). Among developed nations, American gun culture is unparalleled. In 2017, the number of firearms in the United States was greater than the total U.S. population, with 393 million firearms among 326 million people (Ingraham 2018). In the late 2010s, Americans owned 46 percent of all estimated worldwide firearms, reflecting the fact that the United States has the highest gun ownership rate in the world (Fox 2019).

According to the Centers for Disease Control and Prevention (CDC), there were 39,733 firearms-related deaths in the United States in 2017. Accounting for 16.4 percent of all injury deaths, more Americans died from firearms than incidents related to motor vehicle traffic (Kochaneck et al. 2019). Public perceptions of gun violence differ according to political party identification, however. In one 2017 Pew poll, 65 percent of Democrats considered gun violence to be a "very big" problem in the United States compared to 32 percent of Republicans (Oliphant 2017).

For the past 50 years, American policy makers have deliberated about how to regulate firearms. In 1968, Congress passed the Gun Control Act, which barred certain individuals from gun ownership or possession. However, as written, the Gun Control Act lacked enforcement powers and was thus relatively toothless. In 1993, President Bill Clinton signed the Brady Handgun Violence Protection Act (commonly known as the Brady Bill), which required individuals purchasing guns from licensed dealers to submit to background checks. The bill had been named after former President Ronald Reagan's press secretary, James Brady, who had been left paralyzed after an assassination attempt on Reagan in 1981. Indeed, Reagan praised the bill in a 1991 *New York Times* editorial: "If the passage of the Brady bill were to result in a reduction of only 10 or 15 percent of those numbers (and it could be a good deal greater), it would be well worth making it the law of the land" (Reagan 1991). In 1994, Clinton also signed the Violent Crime Control and Law Enforcement Act, which included a 10-year federal ban on assault weapons. The bill passed the Senate by a 95–4 margin, with two Democrats and two Republicans voting nay. However, political commentators suggested that Clinton's signing of both bills was a factor in the Republican resurgence during the 1994 midterm elections that enabled the GOP to recapture control of the House of Representatives, and the Assault Weapons Ban expired under George W. Bush's Republican administration in 2004. These actions occurred amid a decades-long evolution in voting patterns, between the 1970s and 2000s, in which gun owners became increasingly more likely to vote for Republican candidates and gun nonowners (and gun control advocates) for Democratic candidates (Joslyn et al. 2017).

U.S. Supreme Court decisions have reaffirmed Second Amendment rights in several cases. In *District of Columbia v. Heller* (2008), the court struck down a Washington, DC, law that banned handguns, ruling that the Second Amendment guaranteed an individual right to firearm possession for self-defense. The *Heller* decision marked the first time that the Supreme Court held that the Second Amendment protected an individual right to self-defense. The decision came after years of Supreme Court jurisprudence that did not directly interpret whether the Second Amendment conferred an individual right (the right to firearm possession for private use) or a collective right (the right of the state to arm its militia). Two years later, in *McDonald v. City of Chicago* (2010), the Supreme Court struck down a similar gun ban in Chicago, Illinois, ruling that the Second Amendment applied to state and local laws as well as federal law. More recently, in April 2020, the Supreme Court declined to issue an opinion in *New York Rifle & Pistol Association v. City of New*

Gun Safety Research Will Save Lives

On June 19, 2019, Rep. Lucy McBath (D-GA) spoke in favor of allocating funds to the CDC and NIH for firearms-related research. McBath became a gun control advocate and entered politics following the 2012 murder of her 17-year-old son, Jordan Davis.

Mr. Speaker, I rise today to urge action to end the public health crisis of gun violence.

Every day, nearly 100 people are killed in suicides, homicides, and accidents involving guns, but we have not invested nearly enough in preventing these deaths. Of the top 30 causes of death, 29 received more research funding than guns. But today, this body will vote to invest in gun violence research at the Centers for Disease Control and the National Institutes of Health.

I recently visited the Centers for Disease Control Injury Center which is in my district. With this critical funding, they will learn how we can prevent gun tragedies. This investment is long overdue, and I was proud to lead my colleagues in asking for this funding.

We have the responsibility to pursue life-saving research, and today we vote to end gun violence.

As a survivor of gun violence, I could not be more proud of the measures that we have taken to save the countless numbers of lives that may be affected by gun violence in the future. The time has passed for my son. The time has passed for others like my son who was killed unnecessarily due to gun violence, but I am so grateful for this day.

I am so grateful for the funding for the research that will save many, many lives for generations to come.

Source

Congressional Record, vol. 165, no. 103 (June 19, 2019): H4776. Washington, DC: Government Printing Office. Accessed May 15, 2020. https://www.congress.gov/116/crec/2019/06/19/CREC-2019-06-19-pt1-PgH4776.pdf.

York, New York (2019). The case challenged New York City's ban on the transport of licensed handguns outside the city, but the court sent the case back to the lower court after the city repealed the regulation. Two months later, the court declined to hear arguments in 10 other gun rights cases (Higgins and Mangan 2020).

The partisan divide on stricter gun legislation has become increasingly polarized. Between 2001 and 2019, a 17-point gap between Democratic and Republican support for stricter gun legislation grew to more than 50 points according to public opinion surveys (McCarthy 2019). As President Barack Obama observed in 2011, "I know that every time we try to talk about guns, it can reinforce stark divides. People shout at one another, which makes it impossible to listen. We mire ourselves in stalemate, which makes it impossible to get to where we need to go as a country" (Obama 2011). That same year, a Pew poll indicated that 70 percent of Republicans preferred "to protect the right of Americans to own guns," while 67 percent of Democrats preferred "to control gun ownership" (Pew Research Center 2010).

These patterns held true in the 2016 presidential election. One survey found that 63 percent of gun owners supported Republican candidate Donald Trump, while 65 percent of non–gun owners supported Democratic candidate Hillary Clinton (Cohn and Quealy 2017). These increasingly entrenched voting behaviors coincided with notable shifts in political advertising during the 2012, 2014, 2016, and 2018 election cycles. As one study demonstrated, overall gun-related political advertising increased over those four election cycles; however, pro-regulation advertising increased while pro–gun rights advertising decreased (Barry et al. 2020). Accordingly, by 2019, another poll found that 86 percent of Democrats felt that gun laws should be more strict, while 49 percent of Republicans considered existing laws to be "about right" (Schaeffer 2019).

While gun control became subject to partisan discord, so too did questions about public health research on matters of gun safety. In 1992, the CDC launched the National Center on Injury Prevention and Control, which was charged with conducting public health research on gun violence. The following year, a landmark study in the *New England Journal of Medicine* found that the risk of homicide was three times higher when guns were present in the home (Leary 1993). The National Rifle Association (NRA) challenged the study's findings, and as part of its broader legislative agenda, it lobbied to abolish the National Center on Injury Prevention and Control. In 1995, Dr. David Satcher, the CDC director under Clinton, published an editorial in the *Washington Post* responding to the NRA's lobbying efforts. Satcher argued, "Here is a charge that not only casts doubt on the ability of scientists to conduct research involving controversial issues but also raises basic questions about the ability, fundamental to any democracy, to have honest, searching public discussions of such issues" (Satcher 1995).

In the 1996 omnibus spending bill, Rep. Jay Dickey (R-AR) authored a provision that mandated that "none of the funds made available for injury prevention and control at the Centers for Disease Control (CDC) may be used to advocate or promote gun control" (U.S. Public Law 104-208 1996). Although the provision did not explicitly prohibit government-funded gun safety research, federal health agencies essentially ceased funding and conducting research into firearm-related violence in the United States. The 2012 appropriations bill extended the provision to also apply to the National Institutes of Health (NIH) and other federal agencies. The NRA championed the move, arguing that "junk science studies and others like them are designed to provide ammunition for the gun control lobby by advancing the false notion that legal gun ownership is a danger to the public health instead of an inalienable right" (National Rifle Association, Institute for Legislative Action 2011). In 2015, Dickey announced regret for the eponymous provision. As he observed in one interview, "It just couldn't be the collection of data so that they can advocate gun control. That's all we were talking about. But for some reason, it just stopped altogether" (National Public Radio 2015). In a complete reversal, Dickey affirmed that "doing nothing is no longer an acceptable solution" (Diamond 2015).

Following Dickey's reversal, Democrats led by Rep. Robin Kelly (D-IL) called for an end to the Dickey Amendment in 2016, while Republicans led by Rep. Thomas Massie (R-KY) formed the congressional Second Amendment Caucus to rally support for pro-gun reforms.

Democrats advocated for policy action on gun safety for the duration of the Obama administration. Following the 2012 Sandy Hook Elementary School shooting in Newtown, Connecticut, President Barack Obama issued an executive order that asked for $10 million for CDC and other agencies to conduct gun violence research. The White House asserted that "research on gun violence is not advocacy; it is critical public health research that gives all Americans information they need" (Ohlheiser 2013). After NIH-funded firearms research gained public attention early in the Obama administration, Republicans voiced displeasure. Rep. Joe Barton (R-TX) remarked, "It's almost as if someone's been looking for a way to get this study done ever since the Centers for Disease Control was banned from doing it 10 years ago" (McElhatton 2009).

Health policy and gun rights intersected in another way during the Obama administration. The Affordable Care Act (ACA), Obama's signature health reform legislation, included two provisions favored by the gun lobby and requested by Sen. Harry Reid (D-NV). Although the ACA did not prohibit physicians from asking patients about firearms, it prohibited the disclosure of gun ownership to wellness programs as well as the incorporation of gun ownership into the setting of health insurance premiums. Though not well publicized during the partisan debates leading to passage of the ACA, these provisions represented variations on previous state-level efforts to bridge health privacy concerns and gun ownership. In 2006, policy makers in Virginia and West Virginia introduced bills intended to regulate what physicians could ask patients about firearms. Neither bill passed. In 2011, the Republican-led state legislature passed and Gov. Rick Scott (R) signed Florida's Firearm Owner's Privacy Act (FOPA), which banned physicians from asking patients about gun ownership. The bill's sponsor, Rep. Jason Brodeur (R), argued that "the bill addresses a violation of privacy rights concerning firearms and seeks to prevent future occurrences of such violations" (Moisse 2011).

Following passage of Florida's law, other state legislatures, including those in Alabama, Minnesota, North Carolina, Oklahoma, South Carolina, and Tennessee, introduced similar pieces of legislation that subsequently died before adjournment. In 2013, the Republican-led Montana State Legislature passed MCA 50-16-108, which prohibited patients from having to disclose gun information to receive medical care. In 2014, the Republican-led Missouri General Assembly passed S.B. 656, which did not prohibit medical professionals from asking patients about gun safety practices but did prohibit disclosure of any such information unless by court order, in response to direct threat, or with patient consent. Missouri's Gov. Jay Nixon (D) vetoed the measure, which the legislature then overrode, virtually along party lines. In a 112–41 vote in the House, only one Democrat voted aye, and only one Republican voted nay; in the Senate, all Republicans voted aye and all Democrats nay.

Florida's FOPA remained the nation's only active physician gag rule at that point, but it was ultimately struck down in 2017 following a unanimous federal appeals court ruling (Hersher 2017). Democrats and professional physician organizations argued that physicians had the legal right to engage in conversations with patients about household gun access and gun safety practices. In January 2020, Massachusetts state representative Jon Santiago (D) introduced bill H.2005, which proposed implementing a screening program to permit physicians to ask patients about gun safety practices in the home (Corpuz 2020).

Although evidence suggests that mentally ill individuals are more likely to be victims rather than perpetrators of violent crimes, there has been recent bipartisan agreement regarding enhanced mental health reporting as one way to reduce firearms-related violence (Doroshow 2019). For Republicans, emphasizing that mental illness can be a cause of gun violence still preserves the gun rights of law-abiding citizens. For Democrats, enhanced mental health reporting and Extreme Risk Protection Orders (ERPOs, often described as "red flag" laws) allow family members or law enforcement agencies to petition the courts to temporarily confiscate firearms from individuals at risk of harming themselves or others. As health policy scholars have demonstrated, this contemporary policy emphasis on mental illness has followed several decades of media coverage that overemphasized interpersonal violence committed by individuals with mental illness and minimized successful treatment and recovery from mental illness, despite the fact that most individuals with mental illness are not violent (McGinty et al. 2016).

The Dickey Amendment did not explicitly prohibit federal agencies from conducting gun safety research. At one 2018 U.S. House hearing, U.S. Health and Human Services Secretary Alex Azar stated, "My understanding is that the rider does not in any way impede our research mission. It is simply about advocacy" (Christensen 2018). The subsequent 2018 appropriations bill did not include funding for gun violence research. The following year, the House voted to approve a spending bill that included $25 million split evenly between the CDC and the NIH for firearm violence research, the first such funding allocation since the 1996 introduction of the Dickey Amendment (Stracqualursi 2019).

The CDC tracks overall firearms-related deaths (due to accidents, homicides, or suicides), but there exists no standard definition of what constitutes a *mass shooting*. Law enforcement agencies and academic researchers adopt Federal Bureau of Investigation (FBI) terminology to classify mass murders as single incidents in at least one location during which at least four victims are murdered with firearms (Krouse and Richardson 2015). In 2013, the Obama administration revised the definitional threshold for mass shootings to three or more victims. In 2015, the Congressional Research Service concluded that the prevalence of mass shootings increased during each decade from the 1970s onward (Krouse and Richardson

2015). According to one nonprofit that tracks gun violence, 2019 had more mass shootings than the preceding five years (Silverstein 2020). As public tragedies, mass shootings garner significant media attention and renew partisan debate regarding gun rights, public health, and public safety.

Democrats on Guns and Public Health

Democratic responses to gun violence reflect core liberal values. In particular, Democrats maintain that the role of the government is to protect citizens. They hold that governments at the federal, state, and local levels should more effectively regulate firearms to limit the availability of guns (especially high-powered weapons) and thus reduce gun violence, thereby protecting the health and welfare of the American public.

Democrats argue that mass shootings require immediate political action, often emphasizing their view of gun violence as a public health emergency of "epidemic" proportions. Days after a 1999 school shooting in Columbine, Colorado, claimed the lives of 13 victims and both perpetrators, Democrats called for a legislative response. Sen. Chuck Schumer (D-NY) argued, "It's not enough to wring our hands and pray it won't happen again. We need to act" (Schumer 1999). President Bill Clinton later told high school students, "All I'm trying to do is keep more people alive" (CNN 1999). As mass shootings continued during the Obama administration, President Obama and many fellow Democrats advocated for immediate action to pass new gun control regulations, but to no avail, as Republicans remained mostly unified in opposition to such proposals. After more than a dozen people died in a shooting at an Aurora, Colorado, movie theater in July 2012, Sen. Sherrod Brown (D-OH) lamented, "I don't expect anything to happen" (Kane 2012). After 27 adults and children died in a mass shooting at a school in Newtown, Connecticut, in December 2012, President Barack Obama asked, "Are we really prepared to say that we're powerless in the face of such carnage? That the politics are too hard?" (Lander and Baker 2012).

When describing gun violence as a public health emergency, Democrats often frame it in stark terms. Following an October 2015 mass shooting at Umpqua Community College in Oregon, President Obama asserted, "This is something we should politicize. It is relevant to our common life together, to the body politic" (White House, Office of the Press Secretary 2015). After a June 2016 mass shooting at the Pulse nightclub in Orlando, Florida, claimed 49 lives, Sens. Richard Blumenthal (D-CT) and Chris Murphy (D-CT) lamented, "The Senate's inaction on commonsense gun violence prevention makes it complicit in this public health crisis" (Blumenthal 2016). Almost two years later, Rep. Debbie Wasserman Schultz (D-FL) similarly responded after 17 victims died in a shooting at Marjory Stoneman Douglas High School in Parkland, Florida, that "we must do something about this senseless epidemic of gun violence and we must do it now" (Leary 2018a). In July

2019, New Jersey State Assembly member Joann Downey (D) insisted that "we're keeping our society free from the tyranny that is gun violence" after Gov. Phil Murphy (D) of New Jersey signed a "smart gun" bill (Flanagan 2019). The following month, Speaker Nancy Pelosi (D-CA) asserted that "the Republican Senate's continued inaction dishonors our solemn duty to protect innocent men, women and children and end this epidemic [of gun violence] once and for all" (Sarat and Obert 2019). A sense of urgency among Democratic policy makers mirrored that among Democratic voters. In one Pew poll conducted in 2017, 65 percent of self-identified Democrats considered gun violence to be a "very big" problem (Oliphant 2017).

To address gun violence, Democrats argue that the government should fund evidence-based public health research on gun violence and safety. As Rep. William Lacy Clay (D-MO) insisted, "We need to do everything humanly possible to avert this carnage, to stop it, to study it and to recommend to policymakers what we can do to stem the rising tide of murders" (Lowry 2019). Democrats maintain that funding restrictions have led to a scarcity of evidence-based research on gun violence, thus raising questions about the veracity of CDC data (Campbell, Nass, and Nguyen 2018).

In a January 2019 press release introducing the Gun Violence Prevention Research Act with Rep. Carolyn Maloney (D-NY), Sen. Ed Markey (D-MA) stated, "No one should fear non-partisan, scientific research, not Democrats, not Republicans, and not the NRA" (Markey 2019). Several months later, eleven senators—10 Democrats and 1 Independent who caucuses with the Democrats—submitted a letter to U.S. Health and Human Services Secretary Alex Azar asking what methods the CDC employed when tracking gun injury data and to what degree, if any, the Dickey Amendment had impacted data collection. As Sen. Bob Menendez (D-NJ) suggested, "We as lawmakers, as every American citizen, should be able to follow and understand the latest trends on firearms injuries without the concern of coming across 'unstable and potentially unreliable' data" (Campbell and Nass 2019).

Because "the federal government has sat on the sidelines for too long," as Reps. Nita Lowey (D-NY) and Rosa DeLauro (D-CT) argued, local and state governments across the country announced their own firearm safety initiatives and consortia (Lowey and DeLauro 2019). As David Frockt (D), a Washington state senator, observed, "I think we've seen that the federal government can't be a reliable partner in any kind of public health research" (Van Brocklin 2019). Democratic-led states, including California, New Jersey, Rhode Island, and Washington, announced their own efforts to study gun violence (Ranney and Betz 2019). In early 2018, New Jersey State Assembly member Eric Houghtaling (D) suggested, "If we will not allow the CDC to research this important issue, then we will empower our institutions of higher education to do so" (Stainton 2018).

After California established the first state-funded center for firearm violence research at the University of California in July 2017, New Jersey's Gov. Phil Murphy

(D) included $2 million for a gun violence research center at Rutgers University in his 2019 fiscal year budget. Once the U.S. House approved a spending bill in December 2019 that included funding for firearms violence research at the CDC, Rep. Nita Lowey (D-NY) proclaimed, "With this investment, the best public health researchers in the country will be put to work to identify ways to reduce injury and death due to firearms" (Stracqualursi 2019).

In addition to advocating for an end to the Dickey provision, Democrats also sought to expand the federal infrastructure dedicated to studying firearms-related violence. In August 2019, Rep. Mark DeSaulnier (D-CA) introduced H.R. 4177, the Gun Safety Board and Research Act, which proposed establishing a Gun Safety Board under the U.S. Department of Health and Human Services. In a press release, DeSaulnier argued that "creating a way to re-introduce quality research into the gun violence prevention debate will help us rise above partisan politics and get to the roots of the problem" (DeSaulnier 2019).

Democrats also argue that it is important to implement reasonable reform measures, such as gun safety technology and comprehensive background checks that include mental health reporting. In January 2013, Gov. Andrew Cuomo (D) signed the New York Secure Ammunition and Firearms Enforcement (NY SAFE) Act. New York was the first state to pass gun legislation following the Sandy Hook shooting. The NY SAFE Act passed on a bipartisan vote and broadened a ban on assault weapons, included a mental health reporting requirement, and established a universal background check process. In January 2016, President Obama announced a series of executive actions to reduce gun violence that included the licensing of all gun sellers and mental health reporting to the background check system (White House, Office of the Press Secretary 2016). In February 2019, the Democratic-led U.S. House of Representatives passed HR 8, the Bipartisan Background Checks Act of 2019, by a 240–190 margin. All but two Democrats supported the bill, as did eight Republicans. Upon passage, Rep. Mike Thompson (D-CA), the bill's sponsor, remarked, "For six long years, we worked on this issue and the previous [Republican] majority would not even let us have a hearing, let alone a vote to expand background checks" (Thompson 2019). However, Senate Majority Leader Mitch McConnell (R-KY) indicated that he would not bring the bill up for a vote in the Senate; the Trump administration also opposed the measure (Trump 2019).

Democrats point to public polling that indicates some common ground for gun safety policies among Democrats and Republicans. In one 2017 Pew poll, for example, 89 percent of Democrats and Republicans agreed with "preventing the mentally ill from purchasing guns," and 90 percent of Democrats and 77 percent of Republicans agreed with "background checks for private sales and at gun shows" (Oliphant 2017). Another 2019 poll indicated that 95 percent of Democrats and 89 percent of Republicans favored requiring universal background checks (Quinnipiac University Poll 2019). Democrats have also drawn attention to polls that indicated that a majority of Republican voters support "banning assault-style weapons" and "creating a federal database to track gun sales," two measures that Republican policy makers have historically opposed (Oliphant 2017). Following mass shootings in Ohio and Texas in August 2019, Sen. Chris Murphy (D-CT) argued that "if we want to stop gun violence—the kind that happens every day in this nation—we can start with universal background checks, and it's heartbreaking that the President is still so controlled by the gun lobby that he refuses to do what more than 90 percent of Americans want" (Murphy 2019).

Republicans on Guns and Public Health

Republican responses to gun violence reflect long-standing conservative principles. In particular, Republicans argue that individuals have the right to defend themselves, and the U.S. Constitution enshrines the right for American citizens to bear arms. The GOP generally contends that governmental authorities at the federal, state, and local levels must better enforce existing criminal law rather than infringe on the rights of law-abiding citizens.

Republicans argue that while gun violence is tragic, Americans must neither politicize mass shootings nor impose unconstitutional constraints on law-abiding gun owners. In response to Obama's 2016 executive actions on gun reform, former Gov. Jeb Bush (R) of Florida asserted, "I will oppose legislative actions that impose unnecessary burdens on law-abiding gun owners" (Bush 2016). Bush's retort aligned with a subsequent 2017 poll that indicated that 91 percent of Republican gun owners agreed with the statement that gun ownership was essential to their freedom (Parker et al. 2017). After 58 people died in a mass shooting at an October 2017 concert in Las Vegas, Nevada, Trump White House Press Secretary Sarah Huckabee Sanders insisted that "there's a time and place for a political debate, but now is the time to unite as a country" (Davis 2017). Similarly, in the days after the February 2018 mass shooting at Marjory Stoneman Douglas High School, Sen. Marco Rubio (R-FL) remarked, "To be honest, [new gun legislation] isn't going to stop this from happening" (Leary 2018b). In 2019, Rep. Steve Scalise (R-LA) explained that "if our goal is to reduce gun violence, then we should focus on penalizing criminals, not law-abiding citizens" (Scalise 2019). Rep. Andy Barr (R-KY) distinguished the Republican position on guns and gun violence from Democrats as follows: "While some in Congress want to restrict gun rights for everyone, including law-abiding citizens, Republicans are trying to get to the core of the problem—keeping firearms out of the hands of those who, based on criminal background, threatening behavior or mental illness, should not have access to them in the first place" (Barr 2019).

Republicans have insisted that government-funded gun safety research is tantamount to public advocacy for gun control. This line of reasoning was a leading factor in the 1996 implementation of the Dickey Amendment, and it has remained a strongly held belief ever since. In 2015, then House Speaker John Boehner (R-OH)

Mental Illness Is the Underlying Cause of Gun Violence, but Red Flag Laws Are Unconstitutional

On December 9, 2019, Rep. Roger Marshall (R-KS) spoke in support of Second Amendment rights and in opposition to red flag laws.

> Whether it be a handgun, rifle, or shotgun, whatever a citizen's firearm of choice, the right to defend ourselves must not be infringed upon. As I represent Kansas in Congress, I remain staunchly opposed to any laws restricting what kind of firearms a law-abiding citizen can buy or keep in their possession.
>
> Any politician trying to implement mandatory buyback programs, which I really call gun confiscations, or unconstitutional red flag laws in Congress will be met with a groundswell of opposition because these types of laws violate our Second Amendment rights.
>
> In Congress, we need to keep fighting for programs that address the underlying cause of gun violence, which is mental illness, to reach out to those who are struggling so they can get the proper care and attention early so they don't fall through the cracks and harm themselves or others.
>
> We also need to make sure our existing background check system is working properly to continue to prevent tragedies, while not infringing on the rights of mentally stable, law-abiding citizens.
>
> The solutions to preventing gun violence can be found at dinner tables, in our churches, and in our communities. Individually, we must practice and promote responsible gun ownership while collectively ensuring every law-abiding citizen's Second Amendment right is upheld with due process.

Source

Congressional Record, vol. 165, no. 193 (December 4, 2019): H9226. Washington, DC: Government Printing Office. Accessed May 15, 2020. https://www.congress.gov/116/crec/2019/12/04/CREC-2019-12-04-pt1-PgH9226.pdf.

argued that gun research fell outside the CDC's mandate, asserting, "I'm sorry, but a gun is not a disease" (Bertrand 2015). Rep. Jack Kingston (R-GA) rejected President Obama's 2015 proposal to allocate CDC funds for gun research by claiming that "the President's request to fund propaganda for his gun-grabbing initiatives through the CDC will not be included" (Beckett 2014). In 2018, when Democrats again proposed allocating funds toward gun research, Rep. Ken Buck (R-CO) disagreed with removing the CDC restriction. As he explained, "I think it really politicizes an organization that does a really good job of staying out of a political sphere" (Matthews 2018). A year later, Rep. Tom Cole (R-OK) argued that any funding allocation for gun research was unwise: "The money we spend needs to make a difference, not just prove a political point" (Voght 2019).

After the Democratic-led U.S. House passed a spending bill in 2019 that allocated funding for gun violence research, Sen. Roy Blunt (R-MO) condemned it as an "attempt to fund partisan priorities" (Siddons 2019). Blunt's Senate version of the spending bill omitted that funding because "it's clearly controversial," as Blunt explained (Lowry 2019). Blunt also dismissed Democratic complaints that the Dickey Amendment had exerted a chilling effect on government sponsorship of gun safety research, pointing out that the bill had not expressly prohibited such research.

As this partisan debate has raged on inconclusively, gun research has increasingly shifted to other nongovernmental entities, such as the RAND Corporation, which conducted an exhaustive 2018 analysis of the effects of gun policies over several decades (RAND Corporation 2018). Just as Democrats pointed to the uncertain veracity of CDC gun violence data—due, in part, to Dickey—so too did Republicans. As Rep. Doug Collins (R-GA) declared when introducing his Mass Violence Prevention Act in February 2019, "It's cruel to advance legislation that ignores the factors contributing to gun violence when tragedies like Columbine, Parkland and Aurora, Illinois, have showed us again and again what we need to do to keep communities safe" (U.S. House of Representatives, Judiciary Committee 2019).

Although conservatives traditionally oppose all restrictions to gun ownership, some Republicans support measures that redirect public debate from restricting firearms to restricting ownership among "dangerous" individuals. Less than a month after the February 2018 mass shooting at Marjory Stoneman Douglas High School, Gov. Rick Scott of Florida signed S.B. 7026, which included $400 million in mental health funding and expanded police authority to request Extreme Risk Protection Orders. Scott later argued that "the actions of a sick and twisted few cannot be allowed to strip away the constitutional rights of law-abiding citizens" (Scott 2019). After mass shootings in El Paso, Texas, and Dayton, Ohio, later in 2019, Trump remarked that "mental illness and hatred pulls the trigger, not the gun" (Johnson 2019). However, despite Trump's 2019 public calls for mental health reform, two years earlier he had signed H.J Res. 40, which nullified an Obama administration regulation that would have added the names of mentally ill Social Security recipients to the national criminal background database (Trump 2017).

Red flag legislation elicits disagreement among Republicans. When Gov. John Rowland (R) signed Connecticut's law in 1999, Connecticut became the first state to allow court-ordered gun seizures from individuals deemed threats to themselves or others. As other states began adopting red flag legislation in 2019, Republican state representative Arthur O'Neill (R-CT) encouraged lawmakers across the country to follow suit. As he explained, "This piece of legislation was very carefully crafted to protect [the] constitutional rights of the individual who is the possessor of the firearms and at the same time provide us with a way to deal with the problem that is a real threat" (Lawlor 2019). Supporters said that by only removing guns from individuals deemed dangerous by the court system, red flag legislation did not impose upon otherwise mentally stable law-abiding gun owners. Other Republican critics disagree with that assessment. Although Kansas and Oklahoma are not among the states with red flag laws, in 2019, state lawmakers introduced anti–red flag bills with the intention of prohibiting local enactment of any future gun removal orders. Kansas state senator Richard Hilderbrand, the sponsor of one such bill, argued that "the hate in that person's heart is what caused it, so until we start addressing that, you know, we're just going down these rabbit holes that lead to nowhere" (Hanna 2019). In January 2020, Georgia state representative Ken Pullin introduced an anti–red flag bill that asserted "it is the responsibility of the General Assembly to protect the people of Georgia when unconstitutional legislation is passed and signed into law" (Pereira 2020).

Following mass shootings in Dayton, Ohio, and El Paso, Texas, in August 2019, Sen. Mike Braun (R-IN) remarked, "When you have two incidents like that in the same weekend, I think conservatives and Republicans lose in the long run if we don't do something to change the dynamic. And I'm about as hard a Second Amendment guy as there is" (Everett and Levine 2019). That same month, opinion polls indicated that 70 percent of Republicans supported red flag laws that allowed family members to petition a court for a gun removal order, and 66 percent of Republicans supported laws that allowed police to make that petition (Bowden 2019). By August 2020, 19 states and Washington, DC, had passed red flag laws allowing law enforcement officials, medical professionals, lawyers, and family members, among others, to petition to remove a firearm from individuals deemed threats to themselves or others.

Todd M. Olszewski

Further Reading

Barr, Andy. 2019. "A 'False Accusation' That Republicans Aren't Working to Curb Gun Violence." *Lexington Herald Leader*, September 6. Accessed July 13, 2020. https://www.kentucky.com/opinion/op-ed/article234787242.html.

Barry, Colleen, Sachini Bandara, Erika Franklin Fowler, Laura Baum, Sarah Gollust, Jeff Niederdeppe, and Alene Kennedy Hendricks. 2020. "Guns in Political Advertising over Four US Election Cycles, 2012–18." *Health Affairs* 39: 327–333. Accessed February 18, 2021. https://www.healthaffairs.org/doi/10.1377/hlthaff.2019.01102.

Beckett, Lois. 2014. "Republican Say No to CDC Gun Violence Research." ProPublica, April 21. Accessed July 13, 2020. https://www.propublica.org/article/republicans-say-no-to-cdc-gun-violence-research.

Bertrand, Natasha. 2015. "Congress Quietly Renewed a Ban on Gun-Violence Research." Business Insider, July 7. Accessed July 13, 2020. https://www.businessinsider.com/congressional-ban-on-gun-violence-research-rewnewed-2015-7.

Blumenthal, Richard. 2016. "Blumenthal Statement on Orlando Shooting." June 12. Accessed July 27, 2020. https://www.blumenthal.senate.gov/newsroom/press/release/blumenthal-statement-on-orlando-shooting.

Bousquet, Steve. 2018. "Gov. Rick Scott Signs Gun, School Security Legislation over NRA Opposition." *Tampa Bay Times*, March 9. Accessed July 13, 2020. https://www.tampabay.com/florida-politics/buzz/2018/03/09/gov-rick-scott-signs-gun-school-security-legislation-over-nra-opposition/.

Bowden, John. 2019. "Two-Thirds of Republicans Support 'Red Flag' Gun Laws: Poll." The Hill, August 20. Accessed October 30, 2020. https://thehill.com/blogs/blog-briefing-room/news/458039-two-thirds-of-republicans-support-red-flag-gun-laws-npr-poll.

Bush, Jeb. 2016. "Barack Obama's Executive Orders Trample on the Second Amendment." *The Gazette* (Cedar Rapids, IA), January 5. Accessed July 13, 2020. https://www.thegazette.com/subject/opinion/guest-columnists/barack-obamas-executive-orders-trample-on-the-second-amendment-20160105.

Campbell, Sean, and Daniel Nass. 2019. "11 Senators Want to Know Why the CDC's Gun Injury Estimates Are Unreliable." FiveThirtyEight, March 29. Accessed July 13, 2020. https://fivethirtyeight.com/features/11-senators-want-to-know-why-the-cdcs-gun-injury-estimates-are-unreliable/.

Campbell, Sean, Daniel Nass, and Mai Nguyen. 2018. "The CDC Is Publishing Unreliable Data on Gun Injuries. People Are Using It Anyway." FiveThirtyEight, October 4. Accessed July 13, 2020. https://fivethirtyeight.com/features/the-cdc-is-publishing-unreliable-data-on-gun-injuries-people-are-using-it-anyway/.

Christensen, Jen. 2018. "Will a Signal from the Top Mean More Gun Violence Research?" CNN, February 16. Accessed July 13, 2020. https://www.cnn.com/2018/02/16/health/gun-violence-government-research/index.html.

CNN. 1999. "Clinton Discusses School Violence with High Schoolers." April 22. Accessed July 27, 2020. https://www.cnn.com/ALLPOLITICS/stories/1999/04/22/clinton.shooting/.

Cohn, Nate, and Kevin Quealy. 2017. "Nothing Divides Voters Like Owning a Gun." *New York Times*, October 5. Accessed July 13, 2020. https://www.nytimes.com/interactive/2017/10/05/upshot/gun-ownership-partisan-divide.html.

Corpuz, Mina. 2020. "Bill Could Put Doctors 'On the Front Lines' of Addressing Gun Injuries, Deaths." *The Enterprise*, January 2. Accessed July 13, 2020. https://www.enterprisenews.com/news/20200102/bill-could-put-doctors-on-front-lines-of-addressing-gun-injuries-deaths.

Davis, Susan. 2017. "A Familiar, Partisan Response in Congress to Las Vegas Massacre." NPR, October 2. Accessed July 27, 2020. https://www.npr.org/2017/10/02/555099794/a-familiar-partisan-response-in-congress-to-las-vegas-massacre.

DeSaulnier, Mark. 2019. "Congressman DeSaulnier Introduces Bill to Develop Evidence-Based Solutions to Gun Violence." August 12. Accessed July 13, 2020. https://desaulnier.house.gov/media-center/press-releases/congressman-desaulnier-introduces-bill-develop-evidence-based-solutions.

Diamond, Jeremy. 2015. "Former GOP Congressman Flips on Support for Gun Violence Research." CNN, December 3. Accessed July 13, 2020. https://www.cnn.com/2015/12/02/politics/jay-dickey-gun-violence-research/index.html.

Doroshow, Deborah. 2019. "We Need to Stop Focusing on the Mental Health of Mass Shooters." *Washington Post*, May 20. Accessed July 13, 2020. https://www.washingtonpost.com/outlook/2019/05/20/we-need-stop-focusing-mental-health-mass-shooters/.

Everett, Burgess, and Marianne Levine. 2019. "Susan Collins and the GOP Court Trump on Guns." Politico, August 14. Accessed July 13, 2020. https://www.politico.com/story/2019/08/14/susan-collins-gop-trump-guns-1463596.

Flanagan, Brenda. 2019. "Murphy Signs 'Smart Gun' Bill, Calls for More Gun Control." NJTV, July 16. Accessed July 13, 2020. https://www.njtvonline.org/news/video/murphy-signs-smart-gun-bill-calls-for-more-gun-control/.

Fox, Kara. 2019. "How US Gun Culture Compares with the World." CNN, August 6. Accessed July 27, 2020. https://www.cnn.com/2017/10/03/americas/us-gun-statistics/index.html.

Gramlich, John, and Katherine Schaeffer. 2019. "7 Facts about Guns in the U.S." Pew Research Center, October 22. Accessed July 27, 2020. https://www.pewresearch.org/fact-tank/2019/10/22/facts-about-guns-in-united-states/.

Hanna, John. 2019. "GOP Lawmakers in 2 States Seek Anti-Red Flag Laws on Guns." Associated Press, December 30. Accessed April 19, 2021. https://apnews.com/article/852cd866a0272abe993363cbc375e2e7.

Hersher, Rebecca. 2017. "Court Strikes Down Florida Law Barring Doctors from Discussing Guns with Patients." NPR, February 17. Accessed July 13, 2020. https://www.npr.org/sections/thetwo-way/2017/02/17/515764335/court-strikes-down-florida-law-barring-doctors-from-discussing-guns-with-patient.

Higgins, Tucker, and Dan Mangan. 2020. "Supreme Court Decides Not to Hear Big Gun-Rights Cases, Dealing Blow to Second Amendment Activists." CNBC, June 15. Accessed July 27, 2020. https://www.cnbc.com/2020/06/15/supreme-court-will-not-hear-gun-cases-blow-to-2nd-amendment-backers.html.

Ingraham, Christopher. 2018. "There Are More Guns Than People in the United States, according to a New Study of Global Firearm Ownership." *Washington Post*, June 19. Accessed July 27, 2020. https://www.washingtonpost.com/news/wonk/wp/2018/06/19/there-are-more-guns-than-people-in-the-united-states-according-to-a-new-study-of-global-firearm-ownership/.

Johnson, Carla. 2019. "Experts: Mental Illness Not Main Driver of Mass Shootings." Associated Press, August 5. Accessed March 7, 2021. https://apnews.com/article/b8ce29d88543479bbd4894f5a39cc686

Joslyn, Mark, Donald Haider-Markel, Michael Baggs, and Andrew Bilbo. 2017. "Emerging Political Identities? Gun Ownership and Voting in Presidential Elections." *Social Science Quarterly* 98: 382–396. Accessed July 13, 2020. https://onlinelibrary.wiley.com/doi/abs/10.1111/ssqu.12421.

Kane, Paul. 2012. "After Colorado Shooting, Democrats Reluctant to Talk Gun Control." *Washington Post*, July 24. Accessed July 27, 2020. https://www.washingtonpost.com/politics/after-colorado-shooting-democrats-reluctant-to-talk-gun-control/2012/07/24/gJQABeaa7W_story.html.

Kochaneck, Kenneth, Sherry Murphy, Jiaquan Xu, and Elizabeth Arias. 2019. "Deaths: Final Data for 2017." National Vital Statistics Reports, June 24. Accessed July 13, 2020. https://www.cdc.gov/nchs/data/nvsr/nvsr68/nvsr68_09-508.pdf.

Krouse, William, and Daniel Richardson. 2015. "Mass Murder with Firearms: Incidents and Victims, 1999–2013." *Congressional Research Service*, July 30. Accessed July 27, 2020. https://fas.org/sgp/crs/misc/R44126.pdf.

Lander, Mark, and Peter Baker. 2012. "'These Tragedies Must End,' Obama Says." *New York Times*, December 16. Accessed July 27, 2020. https://www.nytimes.com/2012/12/17/us/politics/bloomberg-urges-obama-to-take-action-on-gun-control.html.

Lawlor, Mike. 2019. "Connecticut's 'Red Flag Law' Was the First in the Nation. Twenty Years Later, It's Saved Many Lives." *Hartford Courant*, June 28. Accessed July 13, 2020. https://www.courant.com/opinion/op-ed/hc-op-lawlor-red-flag-law-0630-20190628-nb4wss26ebd63h3zbatwgr7g4e-story.html.

Leary, Alex. 2018a. "Florida Democrats Say School Massacre a Call for Gun Control." *Tampa Bay Times*, February 15. Accessed July 27, 2020. https://www.tampabay.com/florida-politics/buzz/2018/02/15/florida-democrats-say-school-massacre-a-call-for-gun-control/.

Leary, Alex. 2018b. "Rubio Faces Pressure after Parkland: 'It's Not Our Job to Tell You, Senator Rubio, How to Protect Us." *Tampa Bay Times*, February 19. Accessed July 27, 2020. https://www.tampabay.com/florida-politics/buzz/2018/02/19/rubio-faces-pressure-after-parkland-its-not-our-job-to-tell-you-senator-rubio-how-to-protect-us/.

Leary, Warren. 1993. "Gun in Home? Study Finds It a Deadly Mix." *New York Times*, October 7. Accessed July 13, 2020. https://www.nytimes.com/1993/10/07/us/gun-in-home-study-finds-it-a-deadly-mix.html.

Lowey, Nita, and Rosa DeLauro. 2019. "Letter to the Editor." *New York Times*, August 9. Accessed July 13, 2020. https://www.nytimes.com/2019/08/09/opinion/letters/gun-safety-china-trade.html.

Lowry, Bryan. 2019. "Blunt's Budget Bill Omits $50 Million for Gun Violence Study Favored by Democrats." McClatchy DC, September 18. Accessed July 13, 2020. https://www.mcclatchydc.com/news/politics-government/congress/article235215502.html.

Markey, Ed. 2019. "Sen. Markey, Rep. Maloney Reintroduce Bill to Fund Gun Violence Prevention Research." January 17. Accessed July 13, 2020. https://www.markey.senate.gov/news/press-releases/sen-markey-rep-maloney-reintroduce-bill-to-fund-gun-violence-prevention-research.

Matthews, Mark. 2018. "Federal Gun-Violence Research All but Halted 2 Decades Ago. And if Colorado Republicans in Congress Are a Sign, That's Not Going to Change." *Denver Post*, March 4. Accessed July 13, 2020. https://www.denverpost.com/2018/03/04/federal-gun-violence-research/.

McCarthy, Justin. 2019. "64% of Americans Want Stricter Laws on Gun Sales." Gallup, November 4. Accessed July 13, 2020. https://news.gallup.com/poll/268016/americans-stricter-laws-gun-sales.aspx.

McElhatton, Jim. 2009. "U.S. Quietly Begins to Study Gun Safety." *Washington Times*, October 19. Accessed July 13, 2020. https://www.washingtontimes.com/news/2009/oct/19/nih-funds-study-of-teen-firearms/.

McGinty, Emma, Alene Kennedy-Hendricks, Seema Choksy, and Colleen Barry. 2016. "Trends in News Media Coverage of Mental Illness in the United States: 1995–2014." *Health Affairs* 6: 1121–1129. Accessed July 13, 2020. https://www.healthaffairs.org/doi/pdf/10.1377/hlthaff.2016.0011.

Moisse, Katie. 2011. "A Crime for Doctors to Ask about Guns?" ABC News, January 26. Accessed July 13, 2020. https://abcnews.go.com/Health/w_ParentingResource/pediatricians-parents-guns-home/story?id=12770294.

Murphy, Chris. 2019. "Murphy Statement following President Trump's Remarks after Mass Shootings in Texas and Ohio." August 5. Accessed July 13, 2020. https://www.murphy.senate.gov/newsroom/press-releases/murphy-statement-following-president-trumps-remarks-after-mass-shootings-in-texas-and-ohio.

National Public Radio. 2015. "Ex-Rep. Dickey Regrets Restrictive Law on Gun Violence Research." October 9. Accessed July 13, 2020. https://www.npr.org/2015/10/09/447098666/ex-rep-dickey-regrets-restrictive-law-on-gun-violence-research.

National Rifle Association, Institute for Legislative Action. 2011. "Three More Wins in Congress for Gun Owners." December 22. Accessed July 13, 2020. https://www.nraila.org/articles/20111222/three-more-wins-in-congress-for-gun-owners.

Obama, Barack. 2011. "President Obama: We Must Seek Agreement on Gun Reforms." *Arizona Daily Star*, March 13. Accessed July 13, 2020. https://tucson.com/article_011e7118-8951-5206-a878-39bfbc9dc89d.html.

Ohlheiser, Abby. 2013. "CDC Will Now Be Free to Research Gun Violence for First Time in 17 Years." Slate, January 16. Accessed July 13, 2020. https://slate.com/news-and-politics/2013/01/obama-gun-control-executive-orders-call-for-cdc-gun-violence-research-17-years-after-1996-nra-supported-freeze.html.

Oliphant, J. Baxter. 2017. "Bipartisan Support for Some Gun Proposals, Stark Partisan Divisions on Many Others." Pew Research Center, June 23. Accessed July 13, 2020. https://www.pewresearch.org/fact-tank/2017/06/23/bipartisan-support-for-some-gun-proposals-stark-partisan-divisions-on-many-others/.

Parker, Kim, Juliana Menasce Horowitz, Ruth Igielnik, J. Baxter Oliphant, and Anna Brown. 2017. "America's Complex Relationship with Guns." Pew Research Center, June 22. Accessed July 13, 2020. https://www.pewsocialtrends.org/2017/06/22/americas-complex-relationship-with-guns/.

Pereira, Ivan. 2020. "Lawmaker Introduces 'Anti-Red Flag' Bill in Georgia to Combat Gun Control." ABC News, January 15. Accessed October 30, 2020. https://abcnews.go.com/US/lawmaker-introduces-anti-red-flag-bill-georgia-combat/story?id=68299434.

Pew Research Center. 2010. "Gun Rights and Gun Control—September 2010." Accessed July 13, 2020. https://assets.pewresearch.org/wp-content/uploads/sites/12/old-assets/pdf/gun-control-2011.pdf.

Quinnipiac University Poll. 2019. "U.S. Voters Back Dem Plan to Reopen Government 2-1, Quinnipiac University National Poll Finds; More U.S. Voters Say Trump TV Address Was Misleading." January 14. Accessed July 13, 2020. https://poll.qu.edu/national/release-detail?ReleaseID=2592.

RAND Corporation. 2018. "What Science Tells Us About the Effects of Gun Policies." Updated April 22, 2020. Accessed July 13, 2020. https://www.rand.org/research/gun-policy/key-findings/what-science-tells-us-about-the-effects-of-gun-policies.html.

Ranney, Megan L., and Marian E. Betz. 2019. "How Doctors Can Help Prevent Gun Violence." *Harvard Business Review*, October 24. Accessed July 13, 2020. https://hbr.org/2019/10/how-doctors-can-help-prevent-gun-violence.

Reagan, Ronald. 1991. "Why I'm for the Brady Bill." *New York Times*, March 29. Accessed July 13, 2020. https://www.nytimes.com/1991/03/29/opinion/why-i-m-for-the-brady-bill.html.

Saad, Lydia. 2019. "What Percentage of Americans Own Guns?" Gallup, August 14. Accessed July 27, 2020. https://news.gallup.com/poll/264932/percentage-americans-own-guns.aspx.

Sarat, Austin, and Jonathan Obert. 2019. "What Both Sides Don't Get about American Gun Culture." Politico, August 4. Accessed July 13, 2020. https://www.politico.com/magazine/story/2019/08/04/mass-shooting-gun-culture-227502.

Satcher, David. 1995. "Gunning for Research." *Washington Post*, November 5. Accessed July 13, 2020. https://www.washingtonpost.com/archive/opinions/1995/11/05/gunning-for-research/05b6584f-5c26-4a80-b564-cccf5f1c2ddd/.

Scalise, Steve. 2019. "Scalise in Fox News Op-Ed: Democrats Don't Want You to Hear What I Have to Say about Guns." February 6. Accessed July 13, 2020. https://scalise.house.gov/press-release/scalise-fox-news-op-ed-democrats-dont-want-you-hear-what-i-have-say-about-guns.

Schaeffer, Katherine. 2019. "Share of Americans Who Favor Stricter Gun Laws Has Increased since 2017." Pew Research Center, October 16. Accessed July 13, 2020.

https://www.pewresearch.org/fact-tank/2019/10/16/share-of-americans-who-favor-stricter-gun-laws-has-increased-since-2017/.

Schumer, Charles. 1999. "Statement of Sen. Charles Schumer Response to the Shootings at Columbine High School April 21, 1999." April 21. Accessed July 27, 2020. https://www.schumer.senate.gov/newsroom/statements/statement-of-sen-charles-schumer-response-to-the-shootings-at-columbine-high-school-april-21-1999.

Scott, Rick. 2019. "I'm a Gun Owner and NRA Member. I Support Red-Flag Laws to Help Stop Mass Shootings." *Washington Post*, August 9. Accessed October 30, 2020. https://www.washingtonpost.com/opinions/2019/08/09/im-gun-owner-nra-member-i-support-red-flag-laws-help-stop-mass-shootings/.

Siddons, Andrew. 2019. "Gun Research Funding Push Faces Challenge in Senate Even after Shootings." Roll Call, August 9. Accessed July 13, 2020. https://www.rollcall.com/2019/08/09/gun-research-funding-push-faces-challenge-in-senate-even-after-shootings/.

Silverstein, Jason. 2020. "There Were More Mass Shootings Than Days in 2019." CBS News, January 2. Accessed July 27, 2020. https://www.cbsnews.com/news/mass-shootings-2019-more-than-days-365/.

Smith, Tom, and Jaesok Son. 2015. *General Social Survey Final Report: Trends in Gun Ownership in the United States, 1972–2014*. Chicago: NORC.

Stainton, Lilo. 2018. "New Jersey Looks to California for Gun-Violence Research Model." NJ Spotlight, April 3. Accessed July 13, 2020. https://www.njspotlight.com/2018/04/18-04-02-new-jersey-looks-to-california-for-gun-violence-research-model/.

Stracqualursi, Veronica. 2019. "Congress Agrees to Millions in Gun Violence Research for the First Time in Decades." CNN, December 17. Accessed July 13, 2020. https://www.cnn.com/2019/12/17/politics/gun-research-congress-spending-bill-cdc-trnd/index.html.

Thompson, Mike. 2019. "Chairman Thompson Lauds Passage of HR8, His Bipartisan Background Checks Act of 2019." February 27. Accessed July 13, 2020. https://mikethompson.house.gov/newsroom/press-releases/chairman-thompson-lauds-passage-of-hr8-his-bipartisan-background-checks-act.

Trump, Donald J. 2017. "President Donald J. Trump Signs H.R. 255, and H.R. 321 and H.J.Res. 40." Online by Gerhard Peters and John T. Woolley, the American Presidency Project. Accessed March 7, 2021. https://www.presidency.ucsb.edu/node/323739.

Trump, Donald J. 2019. "Statement of Administration Policy: H.R. 8—Bipartisan Background Checks Act of 2019 & H.R. 1112—Enhanced Background Checks Act of 2019." Online by Gerhard Peters and John T. Woolley, the American Presidency Project. Accessed March 7, 2021. https://www.presidency.ucsb.edu/node/335324.

U.S. House of Representatives, Judiciary Committee. 2019. "Collins Introduces Mass Violence Prevention Act." February 25. Accessed July 13, 2020. https://republicans-judiciary.house.gov/press-release/collins-introduces-mass-violence-prevention-act/.

U.S. Public Law 104-208. 1996. 104th Cong., 2d sess., September 30. Accessed July 13, 2020. https://www.govinfo.gov/content/pkg/PLAW-104publ208/pdf/PLAW-104publ208.pdf.

Van Brocklin, Elizabeth. 2019. "States Are Funding the Gun Violence Research the Feds Won't." The Trace, January 29. Accessed July 13, 2020. https://www.thetrace.org/2019/01/state-gun-violence-research-california-new-jersey/.

Voght, Kara. 2019. "A Year after Parkland, Republicans Still Don't Want to Fund Gun Violence Research." *Mother Jones*, March 7. Accessed July 13, 2020. https://www.motherjones.com/politics/2019/03/a-year-after-parkland-republicans-still-dont-want-to-fund-gun-violence-research/.

White House. 2018. "President Donald J. Trump Is Taking Immediate Actions to Secure Our Schools." March 12. Accessed March 7, 2021. https://trumpwhitehouse.archives.gov/briefings-statements/president-donald-j-trump-taking-immediate-actions-secure-schools.

White House, Office of the Press Secretary. 2015. "Statement by the President on the Shootings at Umpqua Community College, Roseburg, Oregon." October 1. Accessed July 13, 2020. https://obamawhitehouse.archives.gov/the-press-office/2015/10/01/statement-president-shootings-umpqua-community-college-roseburg-oregon.

White House, Office of the Press Secretary. 2016. "Fact Sheet: New Executive Actions to Reduce Gun Violence and Make Our Communities Safer." January 4. Accessed July 13, 2020. https://obamawhitehouse.archives.gov/the-press-office/2016/01/04/fact-sheet-new-executive-actions-reduce-gun-violence-and-make-our.

Health Care: Right or Commodity?

At a Glance

Democrats and Republicans have fundamentally disagreed about what role the government should play in the financing, regulation, and delivery of health care in the United States. Guided by their respective interpretations of responsibility, equity, and liberty, Democrats and Republicans have historically held different positions on whether health care access should be defined as a basic human right or as a market commodity that is the personal responsibility of all citizens. Democrats have traditionally considered health care as a human right. In this context, Democrats contend that the role of the government is to promote and regulate a "just" health care system that ensures access to care for all citizens. Republicans have traditionally insisted that health care access is a matter of personal responsibility, one in which the government should accede to the individual liberty of patients and health care providers. In this context, Republicans maintain that market-oriented reforms will improve health care access by delivering improved choice to informed consumers. Partisan rhetoric and policy records illuminate how Democrats and Republicans have debated the economic and medical implications of unequal access to health care: whether insurance status is synonymous with health status, whether rising health care costs are minimized by providing coverage to all citizens, and whether higher taxes are a necessary condition to funding universal coverage.

According to Many Democrats . . .

- Health care should be regarded as a basic human right.
- Federal and state governments have a responsibility to protect health care access as a basic right.
- Health entitlement programs such as Medicaid provide necessary access to citizens who are unable to afford health care, and eligibility should be expanded.
- Health reform efforts should focus on expanding entitlement programs that are funded via increased taxes on the wealthy.
- Universal health care coverage is an important and long-standing policy goal.

According to Many Republicans . . .

- Health care is not a fundamental human right.
- State governments, not the federal government, should be able to mandate health insurance coverage at their discretion.
- Health entitlement programs such as Medicaid contribute to the budget deficit; government health care spending should be reduced by cutting budgets and imposing stricter eligibility requirements.
- Free market-oriented reforms will lower health care costs, encourage competition, and improve consumer choice.
- Universal health care coverage is associated with socialism, which threatens individual liberty.

Overview

The question of whether health care should be regarded as a basic human right or as a market commodity has been a long-standing political question in the United States since the early 20th century. Guided by their respective interpretations of responsibility, equity, and liberty, Democrats and Republicans have historically held different positions on this question—the nuances of which have shifted at different periods in time. The past decade, for example, highlights the widening distance between Democratic and Republican perceptions of the role of government involvement in ensuring health care access to Americans. Between 2008 and 2019, the percentage of Republicans favoring the federal government "doing more to help provide health insurance" declined from 49 to 40 percent, while the percentage of Democrats who answered in the affirmative rose from 92 to 94 percent (Kaiser Family Foundation 2020b).

American conservatives have advanced a market-oriented position that acknowledges the rights of health care professionals, hospitals, insurance companies, and pharmaceutical companies to invest and innovate in health care delivery as well as the rights of American citizens to choose their health insurance coverage. American liberals, on the other hand, have emphasized the rights of citizens they deem as vulnerable, such as the poor and elderly, who may lack economic security and, thus, health security. As sociologist Paul Starr has remarked, "For American liberals in the twentieth century, health insurance for all was a persistent dream and a perennial disappointment, often on the horizon but always seemingly out of reach" (Starr 2011b).

The philosophical divide between Democrats and Republicans has its roots in early 20th-century debates about health insurance and whether the government is responsible for providing health insurance to American citizens. During the first decades of the 20th century, Progressive-era reformers found inspiration from social welfare reform efforts in Europe. In 1911, Britain instituted a national insurance program. Soon thereafter, the American Association for Labor

Legislation distributed a model bill to state legislatures across the country, patterned in part after the British program. Progressive reformers and labor organizations generally supported national insurance legislation and introduced the idea into the American political arena (Numbers 1978). After the United States entered World War I, opponents of government health insurance, who were wary of European social reforms, condemned national health insurance as un-American. In 1925, the New York State Medical Society proclaimed that national health insurance "is a dead issue in the United States. . . . It is not conceivable that any serious effort will again be made to subsidize medicine as the hand-maiden of the public" (Numbers 1997).

The Great Depression of the 1930s brought renewed attention to what role the government should play in ensuring the health and social welfare of American citizens. In 1934, Democratic President Franklin D. Roosevelt sent an economic security bill to Congress that would become the Social Security Act of 1935. Roosevelt had considered including a health insurance provision in the bill, but opposition from the American Medical Association (AMA) led to its removal. Despite his reelection in 1936 and Democratic control of both houses of Congress throughout his presidency, Roosevelt was unable to move national health insurance forward—especially after the 1939 arrival of World War II, which raged for the next six years. For the remainder of his time as president, Roosevelt indicated that he would advocate for national health insurance during peacetime, but he died in April 1945, several months before the war finally came to an end.

After World War II, most urban Americans had private health insurance (Numbers 1997). However, many other unemployed and poor Americans remained uninsured. Roosevelt's successor, Harry Truman, lent his support to a national health insurance program. Following Truman's election to a new term in 1948, the AMA mobilized another public campaign against national health insurance in the United States, which led public support to drop from 75 percent in 1945 to 21 percent by 1949 (Quadagno 2005). Truman ultimately abandoned national health insurance, and the United States turned to the two-tiered system that characterizes the modern American health care system: private health insurance for those who can afford it and public welfare services for those who cannot.

The 1952 election of Republican Dwight Eisenhower ended the debate over national health insurance, at least temporarily. On the one hand, opponents of national health insurance proposals were effective in deriding any national insurance efforts as specters of socialism. On the other hand, the private health insurance system enjoyed considerable growth, reflecting the hard-earned efforts of labor unions as well as the national stature of Blue Cross and Blue Shield. Founded in 1929, Blue Cross guaranteed prepaid hospital care; Blue Shield began as an insurance plan that guaranteed prepaid physicians' services, laying the groundwork for private health insurance in the United States. However, as health care historian Beatrix Hoffman has demonstrated, "a land of limitless health care never existed" after

World War II (Hoffman 2012). Even if private insurance coverage did not provide health security for all, Republicans insisted that it protected against the prospect of socialism. In 1953, the Eisenhower administration determined that employer contributions to health insurance plans were nontaxable benefits, thereby forging a clear connection between employment status and health insurance coverage. No other substantive health reform efforts occurred during Eisenhower's Republican presidential administration, which was defined by six years of Democratic control of both houses of Congress.

The linkage of employment status and insurance coverage brought health coverage to millions of Americans, but it also left low-income Americans and senior citizens without. The Truman and Kennedy administrations both advocated for national health insurance for elderly Americans. Conservative opponents, however, continued to maintain that government-subsidized insurance for the elderly would bring about socialized medicine in the United States. The AMA recruited Hollywood actor Ronald Reagan to serve as the spokesman for "Operation Coffeecup," a campaign to defeat Medicare. As scholar Jeffrey St. Onge has argued, although the campaign was ultimately unsuccessful, it further solidified the specter of socialized medicine as an ongoing concern of the national conservative movement and established Reagan as a future leader of that movement (St. Onge 2017).

Following passage of the landmark Civil Rights Act of 1964, Democratic President Lyndon B. Johnson and a Democratic Congress implemented a national program of government-subsidized insurance for elderly Americans. In 1965, Johnson signed two programs of national health insurance for certain vulnerable members of American society into law. Medicare provided government financing of health care for the elderly, and Medicaid did so for the poor (Cohen et al. 2015). When Johnson announced Medicare's passage, he emphasized the community's obligation to its older citizens: "For the Nation it will bring the necessary satisfaction of having fulfilled the obligations of justice to those who have given a lifetime of service and labor to their country" (Centers for Medicare and Medicaid Services n.d.).

The federal government financed and structured Medicare and Medicaid differently, which in turn shaped public perceptions of the two programs. Medicare, framed as an entitlement earned through payroll contributions, received relatively widespread social support. On the other hand, because Medicaid employed means testing to determine eligibility and provided health coverage to poor Americans, it came to be seen in some quarters as a stigmatized form of public assistance (Cohen et al. 2015). As health care scholar Robert Hackey noted, "The very success of Medicare and Medicaid planted the seeds of discontent with the health care system in the late 1960s" (Hackey 2012). Newly insured Americans exercised their newfound access to care, which raised concerns about whether the federal government could afford to meet its new obligations. Conservative opposition to Johnson's Great Society programs led to significant Republican gains during the 1966 midterm elections. These results marked a political turning point for the nation, with the postwar liberal consensus gradually giving way to a more conservative one that held considerable sway for decades to come.

The ascendant conservative movement brought about the election of Republican Richard Nixon in 1968, who quickly realized that fast-rising health care costs were a potentially serious vulnerability for his administration. Controlling rising health care costs thus became policy priorities for Republicans and Democrats alike—but their proposed solutions followed different guiding principles. While Sen. Ted Kennedy (D-MA) cosponsored a bill that called for government financing of health care, Nixon supported one that called for private financing through an employer mandate: that is, employers, not the federal government, would provide health insurance for employees (Hoffman 2012). In addition to the employer mandate, Nixon also introduced the health maintenance organization as a model for cost control. The Watergate scandal and Nixon's subsequent resignation prevented further legislative action on health rights and health security. During the 1980s and early 1990s, the Reagan and George H. W. Bush administrations continued to emphasize market-based measures to control health costs instead of stricter government regulation.

When Democrat Bill Clinton took office in 1993, he created a task force under the supervision of First Lady Hillary Clinton that was charged with developing a national health reform plan. The Clinton plan that was eventually presented to Congress proposed that states establish publicly financed health alliances through which all state residents would receive their health coverage and that a national board would set requirements for basic plan benefit levels. "Under our plan," said Clinton, "every American would receive a health care security card that will guarantee a comprehensive package of benefits over the course of an entire lifetime" (Starr 2011b). The Clinton plan faced criticism from liberal Democrats, who argued in favor of a single-payer model, and even fiercer opposition from congressional Republicans, who maintained that the Clinton plan represented undue government intrusion into health care.

Although these political forces led to the defeat of the Clinton plan, two other bipartisan achievements during the Clinton administration recast the long-standing debate regarding health care rights and the government. The 1996 Health Insurance Portability and Accountability Act (HIPAA) granted citizens the right to retain their health coverage when they lost or changed jobs, and the 1997 Children's Health Insurance Plan (CHIP) provided health coverage to uninsured children whose families did not qualify for Medicaid.

Several states also explored their own state-level reforms to expand coverage and cut rising costs during the late 1980s and 1990s. For example, in 1990, the New York State Department of Health proposed Universal New York Health Care. Under UNY-Care, the state would have retained the system of private and public insurance, but the government would have served as the sole payer in the state (Beauchamp and Rouse 1990). Although Gov. Mario Cuomo (D) did not move forward with UNY-Care, the proposal signaled willingness by state Democrats to provide a standard package of health benefits to all state residents (Beauchamp 1996).

Oregon also sought to extend insurance coverage to all state residents in 1989. In this case, the Oregon Basic Health Services Act established a standard package of benefits that would vary according to a sliding scale driven by budget considerations (Nelson and Drought 1992). As the plan's architect, Democrat state senator John Kitzhaber argued, "If we can agree that society cannot afford to buy everything for everyone who might conceivably benefit from it, then we have to develop a process to determine what level of care everyone should have access to" (Fox and Leichter 1991). This assumption captured the long-standing tension girding the health rights debate: whether a government has an obligation to ensure health care access as a right and, if so, how that government would distribute limited resources in a fair and equitable manner.

While Democrats and Republicans have differed in opinion on governmental responsibility for ensuring health care, they have also differed in whether the United States should retain or jettison the employment-based insurance coverage model. Former Gov. Howard Dean (D) unsuccessfully sought to introduce a single-payer system in Vermont in 1994, but in 2011, Vermont became the first U.S. state to pass a law for publicly financed universal health care. Passing both state houses almost entirely along party lines and signed into law by Gov. Peter Shumlin (D), the Vermont plan made all Vermont citizens eligible for health benefits through Green Mountain Care, a publicly funded single-payer system (Wallack 2011). As Shumlin explained, "Single-payer coverage will be a right and not a privilege, and will not be connected to employment" (Shumlin 2011).

Critics of the plan responded by forming Vermonters for Health Care Freedom, a nonprofit organization emphasizing market-based reforms over increased government regulation of the health care system. Concerns about prohibitive costs forced Vermont to abandon its single-payer initiative in 2014 (McDonough 2015). Sen. Bernie Sanders (I-VT), however, restoked national debate about single-payer systems during his 2016 and 2020 presidential campaigns.

During the 2020 presidential primary campaign, Democratic members of Congress and several Democratic presidential candidates released different versions of health reform plans that differed in whether they endorsed a single-payer model (in which government enrolls all individuals in a publicly administered plan), eliminated or preserved the private health insurance industry, or expanded access through incremental improvements to the existing Affordable Care Act (ACA). Sens. Bernie Sanders (I-VT) and Elizabeth Warren (D-MA), both of whom endorsed a single-payer model of Medicare for All, emerged as leading challengers for the Democratic presidential nomination. At the same time, however, 55 percent of Democrats indicated a preference for a presidential candidate who would "build upon the existing ACA" (Kaiser Family Foundation 2020b). Former Vice President Joe Biden, the 2020 Democratic nominee, declined to endorse Medicare for All during the campaign.

During the first presidential debate in late September 2020, Trump contended that if Biden was elected, "you're going to extinguish 180 million people with their private health care" and introduce "socialized medicine," to which Biden responded that he instead supported preserving private health insurance and expanding the ACA, not replacing it with Medicare for All (Sullivan 2020). During the final presidential debate in late October, President Trump stated that he intended to "terminate" the ACA whether or not the U.S. Supreme Court struck down the law in the pending Supreme Court case *California v. Texas* challenging its constitutionality. Biden promised that if the ACA was dismantled and he was elected president, he would "pass Obamacare with a public option, [so] it becomes Bidencare" (Hayes 2020).

Democrats on Health Care as a Right

Health care rights took center stage during the 2008, 2012, and 2016 presidential elections when leading Democratic candidates Barack Obama, Hillary Clinton, and Bernie Sanders, respectively, presented differing visions of how they would reform the American health care system. All three candidates employed rights-based language to varying degrees when explaining how they believed that the federal government had a responsibility to ensure coverage to American citizens.

Opinion surveys of likely primary voters during the 2008 presidential campaign highlighted clear philosophical differences between Democratic and Republican voters on Americans' basic right to health care. In one survey, 74 percent of Democrats expressed willingness to pay higher taxes to ensure that all Americans have health insurance compared to 46 percent of Republicans (Blendon, Altman, Deane, et al. 2008). During the second presidential debate with 2008 Republican nominee John McCain, Barack Obama declared that health care "should be a right for every American" (CNN 2008). Obama claimed that the government was responsible for instituting consumer protections for American patients rather than deregulating the health insurance industry. In a subsequent survey taken in the lead up to the general election, 54 percent of those who voted for Obama in the primary indicated that the government should take responsibility for expanding health care access compared to 20 percent of those who voted for McCain (Blendon, Altman, Benson, et al. 2008).

During a September 2009 address to a joint session of Congress, President Obama outlined his health reform proposal not in rights-based language typically embraced by Democrats but rather in terms of economic security as also advanced by Republicans. As he asserted, "My guiding principle is, and always has been, that consumers do better when there is choice and competition. . . . I will not back down on the basic principle that if Americans can't find affordable coverage, we will provide you with a choice" (*New York Times* 2009).

As Obama's reform plan took shape over 2009 and 2010, it developed as a complex political compromise that built upon the existing framework of employer-based coverage while also expanding public support for those lacking coverage or with limited financial means. The Patient Protection and Affordable Care Act (ACA) that was ultimately crafted by the Obama administration and Democrats in Congress contained several key features intended to protect Americans from high health care costs while not specifically conferring a right to health insurance. Most notably, the ACA (also popularly known by both supporters and detractors as Obamacare) included an individual mandate that required individuals to purchase health insurance (an idea initially promoted by conservatives and rejected by Democrats), a system of state health insurance exchanges accompanied by government subsidies for individuals with moderate incomes (a less ambitious version of the regional health alliances proposed under the 1993 Clinton reform plan), and expanded Medicaid eligibility requirements (similar to Gov. Mitt Romney's reform plan in Massachusetts).

The ACA passed the U.S. Senate on December 24, 2009, by a vote of 60–39, with all Democrats and Independents voting for the bill and all Republicans voting against the bill. It passed the U.S. House of Representatives on March 21, 2010, by a vote of 219–212, with 178 Republicans and 34 Democrats voting against the bill. When Obama signed the Affordable Care Act, he proclaimed, "We have just

Health Care Is a Human Right

Rep. Nancy Pelosi (D-CA) made the following remarks on the floor of the U.S. House of Representatives to express her opposition to the American Health Care Act of 2017, a Republican proposal to replace the Affordable Care Act.

> Mr. Speaker, on March 25, 1966—51 years ago, this past Saturday—Dr. King spoke these words: "Of all the forms of inequality, injustice in health is the most shocking and the most inhuman because it often results in physical death."
>
> We came to this floor to fight TrumpCare last week with the moral force of Dr. Martin Luther King's words in our heart. Affordable health care is a civil right; a fundamental right for every American. As we remember Dr. King's wisdom, as we debated this bill: we did so in tribute to our colleague Bobby Rush's late wife, Carolyn Rush. Carolyn was active in the civil rights movement, and she was a champion for Americans' health care. Her funeral was Saturday, the 51st anniversary of Dr. King's words. We were proud to honor Carolyn Rush's memory by saving the Affordable Care Act from repeal and protecting the health of the American people.
>
> Speaker Ryan called this bill an "act of mercy." There is no mercy here. Indeed, inequality and inhumanity is exactly what TrumpCare has in store for the American people.

Source

Congressional Record, vol. 163, no. 53 (March 27, 2017): E393. https://www.congress.gov/115/crec/2017/03/27/CREC-2017-03-27-pt1-PgE393-3.pdf.

enshrined the principle that everybody should have the same basic security when it comes to their health care" (Stolberg and Pear 2010).

In 2012, the U.S. Supreme Court ruled in *National Federation of Independent Business v. Sebelius* that the Medicaid expansion provision of the ACA was unconstitutionally coercive to states, thereby rendering Medicaid expansion optional. Since then, Democratic governors and state legislatures have predominantly enacted Medicaid expansion. When Gov. Pat Quinn (D) of Illinois signed legislation enacting Medicaid expansion, he remarked, "In the home state of President Obama, we believe access to quality health care is a fundamental right and we proudly embrace the Affordable Care Act" (Illinois Department of Human Services 2013). As of November 2020, 38 states and Washington, DC, have expanded Medicaid eligibility requirements.

During the 2016 Democratic presidential primaries, candidates Hillary Clinton and Bernie Sanders made health care rights central to their campaigns. Clinton promised that she would "lead the fight to expand health care access for every American" (Office of Hillary Rodham Clinton n.d.). Sanders, an Independent senator from Vermont, argued later that under his plan, "Americans will benefit from the freedom and security that comes with finally separating health insurance from employment" (Abramson 2017).

Both candidates expressed the importance of expanding access to health care, but they offered different approaches to fulfilling this vision. Sanders's plan represented the views of the Democratic party's progressive wing, and Clinton's plan reflected those of its moderate wing. Sanders, embracing the principles of democratic socialism, advocated replacing the ACA with a national single-payer health insurance system that would be funded through tax increases. Clinton challenged Sanders's vision for universal coverage: "There is no way that can be paid for without raising taxes on the middle class. The arithmetic just doesn't add up" (Bradner and Luhby 2016). Clinton's health plan relied on preserving and expanding the framework of the ACA. In addition to offering a "public option," the government-sponsored insurance option that had been left out of the ACA, Clinton proposed lowering the Medicare eligibility cutoff to 55.

Democrats have maintained that the role of the federal government is to promote and regulate a health care system that ensures access to care for all citizens. The 2016 Democratic party platform explicitly stated that "Democrats believe that health care is a right, not a privilege, and our health care system should put people before profits" (Democratic National Committee 2018). In one 2016 Pew poll, 78 percent of Democratic and Democratic-leaning independents indicated that the federal government should be responsible for health care coverage (Pew Research Center 2016). The 2016 presidential election and Bernie Sanders's Medicare for All proposal brought renewed public attention to single-payer-based universal coverage. By 2017, 81 percent of Democrats and Democratic-leaning independents responding to another Pew poll indicated that the federal government should be responsible for health care coverage; only 30 percent of Republicans and Republican-leaning independents agreed (Pew Research Center 2017).

A majority of Democrats have indicated consistently favorable views of the ACA since its implementation. During Trump's first term as president, one poll found that the percentage of Democrats who reported a favorable view of the ACA grew from 70 percent to 85 percent (Kaiser Family Foundation 2020a). Democrats continue to defend the ACA and interpret its passage as an implicit acknowledgment that health care should be a basic right, particularly as the ACA faces new court challenges to its constitutionality.

Republicans on Health Care as a Commodity

Access to health care took center stage during the 2008, 2012, and 2016 presidential elections when Republican nominees John McCain, Mitt Romney, and Donald Trump, respectively, all presented market-based approaches to health care reform. Romney and Trump also devoted significant attention to repealing the Affordable Care Act.

During the 2008 Republican primary and general election campaigns, both Romney and McCain equated insurance coverage with responsible, informed

Health Care and Consumer Freedom

On July 25, 2017, Sen. Ted Cruz (R-TX) offered these comments in support of the American Health Care Act, a Republican proposal to replace the Affordable Care Act.

> The bill before the Senate includes the consumer freedom amendment—an amendment that I have introduced like the health savings account amendment. It is an amendment that says you, the consumer, should have the freedom to choose the healthcare that is best for your family. You should have the freedom. You shouldn't have to buy what the Federal Government mandates that you must buy; you should choose what meets the needs for you and your family.
>
> The consumer freedom amendment was designed to bring together and serve as a compromise for those who support the mandates in title I. The consumer freedom amendment says that insurance companies, if they offer plans that meet those title I mandates—all the protections for preexisting conditions—they can also sell any other plan that consumers desire. So it takes away nothing. If you like your ObamaCare plans, those are still there. It just adds new options and lets you decide: Do you want the ObamaCare option or do you want something else that is affordable? So rather than getting fined by the IRS, you can actually purchase something you and your family can afford.

Source

Congressional Record, vol. 163, no. 125 (July 25, 2017): S4180. Accessed March 14, 2021. https://www.congress.gov/115/crec/2017/07/25/CREC-2017-07-25-pt1-PgS4168-2.pdf.

consumerism. As a presidential candidate, Romney described his reform vision; "It's the free market way, the private sector way, the individual responsibility way—the American way" (Romney 2007). During one 2008 presidential debate, McCain emphasized that "[Obama] starts talking about government. He starts saying, government will do this and government will do that, and then government will, and he'll impose mandates. . . . The point is that we have got to give people choice in America and not mandate things on them and give them the ability [to purchase health insurance]" (CNN 2008).

The first year of the Obama administration was marked by protracted debates between Democrats and Republicans over health reform. Public opinion of the ACA was deeply divided but remained consistent following its implementation. According to public polling data, 40 percent of Americans held an unfavorable view of the ACA in August 2018—the same percentage of Americans who held that view in April 2010. When viewed along party lines, differences in public opinion were even more pronounced: since its implementation, 65–83 percent of Republicans have held an unfavorable view of the ACA compared to 13–31 percent of Democrats with the same view (Kaiser Family Foundation 2020a).

The ACA became a central focus of the 2012 presidential campaign between Obama and former Massachusetts Gov. Mitt Romney. The ACA's individual mandate had previously formed the basis for Romney's 2006 Massachusetts health care reform. Romney rejected the concept of a national mandate, however, instead insisting that states should be able to innovate at their own discretion (Romney 2011). Romney also claimed that the ACA was fiscally irresponsible, as it "will create a new entitlement even as the ones we already have are bankrupt" (Hamby 2010). Although the conservative-leaning Heritage Foundation introduced the individual mandate during the late 1980s—and it had been a central pillar of "Romneycare" in Massachusetts—conservative perceptions of the mandate soured when Obama incorporated it into his health reform plan (Roy 2012). Political analysts agree that conservative opposition to the individual mandate grew stronger when Obama shifted course from denouncing a mandate to incorporating the concept in his national health reform plan (Starr 2011a).

Today, the majority of Republicans continue to endorse free market–oriented reforms that they assert will encourage competition and improve consumer choice. The 2016 Republican platform stated, "Our goal is to ensure that all Americans have improved access to affordable, high-quality healthcare" (Republican National Committee 2016). Since 2011, Republicans have prioritized repealing the ACA and have held dozens of repeal votes in Congress. During this period, many Republicans contended that the individual mandate is unconstitutional, expressed wariness regarding increased government involvement in the financing and delivery of health care, and condemned the redistributive nature of subsidies offered through insurance exchanges.

After the U.S. Supreme Court issued its 2012 decision in *National Federation of Independent Business v. Sebelius*, Republican governors and state legislatures predominantly rejected their states' participation in Medicaid expansion. Gov. Mary Fallon (R) of Oklahoma offered a typical explanation when she said that accepting Medicaid expansion in her state would "further Oklahoma's reliance on federal money that may or may not be available in the future given the dire fiscal problems facing the federal government" (Cosgrove 2012). While Republican governors like Fallon offered a fiscal justification for not participating in Medicaid expansion, others, such as Florida's Rick Scott, cast their decisions as responses to what they perceived as unconstitutional actions on the part of the federal government. When Scott refused to expand Medicaid in Florida and sued the federal government in 2015 when it threatened to withhold hospital funding if Florida failed to expand Medicaid, Texas's Gov. Greg Abbott (R) praised the move. Although Scott eventually dropped the lawsuit, Abbott said that "when the federal government exceeds its constitutional authority, the states must take action" (Young 2016).

However, other conservative governors did opt to have their states participate in Medicaid expansion. For example, John Kasich, the Republican governor of Ohio, justified his decision during his 2013 State of the State address: "For those that live in the shadows of life, those who are the least among us, I will not accept the fact that the most vulnerable in our state should be ignored. We can help them" (Kasich 2013). As of November 2020, 12 states had not adopted Medicaid expansion. Donald Trump won all of these states during the 2016 presidential election.

Republicans have traditionally reframed health care as an economic choice, one in which citizens have a right to make decisions as informed consumers free from government intervention. In particular, they contended that requiring Americans to purchase health insurance violated citizens' individual rights. Phil Gramm, a retired Republican U.S. senator from Texas, framed his opposition to the ACA as a matter of economic freedom: "Why the Republican majority in Congress has never forced a vote on health-care freedom, giving families the right—promised by President Obama and his Democratic allies—to choose not to participate in Obamacare and to buy the health care of their choice independent of the exchanges, remains the greatest mystery of the 114th Congress" (Gramm 2016). However, Rep. Raul Labrador (R-ID) elicited boos at an April 2017 town hall when he stated, "I just don't think it's a right to have healthcare" (Savransky 2017).

During the 2016 presidential campaign, Republican nominee Donald Trump promised voters that he would immediately repeal and replace the ACA. Following Trump's election, Republicans developed several bills intended to do so; however, Republican efforts to repeal and replace were clouded by uncertainty in terms of what a replacement would entail. Legislative proposals included repealing the individual and employer mandates, deregulating health insurance markets, and allowing states to waive certain federal rules. As Sen. Ron Johnson (R-WI) acknowledged in 2017, "It's way more complex than simply 'repeal and replace.' . . . That's a fun little buzzword, but it's just not accurate" (Sarlin 2017). After Sen. John McCain (R-AZ) cast a dramatic late-night "thumbs-down" vote that proved to be the deciding vote against a Republican "skinny repeal" of portions of the ACA in July 2017, he argued that the bill "offered no replacement to actually reform our health care system and deliver affordable, quality health care to our citizens" (Swanson 2017).

Although the Republican party held majority representation in both houses of Congress, Republican legislators were ultimately unable to pass a bill supported by the party's conservative and moderate wings. While members of the party's conservative wing advocated in favor of full repeal, moderates expressed hesitation if no replacement mechanism was in place. In July 2017, Ted Cruz (R-TX), a prominent member of the party's conservative wing, emphasized that one bill would empower Americans to "choose among more affordable plans that are tailored to their individual healthcare needs" (Cruz 2017), reiterating the prioritization of individual liberty over regulatory action.

On the other hand, moderate Republicans opposed a subsequent reform bill after a September 2017 Congressional Budget Office analysis determined that proposed reductions in Medicaid funding and insurance exchange subsidies would increase the number of uninsured Americans (Congressional Budget Office 2017). As Sen. Susan Collins (R-ME) argued, the "negative impact on millions of Americans who are now insured" was the "final piece of the puzzle" in her decision to vote against the Republicans' final ACA repeal effort of 2017 (Detrow 2017).

In December 2017, President Trump signed into law a tax reform and government spending package that included repeal of the individual mandate. Sen. Orrin Hatch (R-UT) applauded the repeal, declaring that responsibility for health care coverage resided with individual consumers, not the federal government: "Repealing the individual mandate tax restores liberty to the nation's health-care system. Once again, the American people will be back in charge of their health care—not Washington bureaucrats" (Hatch 2017).

Even as the Republican-majority Congress attempted on multiple occasions to repeal the ACA, public opinion polls presented a more complicated and evolving picture of Republican voters' positions. In one 2016 Pew poll, 83 percent of registered Republican voters indicated that health care is not the federal government's responsibility (Pew Research Center 2016). By 2017, the same poll indicated that 32 percent of Republicans and Republican-leaning independents agreed that the federal government should be responsible for health care coverage. Support among Republicans for "government-run" health care thus grew from 19 percent to 32 percent between 2016 and 2017, outpacing an 8-point upswing among Democrats (Pew Research Center 2017).

Following the 2018 midterm elections, Democrats regained control of the House of Representatives, which led Republicans to abandon their efforts to repeal the ACA, albeit temporarily. As Senate Majority Leader Mitch McConnell lamented, the

GOP's failure to repeal and replace was "the one disappointment of this Congress from a Republican point of view" (Sonmez 2018). Throughout Trump's first term as president, opinion polls indicated that 70–82 percent of Republicans held an unfavorable view of the ACA (Kaiser Family Foundation 2020a). In turn, one of Trump's recurring 2020 campaign promises—to eliminate the ACA and unveil his own comprehensive health care plan—led him to claim in September 2020 that "we've really become the health-care party—the Republican Party" (Olorunnipa 2020).

Todd M. Olszewski

Further Reading

Abramson, Alana. 2017. "Bernie Sanders Just Proposed Single-Payer Health Care. What's That?" *Time*, September 13. Accessed March 7, 2021. https://time.com/4939320/bernie-sanders-single-payer-medicare-all-health-care/

Beauchamp, Dan E. 1996. *Health Care Reform and the Battle for the Body Politic*. Philadelphia: Temple University Press.

Beauchamp Dan E., and Ronald L. Rouse. 1990. "Universal New York Health Care: A Single-Payer Strategy Linking Cost Control and Universal Access." *New England Journal of Medicine* 323, no. 10 (September 6): 640–644.

Blendon, Robert J., Drew Altman, John Benson, Mollyann Brodie, Tami Buhr, Claudia Deane, and Sasha Buscho. 2008. "Voters and Health Reform in the 2008 Presidential Election." *New England Journal of Medicine* 359 (November 6): 2050–2061.

Blendon, Robert J., Drew Altman, Claudia Deane, John Benson, Mollyann Brodie, and Tami Buhr. 2008. "Health Care in the 2008 Presidential Primaries." *New England Journal of Medicine* 358 (January 24): 414–422.

Bradner, Eric, and Tami Luhby. 2016. "What's behind the Clinton-Sanders Health Care Fight?" CNN, January 14. Accessed September 5, 2018. https://www.cnn.com/2016/01/14/politics/hillary-clinton-bernie-sanders-medicare-for-all/index.html.

Centers for Medicare and Medicaid Services. n.d. "Presidential Speeches and Addresses on Medicare, 1964–1999." Accessed September 5, 2018. https://www.cms.gov/About-CMS/Agency-Information/History/Downloads/CMSPresidentsSpeeches.pdf.

CNN. 2008. "Transcript of Second McCain, Obama Debate." October 7. Accessed September 5, 2018. http://www.cnn.com/2008/POLITICS/10/07/presidential.debate.transcript/.

Cohen, Alan B., David C. Colby, Keith A. Wailoo, and Julian E. Zelizer. 2015. *Medicare and Medicaid at 50: America's Entitlement Programs in the Age of Affordable Care*. New York: Oxford University Press.

Congressional Budget Office. 2017. "Preliminary Analysis of Legislation That Would Replace Subsidies for Health Care with Block Grants." Accessed September 9, 2018. https://www.cbo.gov/system/files/115th-congress-2017-2018/costestimate/53126-health.pdf.

Cosgrove, Jaclyn. 2012. "Gov. Mary Fallin Says No to Medicaid Expansion in Oklahoma." *The Oklahoman*, November 19. Accessed September 5, 2018. https://newsok.com/article/3730224/gov-mary-fallin-says-no-to-medicaid-expansion-in-oklahoma.

Cruz, Ted. 2017. "Sen. Cruz's Consumer Freedom and HSA Provisions Included in Latest Draft of Senate Health Care Bill." July 13. Accessed September 9, 2018. https://www.cruz.senate.gov/?p=press_release&id=3239.

Democratic National Committee. 2018. "Our Platform." Accessed September 5, 2018. https://www.democrats.org/party-platform#healthcare.

Detrow, Scott. 2017. "3 GOP Senators Oppose Graham-Cassidy, Effectively Blocking Health Care Bill." NPR, September 25. Accessed September 9, 2018. https://www.npr.org/2017/09/25/553429714/3-gop-senators-oppose-graham-cassidy-effectively-blocking-health-care-bill.

Fox, Daniel M., and Howard M. Leichter. 1991. "Rationing Care in Oregon: The New Accountability." *Health Affairs* 10, no. 2 (Summer): 7–27.

Gramm, Phil. 2016. "Where Clinton Will Take ObamaCare." *Wall Street Journal*, October 18, 2016. Accessed March 7, 2021. https://www.wsj.com/articles/where-clinton-will-take-obamacare-1476746073.

Hackey, Robert. 2012. *Cries of Crisis: Rethinking the Health Care Debate*. Reno: University of Nevada Press.

Hamby, Peter. 2010. "Romney on Health Vote: Obama 'Betrayed His Oath to the Nation." CNN, March 22. Accessed September 5, 2018. http://politicalticker.blogs.cnn.com/2010/03/22/romney-on-health-vote-obama-betrayed-his-oath-to-the-nation/?fbid=hihd0TEQQJG.

Hatch, Orrin. 2017. "Senator Orrin Hatch: Repealing the Individual Mandate Tax Is the Beginning of the End of the ObamaCare Era." Fox News, December 20. Accessed September 9, 2018. http://www.foxnews.com/opinion/2017/12/20/sen-orrin-hatch-repealing-individual-mandate-tax-is-beginning-end-obamacare-era.html.

Hayes, Christal. 2020. "Debate: Biden Says He'd Create 'Bidencare' if Supreme Court Strikes Down Affordable Care Act." *USA Today*, October 22. Accessed November 2, 2020. https://www.usatoday.com/story/news/politics/elections/2020/10/22/presidential-debate-bidencare-replace-aca-if-supreme-court-strikes-down/3737892001/).

Hoffman, Beatrix. 2012. *Health Care for Some: Rights and Rationing in the United States Since 1930*. Chicago: University of Chicago Press.

Illinois Department of Human Services. 2013. "Governor Quinn Enacts Largest Increase in Health Care Coverage in State History." Accessed September 5, 2018. http://www.dhs.state.il.us/page.aspx?item=66876&newssidebar=27893.

Jacobs, Lawrence, and Theda Skocpol. 2010. *Health Care Reform and American Politics: What Everyone Needs to Know*. New York: Oxford University Press.

Johnson, Ted. 2017. "Trump Tries to Shift Blame to Democrats after GOP's Repeal-and-Replace Bill Is Pulled from Vote." *Variety*, March 24. Accessed September 5, 2018. https://variety.com/2017/biz/news/donald-trump-healthcare-reform-paul-ryan-1202015804/.

Kaiser Family Foundation. 2020a. "Kaiser Health Tracking Poll: The Public's Views on the ACA." Accessed September 5, 2018. https://www.kff.org/interactive/kaiser-health-tracking-poll-the-publics-views-on-the-aca/#?response=Favorable--Unfavorable&aRange=all.

Kaiser Family Foundation. 2020b. "Public Opinion on Single-Payer, National Health Plans, and Expanding Access to Medicare Coverage." Accessed November 1, 2020. https://www.kff.org/slideshow/public-opinion-on-single-payer-national-health-plans-and-expanding-access-to-medicare-coverage/.

Kasich, John. 2013. "2013 State of the State Address. Lima, Ohio." Accessed September 5, 2018. http://www.governor.ohio.gov/Portals/0/2013%20State%20of%20the%20State%20Transcript.pdf.

McDonough, John E. 2015. "The Demise of Vermont's Single-Payer Plan." *New England Journal of Medicine* 372 (April 23): 1584–1585.

Nelson, Robert M., and Theresa Drought. 1992. "Justice and the Moral Responsibility of Rationing Medical Care: The Oregon Experiment." *Journal of Medicine and Philosophy* 17: 97–117.

New York Times. 2009. "Obama's Health Care Speech to Congress." September 9. Accessed September 5, 2018. https://www.nytimes.com/2009/09/10/us/politics/10obama.text.html.

Numbers, Ronald L. 1978. *Almost Persuaded: American Physicians and Compulsory Health Insurance, 1912–1920*. Baltimore, MD: Johns Hopkins University Press.

Numbers, Ronald L. 1997. "The Third Party: Health Insurance in America." In *Sickness and Health in America: Readings in the History of Medicine and Public Health*, edited by Judith Walzer Leavitt and Ronald L. Numbers, 269–283. Madison: University of Wisconsin Press.

Office of Hillary Rodham Clinton. n.d. "Health Care." Accessed September 5, 2018. https://www.hillaryclinton.com/issues/health-care/.

Olorunnipa, Toluse. 2020. "After Years of Promising His Own Health Care Plan, Trump Settles for Rebranding Rather Than Repealing Obamacare." *Washington Post*, September 24. Accessed November 2, 2020. https://www.washingtonpost.com/politics/trump-health-care-affordable-care-act/2020/09/24/e1cd928a-fe6b-11ea-9ceb-061d646d9c67_story.html.

Pew Research Center. 2016. "Section 3_7. Parties Split on Government's Role in Providing Health Care Coverage." March 31. Accessed September 5, 2018. http://www.people-press.org/2016/03/31/3-views-on-economy-government-services-trade/section-3_7/.

Pew Research Center. 2017. "More Americans Say Government Should Ensure Health Care Coverage." January 13. Accessed September 5, 2018. http://www.pewresearch.org/fact-tank/2017/01/13/more-americans-say-government-should-ensure-health-care-coverage/ft_17-01-13_healthcoverage_govtrole/.

Quadagno, Jill. 2005. *One Nation, Uninsured: Why the U.S. Has No Health Insurance*. New York: Oxford University Press.

Republican National Committee. 2016. "Republican Platform. Great American Families, Education, Healthcare, and Criminal Justice." Accessed September 5, 2018. https://gop.com/platform/renewing-american-values/.

Romney, Mitt. 2007. "Where HillaryCare Goes Wrong." *Wall Street Journal*, September 20, 2007. Accessed March 7, 2021. https://www.wsj.com/articles/SB119025374664933444.

Romney, Mitt. 2011. "If I Were President: Obamacare One Year In." *National Review*, March 23. Accessed September 5, 2018. https://www.nationalreview.com/corner/if-i-were-president-obamacare-one-year-mitt-romney/.

Roy, Avik. 2012. "The Tortuous History of Conservatives and the Individual Mandate." *Forbes*, February 7. Accessed September 5, 2018. https://www.forbes.com/sites/theapothecary/2012/02/07/the-tortuous-conservative-history-of-the-individual-mandate/#2d03c1455fe9.

Sarlin, Benjy. 2017. "What Is 'Repeal and Replace?' A Guide to Trump's Health Care Buzzwords." NBC News, January 28. Accessed November 1, 2020. https://www.nbcnews.com/news/us-news/what-repeal-replace-guide-trump-s-health-care-buzzwords-n713366.

Savransky, Rebecca. 2017. "GOP Rep Booed at Town Hall for Saying Healthcare Isn't a 'Basic Human Right.'" The Hill, April 20. Accessed September 5, 2018. http://thehill.com/homenews/house/329656-gop-rep-booed-at-town-hall-for-saying-healthcare-isnt-a-basic-right.

Shumlin, Peter. 2011. "The Economic Urgency of Health Care Reform." *Huffington Post*, October 5. Accessed September 5, 2018. https://www.huffingtonpost.com/gov-peter-shumlin/health-care-reform-shumlin_b_919900.html.

Snell, Kelsey, and Susan Davis. 2017. "McConnell Ready to 'Move On' from Obamacare Repeal, Others in GOP Say Not So Fast." NPR, December 21. Accessed September 8, 2018. https://www.npr.org/2017/12/21/572588692/mcconnell-wants-bipartisanship-in-2018-on-entitlements-immigration-and-more.

Sonmez, Felicia. 2018. "McConnell: GOP May Take Another Shot at Repealing Obamacare after the Midterms." *Washington Post*, October 17. Accessed November 1, 2020. https://www.washingtonpost.com/politics/mcconnell-gop-may-take-another-shot-at-repealing-obamacare-after-the-midterms/2018/10/17/7a0e7c70-d23c-11e8-8c22-fa2ef74bd6d6_story.html.

St. Onge, Jeffrey. 2017. "Operation Coffeecup: Ronald Reagan, Rugged Individualism, and the Debate over 'Socialized Medicine'." *Rhetoric & Public Affairs* 20, no. 2 (Summer): 223–251.

Starr, Paul. 1982. *The Social Transformation of American Medicine: The Rise of a Sovereign Profession and the Making of a Vast Industry*. New York: Basic Books.

Starr, Paul. 2011a. "The Mandate Miscalculation." *New Republic*, December 14. Accessed September 5, 2018. https://newrepublic.com/article/98554/individual-mandate-affordable-care-act.

Starr, Paul. 2011b. *Remedy and Reaction: The Peculiar American Struggle over Health Reform*. New Haven, CT: Yale University Press.

Stolberg, Sheryl Gay, and Robert Pear. 2010. "Obama Signs Health Care Overhaul Bill, with a Flourish." *New York Times*, March 23. Accessed November 1, 2020. https://www.nytimes.com/2010/03/24/health/policy/24health.html.

Sullivan, Peter. 2020. "Trump, Biden Clash over Health Care as Debate Begins." The Hill, September 29. Accessed November 2, 2020. https://thehill.com/policy/healthcare/518863-trump-biden-clash-over-lawsuit-against-obamacare-as-debate-begins.

Swanson, Kelly. 2017. "McCain Explains His Dramatic Vote against the GOP's Last-Ditch Obamacare Repeal Idea." Vox, July 28. Accessed November 1, 2020. https://www.vox.com/policy-and-politics/2017/7/28/16058488/mccain-skinny-repeal-vote-no-explain-statement.

Wallack, Anya Rader. 2011. "Single-Payer Ahead—Cost Control and the Evolving Vermont Model." *New England Journal of Medicine* 365, no. 7 (August 18): 584–585.

Young, Stephen. 2016. "Texas Facing Medicaid Crunch." *Dallas Observer*, April 11. Accessed September 5, 2018. https://www.dallasobserver.com/news/texas-facing-medicaid-crunch-8198895.

Health Insurance Marketplaces

At a Glance

Before the passage of the Affordable Care Act (ACA) in 2010, individuals who did not purchase health insurance through an employer faced numerous challenges. Insurers typically required prospective subscribers to provide detailed information about their medical history as part of a comprehensive underwriting process. In this "experience-rated" system, individuals deemed to be poor risks—such as persons with chronic or expensive medical conditions or a family history of illness—paid much higher premiums for coverage, if they were able to obtain coverage at all. As a result, patients in the individual health insurance market typically paid higher premiums for less comprehensive coverage. Beginning in 2013, the ACA—also known as Obamacare—reformed the insurance market by limiting the ability of insurers to use individuals' health status to set premiums. The law also established new publicly funded institutions known as health insurance marketplaces that enabled consumers to choose among competing health plans.

Despite a difficult rollout in 2013, Democrats view the marketplaces as a policy success that enabled millions of Americans to obtain affordable individual health insurance plans. Democrats point to the steady growth of enrollment and the number of participating insurers during the Obama administration as evidence that the new marketplaces work well. In addition, since most new enrollees qualified for subsidies (e.g., advanced premium tax credits, or APTCs) based on their family income, the marketplaces made insurance more affordable for most subscribers. Plans sold on the marketplaces could not exclude preexisting conditions from coverage and could no longer establish lifetime caps on benefits. Democrats acknowledge that the marketplaces continue to face challenges, but they argue that the expansion of coverage was a historic policy achievement. For Democrats, the marketplaces remain fundamentally sound.

Democrats have also decried what they see as the Trump administration's efforts to destabilize the marketplaces since 2017. Democrats defined the 2020 presidential election as a pivotal moment for the ACA. As the party's presidential nominee, former Vice President Joe Biden, declared in the first presidential debate, "What's at stake here is, the President's made it clear, he wants to get rid of the Affordable Care Act. He's been running on that. He ran on that and he's been governing on that. He's in the Supreme Court right now trying to get rid of the Affordable Care Act, which will strip 20 million people from having insurance" (*USA Today* 2020).

Republicans tell a very different story. They describe the rollout of the marketplaces in 2013 as an unmitigated disaster characterized by a dysfunctional website (healthcare.gov), long waits, and the disruption of prior coverage. The marketplaces also enrolled far fewer subscribers than expected. Republicans argued that the standardized plans (with more generous benefits) made insurance more expensive for many younger, healthier customers who were less likely to purchase coverage. Insurers also struggled to estimate the risk (and hence cost) of new enrollees in the first two years the marketplaces were operating. Because the marketplaces attracted fewer young and healthy subscribers, the insurance risk pool was skewed toward older, sicker, and more expensive subscribers. Several major insurers lost hundreds of millions of dollars in the first two years. To recoup their losses, many insurers raised premiums by double digits or exited some state marketplaces altogether. Republicans thus advocated for the repeal of the ACA and its replacement by more market-oriented reforms. As President Donald Trump declared in September 2020, the ACA "was terrible and very, very expensive. Hurt a lot of people. Premiums were too high. Deductibles were a disaster" (Trump 2020). The Trump administration supported efforts to repeal and replace the ACA in 2017 and, later, endorsed challenges to the law in court.

In November 2020, a fresh legal challenge to the ACA raised new doubts about the future of the health insurance marketplaces, as the U.S. Supreme Court considered arguments in the case of *California v. Texas* (formerly *Texas v. United States* in the lower courts). The Trump administration declined to defend the constitutionality of the ACA after the passage of the Tax Cuts and Jobs Act of 2017 reset the individual mandate penalty to zero. The initial ruling by the district court in Texas declared that without this penalty, the ACA no longer passed constitutional muster, for in 2012, the Supreme Court had upheld the ACA's individual mandate as a tax on those who chose not to purchase minimum essential coverage. After the Fifth Circuit Court of Appeals upheld the lower court ruling in December 2019, the Supreme Court agreed to hear the latest challenge to the ACA during its 2020–2021 term. The Trump administration argued that nearly all of the ACA should be found invalid (Kaiser Family Foundation 2020c). Democrats made the future of the ACA—and by extension the health insurance marketplaces—a central theme of Joe Biden's 2020 presidential campaign. Democrats warned that millions of Americans would lose health coverage if the Supreme Court overturned the ACA.

According to Many Democrats . . .

- The implementation of the health insurance marketplaces was challenging but ultimately successful.
- The health insurance marketplaces have remained stable despite the departure of some insurers in recent years.
- The ACA marketplaces improved access to affordable health insurance plans.
- Marketplace enrollment remains strong despite continued political opposition at both the federal and state levels.

According to Many Republicans . . .

- The initial rollout of the health marketplaces was a disaster that underscored government's inability to design and manage health care reform.
- Obamacare is collapsing, as health insurance markets face a "death spiral."
- Premiums are skyrocketing; choice is evaporating in health insurance marketplaces.
- Enrollment in ACA marketplaces continues to fall far short of expectations, and far fewer young, healthy customers opted to purchase coverage, resulting in higher costs and ongoing losses for participating insurers.

Overview

The individual health insurance marketplaces created by the Affordable Care Act (ACA) continue to be one of the most contested areas of the 2010 health care reform law. Supporters described the new institutions as "nothing more sinister than an eBay for insurance" (Gawande 2013, 26). Opponents argued that "after four years of ObamaCare, hardworking Americans continue to see their health care costs rise while their coverage choices diminish" (McCain and Barrasso 2015). "Rightly or wrongly, the experience with individual marketplaces has become an acid test for the success or failure of the ACA as a whole" (Blumenthal and Collins 2014, 276). Since 2013, opponents and supporters of the ACA have sparred over their success in enrolling new customers, controlling the cost of premiums, and their impact on patient choice.

The concept of publicly sponsored health insurance marketplaces (also known as exchanges) first emerged in the late 1970s. Alain Enthoven, a health economist at Stanford University, proposed a "consumer choice health plan" in 1978 (Enthoven 1978). Enthoven argued that regulated competition among health insurance plans would reduce health care costs. By the late 1980s, his ideas shaped various proposals for "managed competition." Under managed competition, individuals would purchase affordable coverage through a "public sponsor" that enabled consumers to compare prices and coverage among health plans.

Managed competition also shaped the work of the Jackson Hole group in the early 1990s. This influential group of public and private opinion leaders proposed to use "health insurance purchasing cooperatives" (HIPCs) to purchase health insurance on behalf of small employers and individuals in a defined geographic area (Enthoven 1993). This plan was widely debated during the 1992 presidential campaign; a modified version became a cornerstone of the Clinton administration's proposed Health Security Act, which relied on regional "health alliances" to encourage competition among insurers. The regional alliances "would disseminate information about plans and run the open enrollment" and also make risk-adjusted payments to insurers (Starr 1994).

Reformers hoped that publicly sponsored health insurance marketplaces would have bipartisan appeal. Republicans applauded the virtues of free market competition among private health plans. Democrats hailed new regulations to standardize insurance products and educate consumers. Reformers on both sides of the aisle saw regulated competition among private insurers as a way to bridge the partisan divide over health care reform. Massachusetts incorporated a health insurance exchange into its landmark health reform bill in 2006, as Gov. Mitt Romney—a conservative Republican—worked with liberal Democratic legislators to enact comprehensive reform. The state's new exchange, the Massachusetts Health Connector, offered one-stop shopping for consumers to compare health insurance plans and sign up for coverage. Conservative scholars compared the state's approach to a CarMax auto dealership, where consumers had "many different kinds of cars to choose from, all obtainable though one giant dealership" (Haislmaier 2006). After 2006, Massachusetts emerged as a model for the nation, as the uninsured rate in the state fell from 10.4 percent in 2006 to 4.4 percent in 2009 (Brandon and Carnes 2014).

Health insurance marketplaces emerged as one of the ACA's principal strategies to expand coverage to low- and moderate-income Americans. Former Senate Majority Leader Bill Frist (R-TN) described the marketplaces as "perhaps the most innovative, market-driven, and ultimately constructive part of the law." For Frist, "helping more Americans find and compare the private insurance they need and can afford should be an easy principle both political parties can agree on" (Frist 2012). However, Frist's endorsement did not reflect the view of most Republican governors and members of Congress. Drawing on the experience in Massachusetts, where a similar plan gained bipartisan support, Democrats hoped that the ACA's marketplaces—which were designed to foster competition among private health insurance plans for subscribers—would win over moderate Republicans. During the contentious negotiations over the ACA in 2009–2010, Democrats offered numerous concessions to attract support from Republicans. The buy-in from Republicans in Congress, however, never materialized (Brill 2015). Most Republicans portrayed the new marketplaces created by the ACA as a "government takeover" of the health care system. On the eve of the first open enrollment period, Senate Minority Leader Mitch McConnell (R-KY) condemned the bill as a "monstrosity" and "the single worst piece of legislation passed in the last fifty years" (Gawande 2013, 25).

The Obama administration initially assumed that most (if not all) states would establish their own marketplaces with full funding by the federal government. Fewer than 20 states opted to do so. The remaining states (including nearly all states led by Republican governors) chose to use the federal government's Healthcare.gov website. Regardless of which approach states adopted, marketplaces offered consumers a choice of different health plans organized by "metal" level: bronze plans offered the least coverage and lowest premiums, while silver, gold, and platinum offerings offered enhanced coverage, albeit at a greater cost.

The implementation of the new marketplaces in October 2013 was deeply troubled. The federal government's website (Healthcare.gov) was largely inoperable, leading to extended wait times for millions of frustrated consumers. Enrollment trickled in, even as millions of consumers attempted to shop for coverage. The "troubled launch of the individual marketplaces created an irresistible narrative of government incompetence and seemed to confirm opponents' predictions of the law's failure" (Blumenthal and Collins 2014, 276). A CBS News poll conducted in October 2013 found that only 12 percent of Americans thought the sign-up process through the new marketplaces was "going well" (Dutton et al. 2013). At a news conference in November 2013, President Barack Obama apologized to the nation: "We fumbled the roll-out on this health care law" (Page 2013, 1A).

In response to these early struggles, the Obama administration assembled a team of programmers from tech companies such as Google and Oracle to tackle the website's woes (Brill 2015). With seasoned programmers and tech executives tasked with addressing the technical glitches that plagued Healthcare.gov, the pace of enrollment had picked up by year's end. The first open enrollment period ended with roughly eight million Americans having signed up for a marketplace plan.

After surviving technical obstacles during its first year of implementation, the health insurance marketplaces faced a new legal threat in 2014. The case of *King v. Burwell* challenged the constitutionality of subsidies for individuals who purchased health insurance through the marketplaces. The language of the ACA stated that individuals could qualify for advanced premium tax credits if they enrolled in a health plan "through an exchange established by the State." Because most states did not establish their own exchanges, the case threatened to end subsidies for any individuals purchasing coverage through the federal marketplace. In a 6–3 decision handed down in June 2015, the Supreme Court declared, "Congress passed the Affordable Care Act to improve health insurance markets, not to destroy them. If at all possible, we must interpret the Act in a way that is consistent with the former, and avoids the latter" (*King v. Burwell* 2015, 21). Once again, the marketplaces survived.

More than seven million Americans qualified for cost-sharing reductions in 2016 (Gabel et al. 2016). The ACA provided that the Department of Health and Human

Services "shall make periodic and timely payments to the issuer equal to the value of the reductions" that insurers provided low-income enrollees. In the case of *House v. Burwell*, the House of Representatives mounted yet another legal challenge to the ACA, suing the Obama administration to challenge the cost-sharing reductions (CSRs) paid to insurers. The Obama administration asked for the case to be dismissed for lack of jurisdiction, but a federal judge allowed the case to proceed (Jost 2016). The House argued that it did not explicitly appropriate funding for the cost-sharing reductions and that the Constitution prohibits the expenditure of public funds without an explicit appropriation. In late 2017, President Trump chose to stop CSR payments, "throwing a bomb into the insurance marketplaces created under the Affordable Care Act" (Goldstein and Eilperin 2017). "Insurers have said that stopping the cost-sharing payments would be the single greatest step the Trump administration could take to damage the marketplaces—and the law" (Goldstein and Eilperin 2017). The Trump administration's decision to suspend CSR payments spurred more than 20 lawsuits by insurers. In August 2020, the federal Circuit Court of Appeals ruled that insurers were entitled to reimbursement for 2017 but did not require the federal government to resume CSR payments without congressional appropriations (Jost 2020).

In addition, the suspension of the ACA's "risk corridor" program also contributed to growing instability in individual health insurance markets. The ACA promised to reimburse insurers who enrolled sicker-than-expected subscribers to address the uncertainty inherent in the risk pool (Luthi 2020). After Republicans regained control of Congress in 2014, these supplemental payments to insurers who lost money selling marketplace plans were not extended. The suspension of risk corridor payments led some insurers to withdraw from the marketplaces, while a majority of newly formed "co-op" insurers went out of business after premiums failed to cover the cost of claims for sicker-than-expected subscribers. The federal government's decision to end the risk corridor program prompted several insurers to sue, alleging that the government had breached its promise to compensate participating plans for the risks of selling in the new marketplaces. In April 2020, insurers won a major victory, as the U.S. Supreme Court upheld their challenge in the case of *Maine Community Health Options v. United States*. As Justice Sonia Sotomayor argued in her majority opinion, "The Government should honor its obligations" (Luthi 2020). The Supreme Court's 8–1 decision paved the way for insurers to claim more than $12 billion in deferred risk corridor payments.

By 2016, the ACA health insurance marketplaces were in turmoil. Several of the nation's largest insurers—Aetna, Anthem, Humana, and United Health Group—reported mounting losses on marketplace plans. Insurers warned that mounting losses were unsustainable. Only 30 percent of insurers earned a profit selling policies on the individual health insurance market in 2014; insurers lost more than $2.7 billion, even after federal risk adjustment payments (McKinsey Center for U.S. Health System Reform 2016). Because the new marketplaces attracted sicker-than-average patients who used more health care services, insurers found it difficult to earn a profit without charging more for coverage (Sanger-Katz 2016). A year earlier, Aetna CEO Mark Bertolini noted, "This business model remained unprofitable in 2015, and we continue to have serious concerns about the sustainability of the public exchanges" (Johnson 2016). His counterpart at Anthem, Joseph Swedish, offered an even bleaker assessment, arguing that "the marketplace has been and continues to be unsustainable" (Abelson 2016). Aetna, Humana, and United HealthCare announced plans to limit their participation in health insurance marketplaces around the nation, and UnitedHealth projected a $650 million annual loss for its marketplace business (Johnson 2016). In early 2017, Bertolini concluded that the Obamacare marketplaces were in a "death spiral" and argued that "it's not going to get any better; it's getting worse" (Demko 2017).

From 2016 to 2018, competition on the health insurance marketplaces declined, as many insurers withdrew from the marketplaces altogether. During the initial 2014 open enrollment period, each state had an average of 5 insurers offering marketplace plans. The average number of insurers in each state peaked at 6 in 2015 before falling to 3.5 in 2018 (Kaiser Family Foundation 2019b). Reduced competition meant fewer choices and higher premiums for consumers. Average premiums for marketplace plans increased from $299 per month in 2016 to $481 per month in 2018, before dropping slightly to $477 in 2019 (Kaiser Family Foundation 2019a). Rising premiums, in turn, raised new concerns that unsubsidized consumers would drop out of the individual market altogether. During the 2018–2019 open enrollment period, five states had only one participating insurer. By 2018, nearly one in four marketplace enrollees reported that only one insurer was selling plans in their area, and more than half of all Americans (53 percent) believed the marketplaces were "collapsing" (Kirzinger et al. 2018).

Since then, public opinion of the ACA, which remains part of the health care insurance landscape, continued to be sharply divided. During the botched rollout of the health insurance marketplaces in October 2013, only one-third of the public (34 percent) approved of the law. However, public support for the ACA improved over time. On the eve of the 2016 presidential election, 45 percent of the Americans held a "generally favorable" view of the ACA, and an equal number (45 percent) harbored a "generally unfavorable" view of the law (Kirzinger, Sugarman, and Brodie 2016). Although public opinion remains split on the ACA itself—with only 46 percent expressing a "generally favorable" view of the law in 2018—a majority of the public holds favorable views of the health insurance marketplaces. More than 80 percent of Americans expressed support for the marketplaces, including 91 percent of Democrats and 71 percent of Republicans (Kirzinger, Muñana, and Brodie 2019). In September 2020, the Kaiser Family Foundation's monthly health tracking poll found that a plurality of Americans (49 percent) held a "generally favorable" view of the ACA, while 42 percent viewed the law unfavorably (Kaiser Family Foundation 2020a). Republicans and Democrats continued to hold polar opposite views of the law, as 82 percent of Democrats had a favorable view of the ACA, while 79 percent of Republicans held an unfavorable view (Kaiser Family Foundation 2020a). More than a decade after its passage, the ACA remained a litmus test for both parties. Despite Republicans' pledge to repeal and replace the ACA, neither the Trump administration nor congressional Republicans advanced a concrete health care reform agenda after their effort to undo the ACA fizzled out in 2017.

The election of President Donald Trump in 2016 marked a fundamental shift in the federal government's support for the health insurance marketplaces. During the 2016 election campaign, Trump pledged to "repeal and replace" Obamacare if elected. After his election, President Trump lent his support to several bills to do just that. In addition, both the president and Tom Price, his secretary of Health and Human Services, mounted a verbal assault on the marketplaces, which they described as "collapsing" or "imploding" in the months leading up to the open enrollment period in 2017. The administration also hampered marketplace enrollment by reducing spending on advertising, supporting a repeal of the individual mandate, and ending cost-sharing reduction payments to insurers (Levitt 2017).

Several other policy actions embraced by the Trump administration—from supporting the repeal of the individual mandate, to ending cost-sharing reduction payments to insurers, to allowing the sale of short-term health plans and steep cutbacks in funding for consumer education and outreach programs—also tended to destabilize the marketplaces. On the other hand, the Trump administration approved several state innovation waiver proposals to create "reinsurance" programs to insulate insurers from unexpected losses from new subscribers (Blumenthal et al. 2018). As another ACA open enrollment period drew near in the fall of 2020, the health insurance marketplaces remained stable, yet vulnerable to future policy disruption.

After overcoming a variety of technical and legal challenges, media attention—and Republican critiques of the marketplaces—shifted to enrollment, which fell far short of initial projections. Critics charged the marketplaces were underperforming. Total marketplace enrollment increased from 8 million in 2014 to a peak of 12.7 million in 2016 (Kaiser Family Foundation 2020b. In recent years, however, enrollment declined amid growing concerns about the future of the ACA and the Trump administration's decisions to reduce marketing and outreach funding. In fact, the number of subscribers fell far short of initial estimates by government agencies and think tanks (Glied, Arora, and Solís-Román 2015). The Congressional Budget Office (CBO) estimated that 25 million Americans would purchase a marketplace plan in 2017 (Congressional Budget Office 2014). Total marketplace enrollment in 2017 was less than half of what was projected (Centers for Medicare and Medicaid Services 2018). Enrollment declined to 12.2 million during the 2017 open enrollment period and fell again—to 11.8 million—in 2018. By the 2020 open enrollment period, marketplace enrollment had fallen to

11.4 million, a decline of roughly 300,000 from the previous year (Kaiser Family Foundation 2020b.

Notably, enrollment among individuals who did not qualify for advanced premium tax credits (APTCs) fell precipitously. As the Centers for Medicare and Medicaid Services (CMS) noted, "Unsubsidized enrollment declined by 2.5 million people, representing a 40 percent drop nationally" (Centers for Medicare and Medicaid Services 2019). While some states, such as Rhode Island, saw little erosion in enrollment, unsubsidized enrollment fell by more than 70 percent between 2017 and 2018 in Arizona, Georgia, Iowa, Nebraska, Oklahoma, and Tennessee (*Wall Street Journal* 2019). The marketplaces also struggled to attract younger (and therefore healthier) subscribers. The result was a classic "adverse selection" problem for insurers; because older and sicker customers were more likely to sign up for coverage, the health care costs for new enrollees rose faster than expected. Notably, more enrollees were over the age of 55 than between the ages of 18 and 34 (Centers for Medicare and Medicaid Services 2018). Before 2017, "the marketplaces were fragile in some places. The political and policy uncertainty has made them fragile everywhere" (Armour, Mathews, and Radnofsky 2017).

Nevertheless, the health insurance marketplaces have stabilized in recent years. Premiums in the individual marketplace actually declined by 2 percent in 2019—the first decline in five years—while the number of insurers participating in the marketplace increased (Verma 2018). On the eve of the 2020 open enrollment period, the individual insurance market was more competitive—and more profitable—for insurers. Oscar Insurance Corp., for example, expanded its marketplace presence to six additional states for the 2020 enrollment period; after years of turmoil and uncertainty, Oscar's CEO, Mario Schlosser, declared that "the market is now clearly stabilizing" (Mathews 2019). Premiums for the benchmark silver plan fell 4 percent in 2020, following a 1.5 percent decline in 2019, while the number of insurers selling plans on Healthcare.gov increased to 175, compared to 132 in 2018 (Armour 2019b). The number of participating insurers on health insurance marketplaces increased from an average of 4.0 in 2019 to 4.5 in 2020. Furthermore, during the 2020 open enrollment period, only 10 percent of all marketplace enrollees had only one marketplace insurer (Fehr, Kamal, and Cox 2020).

Legal challenges continue to pose an existential threat to the health insurance marketplaces and, more broadly, to the ACA itself. In 2018, 20 states, led by the state of Texas, filed a new lawsuit; the plaintiffs argued that by eliminating the tax penalty for failing to purchase health insurance, the passage of the Tax Cuts and Jobs Act of 2017 (Pub. L. 115-97) undercut the legal foundation of the ACA itself (Musumeci 2020). The Trump administration declined to defend the ACA in court, prompting a number of Democratic states to join the litigation as "intervenor defendants" in an effort to save the law. In the case of *Texas v. United States* (2018), Judge Reed O'Connor—a conservative federal district court judge in

Texas—argued that by repealing the penalty, Congress "sawed off the last leg [the ACA] stood on." Without a tax penalty, which yields revenue for the government, O'Connor declared "the Individual Mandate is no longer fairly readable as an exercise of Congress' tax power and continues to be unsustainable under Congress' Interstate Commerce Power. The Court therefore finds the individual mandate, unmoored from a tax, is unconstitutional" (O'Connor 2018).

In December 2019, the U.S. Court of Appeals for the Fifth Circuit upheld O'Connor's ruling but sent the case back to the lower court for further review. The U.S. Supreme Court agreed to hear the case during its 2020–2021 term, but oral arguments were scheduled for November 10, 2020—after the presidential election—with a final decision in the case expected by June 2021. If the Supreme Court upholds lower court rulings and strikes down the ACA in its entirety, the legal foundation for health insurance marketplaces would crumble, and the individual insurance market would return to its pre-2010 condition. All of the ACA's insurance market regulations—such as bans on preexisting conditions, lifetime coverage limits, and subsidies to purchase insurance—would end, as would federal support for health insurance marketplaces. A decade after its passage, the fate of the ACA and the health insurance marketplaces hung in the balance once again.

Democrats on Health Insurance Marketplaces

Democrats view the implementation of the health insurance marketplaces as challenging, but ultimately successful. For supporters, the implementation of the ACA represented a triumph over adversity. Initially, Democrats downplayed the technical problems that bedeviled the launch of the marketplaces in October 2013. As Health and Human Services (HHS) Secretary Kathleen Sebelius noted, "When the Health Insurance Marketplace opened last week, demand was so high, it exceeded even optimists' expectations" (Sebelius 2013a). Although the marketplace was largely inoperable for more than a month after it opened for business in October 2013, the Obama administration sought to reassure the public. President Obama urged patience: "A couple of weeks ago, Apple rolled out a new mobile operating system, and within days, they found a glitch, so they fixed it. I don't remember anybody suggesting Apple should stop selling iPhones or iPads or threatening to shut down the company if they didn't" (Eischen and DelReal 2013).

By early December, a group of "fixers" from Silicon Valley had made substantial progress in addressing the bottlenecks that plagued the enrollment process (Brill 2015). While acknowledging that "these problems are unacceptable," Sebelius reassured consumers that "we've been working 24/7 to make improvements, and more consumers are successfully shopping online and enrolling in a health plan each week" (Sebelius 2013b). President Obama celebrated the results of the first open enrollment period, noting, "There are 7.5 million people across the country that have the security of health insurance, most of them for the first time" (Condon 2014).

Democrats also regard the individual insurance market as stable, despite repeated attempts by Republicans to either repeal the ACA or to limit federal support for the new marketplaces. In 2016, after several large insurers warned that they might pull out of the marketplaces, Obama administration officials expressed "full confidence, based on data, that the Marketplaces will continue to thrive for years ahead. The number of insurers has grown year over year. The Marketplace should be judged by the choices it offers insurers, not the decisions of any one insurer" (Johnson 2016). Democratic voters also expressed confidence in the ACA and supported efforts to improve its performance. For example, 90 percent of Democrats in one poll agreed that it was important for government to "fix the remaining problems with the Affordable Care Act in order to help the marketplaces work better" (Kirzinger et al. 2017).

The passage of the ACA also marked a signature domestic policy achievement—and political triumph—for the Democratic party. Since the 1940s, when Harry

The Undeniable Success of the ACA

On March 25, 2016—the sixth anniversary of the Affordable Care Act's passage—Rep. Nancy Pelosi (D-CA) highlighted the law's impact on the uninsured in the United States. Pelosi, who served as Speaker of the House when the ACA was enacted, painted a bright picture of the law's implementation, drawing upon the experience of Covered California, her state's ACA marketplace.

> This week marked six years since the day President Obama signed the Affordable Care Act into law, taking a giant step toward fulfilling the generations-long struggle to make health care a right, not a privilege, for all Americans. . . . These amazing successes can be seen in California, where Covered California, our state's health insurance marketplace, is establishing a bright and healthy future for the Golden State—the uninsured rate in 2015 was down 10 percent from just two years prior, and more than 4 million Californians have gained Medicaid or CHIP coverage since the first open enrollment period.
>
> Recently I met Anita Hiley, whose story is an incredible example of these benefits. Anita was diagnosed with stage-four uterine cancer, which had metastasized throughout her body. Knowing she needed the best care possible, Anita turned to Covered California. Since it was no longer possible for Anita to be denied coverage due to a pre-existing condition, she was able to obtain health insurance and the lifesaving cancer treatment she desperately needed. As we celebrate the sixth anniversary of the Affordable Care Act, Democrats take pride in its monumental success for the American people, and we recommit ourselves to the historic legislation's great legacy—ensuring that health care will remain a right, not a privilege, for all Americans.

Source

Pelosi, Nancy. 2016. "Six Years Later." March 25, 2016. Accessed August 31, 2018. https://pelosi.house.gov/news/pelosi-updates/six-years-later.

Truman became the first president to publicly endorse a national health insurance plan, successive administrations had tried—and failed—to expand coverage to all Americans. Although the ACA's marketplaces did not guarantee universal coverage, they significantly improved access to affordable health insurance plans for the self-employed, early retirees, and others who did not qualify for employer-sponsored coverage. Peter Lee, the director of Covered California, celebrated the performance of his state's health insurance marketplace: "We are proving that health insurance exchanges can keep prices in check. Residents who enroll through Covered California, our statewide exchange, will see only modest 4 percent increases in 2016. Those selecting the lowest-priced plans actually will save 4.5 percent" (Lee and Robinson 2015). The result, Lee argued, was better choice at a lower cost. "Covered California standardizes the deductibles and other characteristics of plans offered. That empowers consumers, who can make apples-to-apples comparisons" (Lee and Robinson 2015). As Hillary Clinton noted on the eve of the 2016 presidential election, "By securing new coverage for millions of previously uninsured people and providing peace of mind, the Affordable Care Act is an essential step toward universal health care" (Clinton 2016).

During the 2020 presidential campaign, however, Democratic views of the ACA diverged. Sen. Bernie Sanders (D-VT) and other progressives argued that the time had come to move past the ACA toward a single-payer, Medicare for All model that provided public insurance for all Americans. Other candidates, such as former Vice President Joe Biden, sought to improve, not replace, the ACA. As Biden, who eventually won his party's presidential nomination, declared in July 2019, "We should not be scrapping Obamacare, we should be building on it" (Barrow 2019). During the October 2020 vice presidential debate, Sen. Kamala Harris (D-CA) touted Biden's support for the ACA, noting that his support "brought health care to over 20 million Americans and protected people with pre-existing conditions and what it also did is it saved those families, who otherwise were going bankrupt because of hospital bills they could not afford" (Page 2020). Democratic senators used the confirmation hearings for Amy Coney Barrett—President Donald Trump's nominee for the U.S. Supreme Court—to highlight the importance of defending the ACA. As Sen. Dianne Feinstein (D-CA) argued, "Health care coverage for millions of Americans is at stake. The president has promised to appoint justices who will vote to dismantle that law. The bottom line is this: there have been 70 attempts to repeal the ACA, but clearly the effort to dismantle the law continues" (Henney 2020). Sen. Dick Durbin (D-IL) echoed these concerns, noting that "Republicans in Congress have been obsessed with repealing Obamacare for years, but they don't have the votes to do it. They've got to rely on the court to do their work" (Henney 2020).

Democrats point out that enrollment in marketplace plans remains strong despite continued political opposition to the ACA from Republicans at both the federal and state levels. Obama administration officials focused on the number of

Americans visiting the online marketplace and selecting marketplace plans during the first three open enrollment periods. Democrats dismissed concerns that enrollment lagged behind early projections, choosing instead to focus on year-over-year growth. As the Centers for Medicare and Medicaid Services (CMS) noted in 2016, "With millions of Americans insured through the Health Insurance Marketplaces, it's clear that Marketplace coverage is a product that consumers want and need as well as an important business for insurers" (Centers for Medicare and Medicaid Services 2016). In December 2017, Lori Lodes from Get America Covered—a pro-ACA advocacy organization—defended the ACA, despite a modest decline in sign-ups during the first year of the Trump administration: "We've defied expectations when it comes to enrolling new customers. People want health care coverage" (Armour 2017).

Meanwhile, Biden made Obamacare a central element of his successful campaign for his party's 2020 presidential nomination. "I think one of the most significant things we've done in our administration is pass the Affordable Care Act," he declared in July 2019. "I don't know why we'd get rid of what in fact was working and move to something totally new" (Barrow 2019). That same month, a tracking poll conducted by the Kaiser Family Foundation found that a majority of Democrats agreed with Biden; 55 percent of Democrats and Democratic-leaning independents favored "building on the existing ACA," and 39 percent favored "replacing the ACA with a national Medicare-for-All plan" (Kaiser Family Foundation 2019c).

Republicans on Health Insurance Marketplaces

Republican legislators and governors presented a united front of opposition to the implementation of the ACA's health insurance marketplaces. Most Republican-led states decided not to establish their own health insurance marketplaces and instead ceded responsibility to the federal government. Several of the nation's largest states led by Republican governors, including Florida and Texas, refused to accept federal funds to plan and implement the new marketplaces. As Gov. Rick Perry of Texas announced in 2012, "I stand proudly with the growing chorus of governors who reject the Obamacare power grab." He added, "We in Texas have no intention to implement so-called state exchanges or to expand Medicaid under Obamacare. . . . I will not be party to socializing healthcare and bankrupting my state in direct contradiction to our Constitution and our founding principles of limited government" (Ramshaw 2012).

Wisconsin's Gov. Scott Walker echoed these concerns in a letter to HHS Secretary Kathleen Sebelius: "No matter which option is chosen, Wisconsin taxpayers will not have meaningful control over the health care policies and services sold to Wisconsin residents" (Fox News 2012). Republican opposition did not diminish over time. In 2017, for example, more than 60 percent of Republicans polled "believed that President Trump and Congressional Republicans should continue their efforts to 'repeal and replace' the ACA" (Kirzinger et al. 2017). After the December 2018 ruling by Judge O'Connor declared the ACA unconstitutional, Rep. Kevin McCarthy (R-CA) declared, "Obamacare is a broken law. Americans have lost their doctors and seen premiums skyrocket. Yesterday's court decision also underscores what we have believed—it is an unconstitutional law" (McCarthy 2018).

Republicans portrayed the implementation of the health insurance marketplaces in 2013 as an unmitigated disaster. For Republicans, the website's problems—and the widespread frustration among consumers and insurers that accompanied the launch of the new program—were not simply technical hurdles to overcome. Instead, the botched rollout underscored the dangers of a government-run health care system. "The catastrophe that is Healthcare.gov and the 36 insurance exchanges run by the federal government is an insult to the 'glitches' President Obama said were inevitable" (*Wall Street Journal* 2013). For Republicans, the website woes offered a cautionary tale about the inability of government to manage

Repealing and Replacing Obamacare

Senate Majority Leader Mitch McConnell (R-KY), a strident critic of the Affordable Care Act, delivered the following remarks in February 2017 in support of the American Health Care Act, a bill that proposed to repeal and replace the Affordable Care Act.

> ObamaCare is a disaster, an absolute disaster. Just one in five Americans say their families are better off since it went into effect. More actually say they are worse off. And, really, is it any wonder?
>
> Americans were promised that costs would go down, but in fact they skyrocketed. Americans were promised choice, but it shriveled. We have been warning that choices would continue their downward decline under the ObamaCare status quo, and that is just what we saw this very week.
>
> One large national insurer announced it was being forced from the marketplace altogether—meaning thousands, including many in Kentucky, will lose their current health plans, thanks to ObamaCare.
>
> The CEO of another major insurer predicted more insurers would soon follow—meaning thousands could find themselves without a single choice of health coverage, thanks to ObamaCare. This partisan law has entered a "death spiral," the CEO warned, and "it is not going to get any better; it's getting worse." This should be a wake-up call to the do-nothing crowd on the left. ObamaCare isn't working. It isn't sustainable, and it is going to continue attacking the middle class until it is repealed and replaced.

Source

Congressional Record, vol. 163, no. 28 (Thursday, February 16, 2017): S1224. Washington, DC: Government Printing Office. Accessed August 31, 2018. https://www.congress.gov/crec/2017/02/16/modified/CREC-2017-02-16-pt1-PgS1224-2.htm.

health care reform. The Obama administration "likened the exchanges to a new Apple product and asked for forbearance as problems were fixed. But Apple doesn't ship products that don't work and then force everyone to buy them" (*Wall Street Journal* 2013).

The technical problems associated with the initial rollout—and the resulting media firestorm—provided Republican legislators with ample ammunition to attack the new marketplaces. As Rep. Fred Upton (R-MI) declared, "Delays and technical failures have reached epidemic proportions." Rep. Darrell Issa (R-CA) was more direct: "Basically, HHS has screwed this whole thing up" (Eischen and DelReal 2013). Senate Minority Leader Mitch McConnell, meanwhile, declared at the conclusion of the first open enrollment period that "Obamacare has been a rolling disaster. . . . [The resignation of Kathleen Sebelius] is cold comfort to the millions of Americans who were deceived about what it would mean for them and their families" (Condon 2014). Republicans pressed for private, not public, solutions that they claimed would increase access to affordable coverage by unleashing competition in the health insurance marketplace and continued to campaign for the repeal of the ACA. Rep. Kevin McCarthy (R-CA) claimed, "House Republicans acted earlier this Congress to establish a healthcare system that puts patients first. This will offer more choice, reduce costs, and put our country's healthcare system on a sustainable path" (McCarthy 2018).

Republicans described the new Obamacare marketplaces as unstable and unworkable. "All across the country," Senate Minority Leader Mitch McConnell declared, "our constituents are having an unpleasant interaction with Obamacare. Whether they can sign up for a policy or not, they are discovering, of course, higher premiums, a higher deductible" (Mason and Felsenthal 2014). In particular, Republicans zeroed in on surging health insurance premiums as evidence that the marketplaces were not working. In 2015, Sen. John McCain (R-AZ) dismissed the Obama administration's claims that increases in health insurance premiums were "modest." As McCain observed, "In Arizona, 24 exchange plans will see double-digit rate hikes in 2016. In Phoenix, premium increases are projected to top 19 percent. The highest average premium increase in my home state is projected to reach a whopping 78 percent. My constituents in Arizona call and write me daily, daily, begging and pleading that something be done to alleviate the financial hardship of Obamacare" (McCain 2015).

In 2017, Sen. Orrin Hatch (R, UT) argued, "Obamacare has not improved over time, and it doesn't work any better now than it did during the first few years of implementation" (Hatch 2017). One year later, CMS Administrator Seema Verma, an appointee of the Trump White House who was a long-standing opponent of the ACA, declared that "while the ACA's vital signs have stabilized, the patient remains in critical condition. Stabilizing already high rates means you still have high rates. Millions of Americans are priced out of the insurance marketplace" (Verma 2018). Indeed, government data confirmed that about 2.5 million Americans who were ineligible for advanced premium tax credits exited the individual insurance marketplace between 2016 and 2018 (Armour 2019b).

Republicans cited rapid growth in premiums (even though most marketplace subscribers qualify for subsidies) and diminished competition among insurers as evidence the ACA marketplaces were in a state of crisis. Republicans point to spiraling premiums as evidence that the ACA marketplaces are unraveling. As Edward Haislmaier, a conservative analyst with the Heritage Foundation, noted, "We're seeing a fish-or-cut-bait moment for insurers. They now have a couple of years of data, and they're seeing that the market is not particularly good for them" (Edwards 2016). Sen. Orrin Hatch also criticized the "unworkable system" created by the ACA: "Premiums and health care costs have skyrocketed year after year. . . Patients have had fewer and fewer options when choosing providers and insurance plans" (Hatch 2017).

From this vantage point, patients' choice of plans is eroding, placing insurance out of reach for individuals who do not qualify for income-based subsidies. Republicans also pointed to lower than expected enrollment as further evidence of marketplace collapse. After marketplace enrollment declined in 2017, Sen. John Barrasso (R-WY) declared, "I think Obamacare itself is sabotaging enrollment because the costs are so high, the choices are so limited that people realize it's not a good deal for them personally." In 2020, Sen. Joni Ernst (R-IA) concurred with this assessment, noting on her website that "President Obama promised health insurance premiums would go down under ObamaCare. They haven't. Across the country, folks have endured significant health insurance premium increases, as well as increases in out of pocket costs like deductibles and copays" (Ernst 2020).

Republicans argue that the current system is simply unsustainable. "The problems have already been there, and they are just getting worse," asserted Verma in 2017. "We can try to put paint on the walls and wallpaper up, but the foundation we're standing on is crumbing" (Armour, Mathews, and Radnofsky 2017). In 2017, House Speaker Paul Ryan (R-WI) offered a similar assessment: "Obamacare is collapsing and failing, so we won't be able to ignore that problem. We're going to have to revisit the problem of a health insurance marketplace that is collapsing" (Armour 2017).

Republicans have displayed little interest in enacting measures to stabilize the marketplaces. While Sens. Lamar Alexander (R-TN) and Patty Murray (D-WA) sought to broker a compromise bill to strengthen the marketplaces, such bipartisan efforts failed to gain traction in either 2017 or 2018. To date, Congress has yet to enact any reforms to stabilize the marketplaces. Democrats and Republicans remain deadlocked. As Alexander noted ruefully, "I know of nothing the Republicans and Democrats can agree on to stabilize the individual insurance market" (Rovner 2018).

Republicans favor private, market-oriented efforts to increase competition and lower prices in the individual insurance market. Sen. Ted Cruz (R-TX) argued,

"Congress should repeal Obamacare and make meaningful reforms to expand Health Savings Accounts, allow individuals to purchase insurance across state lines, and make health care more personal, portable, and affordable" (Cruz 2020). For Republicans, fewer regulations—and a larger role for states—are necessary to address the shortcomings of the individual insurance market. Sen. Joni Ernst (R-IA) asserted that "health care reform should be focused on choice, not mandates. Patients, families, and doctors know what best meets their needs, and they are the ones who should be in control of health care decisions, not Washington, D.C. Instead of this Washington-centered approach, we need to look for patient-centered alternatives that increase access to quality health care services at an affordable price" (Ernst 2020). Sen. Mike Enzi (R-WY) echoed this view: "We must replace the law with common sense reforms that give states flexibility to address their unique health care needs, promote greater competition in the insurance market, and drive down health care costs. I believe access, affordability, and quality result from a competition-oriented, market-based approach to healthcare" (Enzi 2020).

Robert B. Hackey

Further Reading

Abelson, Reed. 2016. "Cost, Not Choice, Is Top Concern of Health Insurance Customers." *New York Times*, August 12. Accessed September 5, 2018. https://www.nytimes.com/2016/08/13/business/cost-not-choice-is-top-concern-of-health-insurance-customers.html.

Armour, Stephanie. 2016. "Young Adult Health Insurance Sign-Ups Disappoint." *Wall Street Journal*, January 7. Accessed May 28, 2020. https://www.wsj.com/articles/young-adult-health-insurance-sign-ups-disappoint-1452213575.

Armour, Stephanie. 2017. "Affordable Care Act Sign-Ups Bump Up, but Still Fewer Expected This Year." *Wall Street Journal*, December 15. Accessed May 28, 2020. https://www.wsj.com/articles/fewer-people-than-last-year-expected-to-sign-up-for-affordable-care-act-1513353076.

Armour, Stephanie. 2019a. "Affordable Care Act Sign-Ups Total 11.4 Million for This Year." *Wall Street Journal*, March 25. Accessed August 26, 2019. https://www.wsj.com/articles/affordable-care-act-sign-ups-total-11-4-million-for-this-year-11553555429.

Armour, Stephanie. 2019b. "Premiums for ACA Health Plans Are Set to Drop in 2020." *Wall Street Journal*, October 22. Accessed May 27, 2020. https://www.wsj.com/articles/premiums-for-aca-health-plans-are-set-to-drop-in-2020-11571749200.

Armour, Stephanie, Anna Wilde Mathews, and Louise Radnofsky. 2017. "Republicans Lock onto Insurance Troubles in Push to Topple Health Law." *Wall Street Journal*, May 18. Accessed May 28, 2020. https://www.wsj.com/articles/republicans-lock-onto-insurance-troubles-in-push-to-topple-health-law-1495121289.

Barrow, Bill. 2019. "Biden Aggressively Defends the Affordable Care Act." *PBS News Hour*, July 15. Accessed August 26, 2019. https://www.pbs.org/newshour/politics/biden-aggressively-defends-the-affordable-care-act.

Blumenthal, David, and Sara Collins. 2014. "Health Care Coverage under the Affordable Care Act—A Progress Report." *New England Journal of Medicine* 371 (July 17): 275–281. Accessed August 26, 2019. https://www.nejm.org/doi/full/10.1056/NEJMhpr1405667.

Blumenthal, David, Sara Collins, Shanoor Seervai, and Herman Buphal. 2018. "States Take the Lead on Reinsurance to Stabilize the ACA Marketplaces." Commonwealth Fund, May 22. Accessed August 26, 2019. https://www.commonwealthfund.org/blog/2018/states-take-lead-reinsurance-stabilize-aca-marketplaces.

Brandon, William P., and Keith Carnes. 2014. "Federal Health Insurance Reform and 'Exchanges': Recent History." *Journal of Health Care for the Poor and Underserved* 25. Accessed May 28, 2020. https://muse.jhu.edu/article/536602.

Brenan, Megan. 2017. "Affordable Care Act Approval Slips after Record Highs." Gallup, November 27. Accessed September 2, 2018. https://news.gallup.com/poll/222734/affordable-care-act-approval-slips-record-highs.aspx.

Brill, Steven. 2015. *America's Bitter Pill: Money, Politics, Backroom Deals, and the Fight to Fix Our Broken Healthcare System*. New York: Random House.

Centers for Medicare and Medicaid Services. 2016. "Strengthening the Marketplace – Actions to Improve the Risk Pool." June 8. Accessed March 1, 2021. https://www.cms.gov/newsroom/fact-sheets/strengthening-marketplace-actions-improve-risk-pool.

Centers for Medicare and Medicaid Services. 2018. "Health Insurance Exchanges 2018 Open Enrollment Period Final Report." April 3. Accessed September 5, 2018. https://www.cms.gov/newsroom/fact-sheets/health-insurance-exchanges-2018-open-enrollment-period-final-report.

Centers for Medicare and Medicaid Services. 2019. "Trends in Subsidized and Unsubsidized Enrollment." August 12. Accessed August 26, 2019. https://www.cms.gov/CCIIO/Resources/Forms-Reports-and-Other-Resources/Downloads/Trends-Subsidized-Unsubsidized-Enrollment-BY17-18.pdf.

Clinton, Hillary. 2016. "My Vision for Universal, Quality, Affordable Health Care." *New England Journal of Medicine* 375 (October 27): e36. Accessed September 4, 2018. https://www.nejm.org/doi/full/10.1056/NEJMsb1612292.

Condon, Stephanie. 2014. "Obama on Kathleen Sebelius: 'The Final Score Speaks for Itself.'" CBS News, April 11. Accessed September 11, 2018. https://www.cbsnews.com/news/obama-on-kathleen-sebelius-the-final-score-speaks-for-itself/.

Congressional Budget Office. 2014. "Updated Estimates of the Effects of the Insurance Coverage Provisions of the Affordable Care Act." Accessed September 3, 2018. https://www.cbo.gov/publication/45231.

Cruz, Ted. 2020. "Healthcare." Accessed May 28, 2020. https://www.cruz.senate.gov/index.cfm?id=34&p=issue&pg=1.

Demko, Paul. 2017. "Aetna CEO: Obamacare Markets Are in a 'Death Spiral.'" Politico, February 15. Accessed September 11, 2018. https://www.politico.com/story/2017/02/obamacare-market-death-spiral-aetna-mark-bertolini-235041.

Desiderio, Andrew. 2017. "Republican Senator to Constituents: Don't Sign Up for Obamacare." *Daily Beast*, October 3. Accessed September 7, 2018. https://www.thedailybeast.com/republican-senator-to-constituents-dont-sign-up-for-obamacare.

Dutton, Sarah, Jennifer De Pinto, Anthony Salvanto, and Fred Backus. 2013. "Poll: Congress, Tea Party Take Hits from Government Shutdown." CBS News, October 22. Accessed September 3, 2018. https://www.cbsnews.com/news/poll-congress-tea-party-take-hits-from-government-shutdown/.

Edwards, Haley. 2016. "Cracks in the Obamacare Crystal Ball." *Time*, August 29: 14.

Eischen, Trevor, and Jose DelReal. 2013. "Obamacare Online Glitches: 25 Great Quotes." Politico, October 15. Accessed February 13, 2021. https://www.politico.com/gallery/2013/10/obamacare-online-glitches-25-great-quotes-175140.

Enthoven, Alain. 1978. "Consumer Choice Health Plan: A National Health Insurance Proposal Based on Regulated Competition in the Private Sector." *New England Journal of Medicine* 298: 709–720.

Enthoven, Alain. 1993. "The History and Principles of Managed Competition." *Health Affairs* (Suppl.): 24–48.

Enzi, Mike. 2020. "Health Care." Accessed May 28, 2020. https://www.enzi.senate.gov/public/index.cfm/healthcare.

Ernst, Joni. 2020. "Health Care." Accessed May 28, 2020. https://www.ernst.senate.gov/public/index.cfm/health-care.

Fehr, Rachel, Rabah Kamal, and Cynthia Cox. 2020. "Insurer Participation on ACA Marketplaces, 2014–2020." Kaiser Family Foundation, November 21. Accessed October 13, 2020. https://www.kff.org/private-insurance/issue-brief/insurer-participation-on-aca-marketplaces-2014-2020/.

Fingerhut, Hannah. 2017. "For the First Time, More Americans Say 2010 Health Care Law Has Had a Positive Than Negative Impact on U.S." Pew Research Center, December 11. Accessed September 5, 2018. http://www.pewresearch.org/fact-tank/2017/12/11/for-the-first-time-more-americans-say-2010-health-care-law-has-had-a-positive-than-negative-impact-on-u-s/.

Fox News. 2012. "Republican Governors Decide against Setting Up Obamacare Insurance Markets." Accessed September 12, 2018. http://www.foxnews.com/politics/2012/11/16/republican-governors-decide-against-setting-up-obamacare-insurance-markets.html.

Frist, Bill. 2012. "Why Both Parties Should Embrace Obamacare's State Exchanges." The Week, July 18. Accessed August 23, 2018. http://theweek.com/articles/473861/why-both-parties-should-embrace-obamacares-state-exchanges.

Gabel, Jon, Heidi Whitmore, Matthew Green, Adrienne Call, Sam Stromberg, and Rebecca Oran. 2016. "The ACA's Cost-Sharing Reduction Plans: A Key to Affordable Health Coverage for Millions of U.S. Workers." Commonwealth Fund, October 16. Accessed October 12, 2020. https://www.commonwealthfund.org/publications/issue-briefs/2016/oct/acas-cost-sharing-reduction-plans-key-affordable-health-coverage.

Gawande, Atul. 2013. "States of Health." *New Yorker* (October 7): 25–26. Accessed August 31, 2018. https://www.newyorker.com/magazine/2013/10/07/states-of-health.

Glied, Sherry, Anupama Arora, and Claudia Solís-Román. 2015. *The CBO's Crystal Ball: How Well Did It Forecast the Effects of the Affordable Care Act?* Commonwealth Fund. Accessed February 27, 2021. https://www.commonwealthfund.org/sites/default/files/documents/___media_files_publications_issue_brief_2015_dec_1851_glied_cbo_crystal_ball_forecast_aca_rb_v2.pdf.

Goldstein, Amy, and Juliet Eilperin. 2017. "Trump to End Key ACA Subsidies, a Move That Will Threaten the Law's Marketplaces." *Washington Post*, October 13. Accessed February 27, 2021. https://www.washingtonpost.com/national/health-science/trump-to-sign-executive-order-to-gut-aca-insurance-rules-and-undermine-marketplaces/2017/10/11/40abf774-ae97-11e7-9e58-e6288544af98_story.html.

Haislmaier, Edmund. 2006. "Massachusetts Health Reform: What the doctor ordered." Heritage Foundation, May 6. Accessed February 27, 2021. https://www.heritage

.org/health-care-reform/commentary/massachusetts-health-reform-what-the-doctor-ordered.

Hatch, Orrin. 2017. "Obamacare Doesn't Deserve a Bailout." *Washington Post*, September 8. Accessed February 27, 2021. https://www.washingtonpost.com/opinions/obamacare-doesnt-deserve-a-bailout/2017/09/08/99af1838-9344-11e7-aace-04b862b2b3f3_story.html.

Henney, Megan. 2020. "Dems Frame Amy Coney Barrett as Threat to ObamaCare during Confirmation Hearing." Fox Business, October 12. Accessed October 13, 2020. https://www.foxbusiness.com/politics/dems-frame-amy-coney-barrett-as-threat-to-obamacare-during-confirmation-hearing.

Jackson, David. 2013. "Obama: Health Care Website Problems Inexcusable." *USA Today*, October 21. Accessed August 19, 2018. https://www.usatoday.com/story/news/2013/10/21/obama-health-care-internet-glitches-health-and-human-services/3142759/.

Johnson, Carolyn Y. 2016. "United Health Group to Exit Obamacare Exchanges in All but a 'Handful' of States." *Washington Post*, April 19. Accessed August 19, 2018. https://www.washingtonpost.com/news/wonk/wp/2016/04/19/unitedhealth-group-to-exit-obamacare-exchanges-in-all-but-a-handful-of-states/.

Jost, Timothy. 2016. "The House and the ACA—A Lawsuit over Cost-Sharing Reductions." *New England Journal of Medicine* 374 (January 7): 5–7. Accessed September 3, 2018. https://www.nejm.org/doi/full/10.1056/NEJMp1513600.

Jost, Timothy. 2020. "Court Says Marketplace Insurers Are Entitled to Payments for Reducing Cost-Sharing, but Must Offset Premium Tax Credit Increases." Commonwealth Fund, August 18. Accessed February 27, 2021. https://www.commonwealthfund.org/blog/2020/court-marketplace-insurers-payments-reducing-cost-sharing.

Kaiser Family Foundation. 2019a. "Marketplace Average Benchmark Premiums: Timeframe 2014–19." Accessed August 26, 2019. https://www.kff.org/health-reform/state-indicator/marketplace-average-benchmark-premiums/.

Kaiser Family Foundation. 2019b. "Number of Issuers Participating in the Individual Health Insurance Marketplaces." Accessed May 27, 2020. https://www.kff.org/other/state-indicator/number-of-issuers-participating-in-the-individual-health-insurance-marketplace/.

Kaiser Family Foundation. 2019c. "Public Opinion on Single-Payer, National Health Plans, and Expanding Access to Medicare Coverage." July 30. Accessed August 26, 2019. https://www.kff.org/slideshow/public-opinion-on-single-payer-national-health-plans-and-expanding-access-to-medicare-coverage/.

Kaiser Family Foundation. 2020a. "KFF Health Tracking Poll: The Public's Views on the ACA." Accessed May 28, 2020. https://www.kff.org/interactive/kff-health-tracking-poll-the-publics-views-on-the-aca/.

Kaiser Family Foundation. 2020b. "Marketplace Enrollment." Accessed May 27, 2020. https://www.kff.org/health-reform/state-indicator/marketplace-enrollment/.

Kaiser Family Foundation. 2020c. "Potential Impact of *California v. Texas* Decision on Key Provisions of the Affordable Care Act." September 22. Accessed October 12, 2020. https://www.kff.org/health-reform/issue-brief/potential-impact-of-california-v-texas-decision-on-key-provisions-of-the-affordable-care-act/.

King v. Burwell. 2015. No. 14-114. Accessed February 13, 2021. https://www.supremecourt.gov/opinions/14pdf/14-114_qol1.pdf.

Kingsdale, Jon. 2014. "After the False Start: What Can We Expect from the New Health Insurance Marketplaces?" *New England Journal of Medicine* 370, no. 5: 393–396. Accessed August 26, 2019. https://www.nejm.org/doi/full/10.1056/NEJMp1315956.

Kirzinger, Ashley, Bianca DiJulio, Bryan Wu, and Mollyann Brodie. 2017. "Kaiser Health Tracking Poll—August 2017: The Politics of ACA Repeal and Replace Efforts." Kaiser Family Foundation. Accessed September 4, 2018. https://www.kff.org/health-reform/poll-finding/kaiser-health-tracking-poll-september-2017-whats-next-for-health-care/.

Kirzinger, Ashley, Liz Hamel, Cailey Muñana, and Mollyann Brodie. 2018. "Kaiser Health Tracking Poll—March 2018: Non-Group Enrollees." Kaiser Family Foundation. Accessed September 4, 2018. https://www.kff.org/health-reform/poll-finding/kaiser-health-tracking-poll-march-2018-non-group-enrollees/.

Kirzinger, Ashley, Cailey Muñana, and Mollyann Brodie. 2019. "6 Charts about Public Opinion on the Affordable Care Act." Kaiser Family Foundation, July 19. Accessed August 26, 2019. https://www.kff.org/health-reform/poll-finding/6-charts-about-public-opinion-on-the-affordable-care-act/.

Kirzinger, Ashley, Elise Sugarman, and Mollyann Brodie. 2016. "Data Note: Americans' Opinions of the Affordable Care Act." Kaiser Family Foundation, October 27. Accessed September 5, 2018. https://www.kff.org/health-reform/poll-finding/data-note-americans-opinions-of-the-affordable-care-act/.

Lee, Peter, and James Robinson. 2015. "Obamacare Works in California. Here's Why." *Los Angeles Times*, July 27. Accessed September 7, 2018. http://www.latimes.com/opinion/op-ed/la-oe-0728-lee-aca-insurance-prices-20150727-story.html#.

Levitt, Larry. 2017. "Is the Affordable Care Act Imploding?" *JAMA* 317, no. 20. Accessed May 28, 2020. https://newsatjama.jama.com/2017/04/17/jama-forum-is-the-affordable-care-act-imploding/.

Luthi, Susannah. 2020. "Supreme Court Rules Government Must Pay Billions to Obamacare Insurers." Politico, April 27. Accessed May 27, 2020. https://www.politico.com/news/2020/04/27/supreme-court-rules-government-must-pay-billions-to-obamacare-insurers-211184.

Mason Jeff, and Mark Felsenthal. 2014. "Obamacare Enrollment Exceeds Seven Million Target Despite Setback." Reuters, April 2. https://www.reuters.com/article/us-usa-healthcare-enrollment-idUSBREA2U0QW20140402.

Mathews, Anna Wilde. 2019. "Health Insurers Set to Expand Offerings under the ACA." *Wall Street Journal*, August 22. Accessed May 27, 2020. https://www.wsj.com/articles/health-insurers-set-to-expand-offerings-under-the-aca-11566468120.

McCain, John. 2015. "Restoring Americans' Health Care Freedom Reconciliation Act of 2015." Congressional Record, Volume 161 (2015), Part 14 [Senate], pp. 19441-. Accessed April 19, 2021. https://www.govinfo.gov/content/pkg/CRECB-2015-pt14/html/CRECB-2015-pt14-Pg19441-2.htm.

McCain, John, and John Barrasso. 2015. "ObamaCare Opt-Out Act: Let All Americans Make Their Own Health Care Decisions." Fox News, January 13. Accessed September 5, 2018. https://www.foxnews.com/opinion/2015/01/13/why-am-reintroducing-obamacare-opt-out-act.print.html.

McCarthy, Kevin. 2018. "Congressman McCarthy on the Obamacare Ruling." December 15. Accessed May 28, 2020. https://kevinmccarthy.house.gov/media-center/press-releases/congressman-mccarthy-on-the-obamacare-ruling.

McKinsey Center for U.S. Health System Reform. 2016. "Exchanges Three Years In: Market Variations and Factors Affecting Performance." Accessed September 4, 2018. https://healthcare.mckinsey.com/exchanges-three-years-market-variations-and-factors-affecting-performance.

Moffitt, Robert. 2006. "The Rationale for a Statewide Health Insurance Exchange." Heritage Foundation, October 5. Accessed August 19, 2018. https://www.heritage.org/health-care-reform/report/the-rationale-statewide-health-insurance-exchange.

Musumeci, MaryBeth. 2020. "Explaining *Texas v. U.S.*: A Guide to the Case Challenging the ACA." Kaiser Family Foundation, March 10. Accessed May 28, 2020. https://www.kff.org/health-reform/issue-brief/explaining-texas-v-u-s-a-guide-to-the-case-challenging-the-aca/.

Obama, Barack. 2016. "United States Health Care Reform: Progress to Date and Next Steps." *JAMA* 316, no. 5: 525–532. Accessed September 2, 2018. http://jamanetwork.com/journals/jama/fullarticle/2533698.

Oberlander, Jonathan. 2018. "The Republican War on Obamacare—What Has It Achieved? *New England Journal of Medicine* 379 (August 23): 703–705. Accessed August 26, 2019. https://www.nejm.org/doi/full/10.1056/NEJMp1806798.

O'Connor, Reed. 2018. "Memorandum Opinion and Order: *Texas, et al. v. United States of America, et al.*" Civil Action No. 4:18-cv-00167-0. December 14. Accessed May 28, 2020. https://www.documentcloud.org/documents/5629711-Texas-v-US-Partial-Summary-Judgment.html.

O'Keefe, Ed, and Paul Kane. 2013. "Sen. Cruz Ends Anti-Obamacare Talkathon after More Than 21 Hours." *Washington Post*, September 25. Accessed September 2, 2018. https://www.washingtonpost.com/politics/sen-cruz-continues-night-long-attack-on-obamacare/2013/09/25/5ea2f6ae-25ae-11e3-b75d-5b7f66349852_story.html.

Page, Susan. 2013. "Obama Apologizes, but That Might Not Be Enough Now." *USA Today*, November 15–17: 1A.

Page, Susan. 2020. "Read the Full Transcript of Vice Presidential Debate between Mike Pence and Kamala Harris." *USA Today*, October 8. Accessed October 13, 2020. https://www.usatoday.com/story/news/politics/elections/2020/10/08/vice-presidential-debate-full-transcript-mike-pence-and-kamala-harris/5920773002/.

Ramshaw, Emily. 2012. "Perry: Texas Won't Implement Key Elements of Federal Health Reform." Accessed September 12, 2018. https://www.texastribune.org/2012/07/09/perry-tx-wont-implement-key-elements-health-reform/.

Rovner, Julie. 2018. "Consumers Brace for Premiums Hikes while Lawmakers Grasp at Remedies." Kaiser Health News, May 11. Accessed September 9, 2018. https://khn.org/news/consumers-brace-for-premium-hikes-while-lawmakers-grasp-at-remedies/.

Sanger-Katz, Margot. 2016. "Football Team at the Buffet: Why Obamacare Markets Are in Crisis." *New York Times*, September 26. Accessed September 9, 2018. https://www.nytimes.com/2016/09/25/upshot/football-team-at-the-buffet-why-obamacare-markets-are-in-crisis.html.

Sebelius, Kathleen. 2013a. "HealthCare.gov Simple, User-Friendly." *USA Today*, October 7. Accessed September 11, 2018. https://www.usatoday.com/story/opinion/2013/10/07/healthcaregov-kathleen-sebelius-editorials-debates/2939993/.

Sebelius, Kathleen. 2013b. "Improvement Dramatic over Oct. 1." *USA Today*, December 1. Accessed September 11, 2018. https://www.usatoday.com/story/opinion/2013/12/01/kathleen-sebeliushealthcaregov-obamacare-editorials-debates/3799145/.

Semanskee, Ashley, Cynthia Cox, Gary Claxton, Michelle Long, and Rabah Kamal. 2017. "Insurer Participation on ACA Marketplaces, 2014–2018." Kaiser Family Foundation. Accessed September 4, 2018. https://www.kff.org/health-reform/issue-brief/insurer-participation-on-aca-marketplaces/.

Starr, Paul. 1994. *The Logic of Health Care Reform*. New York: Penguin Press.

Trump, Donald J. 2020. "Remarks by President Trump on the America First Healthcare Plan." September 24. Accessed October 13, 2020. https://www.whitehouse.gov/briefings-statements/remarks-president-trump-america-first-healthcare-plan/.

USA Today. 2020. "Read the Full Transcript from the First Presidential Debate between Joe Biden and Donald Trump." September 30. Accessed October 13, 2020. https://www.usatoday.com/story/news/politics/elections/2020/09/30/presidential-debate-read-full-transcript-first-debate/3587462001/.

Verma, Seema. 2018. "Remarks by Administrator Seema Verma at the ALEC Policy Summit." November 29. Accessed August 26, 2019. https://www.cms.gov/newsroom/press-releases/remarks-administrator-seema-verma-alec-policy-summit.

Wall Street Journal. 2013. "ObamaCare's Black Box." October 17. Accessed April 19, 2021. https://www.wsj.com/articles/SB10001424052702304106704579137501568384292.

Wall Street Journal. 2019. "Still Heading for the ObamaCare Exits" August 16. Accessed August 26, 2019. https://www.wsj.com/articles/still-heading-for-the-obamacare-exits-11565911387.

Immigrant Health Coverage

At a Glance

Since 1882, U.S. immigration law has included a "public charge" principle that requires immigration officials to deny entry to individuals who they deem unlikely to be self-sufficient and who thus pose an economic burden to the government. In turn, Democrats and Republicans have long engaged in contentious debates regarding whether and how to extend health coverage to noncitizens. Before 1996, legal immigrants and lawful permanent residents had access to public health benefits comparable to American citizens. After passage of the Personal Responsibility and Work Opportunity Reconciliation Act (PRWORA) in 1996, legal immigrants became subject to a five-year waiting period before qualifying for participation in major federally funded, means-tested assistance programs such as Medicaid, Supplemental Nutrition Assistance Program (SNAP), Supplemental Security Income (SSI), and Temporary Assistance to Needy Families (TANF). Contemporary partisan debates center on the merits of regulating immigration based on the ability to pay for health insurance, limiting health coverage to qualified immigrants, and prohibiting coverage for undocumented immigrants.

Democrats frame their support for extending health coverage to noncitizens as an extension of their long-standing contention that health care is a human right. Moreover, Democrats argue that extending health coverage to noncitizens is fiscally responsible; by providing health care access to all individuals regardless of immigration status, noncitizens will be less likely to seek care at emergency rooms, thereby reducing the nation's emergency care cost burden. From PRWORA's passage in 1996 to the Trump administration's 2020 change to the public charge rule, Democrats have maintained that these policies discriminate against legal, taxpaying immigrants.

Republicans, who have historically opposed extending health coverage to noncitizens, argue that providing health coverage to noncitizens is unfair to American citizens. Countering Democratic claims of potential cost savings, Republicans maintain that providing health care coverage to undocumented immigrants would pose a significant financial burden to the nation and further incentivize illegal entry. They also suggest that regulating immigrant entry and visas according to financial status would further reduce the strain on the national budget.

According to Many Democrats . . .

- Health care is a human right for all, independent of immigration status.
- Providing access to health care to all individuals regardless of immigration status will reduce the cost of emergency care.
- Providing health care to immigrants regardless of immigration status would improve the nation's overall health by ensuring access to care for millions of underserved individuals and families.
- The public charge rule discriminates against legal, taxpaying immigrants.

According to Many Republicans . . .

- It is unfair to provide health coverage to noncitizens and undocumented immigrants.
- Providing health care to undocumented immigrants would impose a significant financial burden on U.S. taxpayers.
- Providing health care to undocumented immigrants would further incentivize illegal entry.
- Regulating immigrant entry and visas according to financial status would reduce the strain on national resources.

Overview

In 2017, the foreign-born population in the United States reached its highest share in over a century: 44.5 million foreign-born individuals, representing 13.7 percent of the American population (Tavernise 2018). By 2018, however, the United States had experienced a sharp drop in immigrant population growth, due in part to restrictive policies introduced by the Trump administration (Tavernise 2018). During his 2016 presidential campaign, Donald Trump promised to build a wall along the Mexican border to stem the influx of migrants across the southern border. The Trump administration subsequently instituted travel bans, narrowed asylum eligibility, sought to limit family chain migration, and revised the public charge rule that applied to individuals applying for green cards. All of these immigration restriction efforts were met with vociferous Democratic opposition.

Democrats and Republicans have long deliberated how to regulate immigration. Since 1882, U.S. immigration law has included a public charge principle.

Congress included language in the Immigration Act of 1882 that required immigration officials to turn away "any person unable to take care of himself or herself without becoming a public charge" (*An Act to Regulate Immigration* 1882). An integral component of recent partisan debates centers on health coverage for noncitizens residing within the United States—both legal and undocumented. Historically, an individual's citizenship status has determined his or her ability to access health care in the United States. In 1971, the U.S. Supreme Court ruled in *Graham v. Richardson* that state restrictions on legal immigrants' eligibility for public benefits violated the Constitution's equal protection clause (*Graham v. Richardson* 1971).

Legal immigrants and lawful permanent residents remained eligible for public health benefits comparable to U.S. citizens until 1996. In 1994, California voters approved Proposition 187, a ballot initiative that would have denied all public services to undocumented immigrants living in the state. Gov. Pete Wilson (R) supported Proposition 187 during his 1994 reelection campaign (Nowrasteh 2016). Subsequent injunctions by federal judges prevented the measure's enactment, however, and scholars have demonstrated how the proposition spurred Latino voters to leave the Republican party for the Democratic party, turning California into a Democratic stronghold ever since (Dyck, Johnson, and Wasson 2012). In 1996, the Illegal Immigration Reform and Immigrant Responsibility Act (Public Law 104-208) allowed immigration officials to deny visas to immigrants deemed to be potential public charges and also required immigrant sponsors to assume financial responsibility for prospective immigrants.

Immigrant health coverage changed significantly when President Bill Clinton signed the Personal Responsibility and Work Opportunity Reconciliation Act (PRWORA) in 1996, fulfilling his earlier welfare reform campaign promise. During the 1994 midterm election campaign, Republicans released the Contract with America, a legislative agenda that detailed a conservative commitment to lowering taxes, reducing the size of the government, and implementing welfare reform. After Republicans retook the U.S. House of Representatives and the U.S. Senate, Clinton employed a "triangulation" strategy, in which he adopted centrist positions on certain policy debates, including welfare reform (Wills 1997). Introduced in the House of Representatives by Rep. John Kasich (R-OH), PRWORA passed the House of Representatives by a 256–120 margin and the Senate by a 74–24 margin. While almost all Republicans in both chambers voted in favor of the final version, Democrats in both chambers split their votes.

At its core, PRWORA replaced Aid to Families with Dependent Children, a federal entitlement program, with the more restrictive Temporary Assistance to Needy Families (TANF), a state-based block grant program. Decades of public opinion polling leading up to the introduction of PRWORA indicated that although most Americans agreed that the government had a responsibility to support those in need, they also believed that the government spent too much on welfare. By 1995, 66 percent of Americans in one public opinion survey agreed that the government was spending too much on welfare (MacLeod, Montero, and Speer 1999).

PRWORA distinguished between qualified immigrants and nonqualified immigrants, though not necessarily between legal and undocumented immigrants, and established a five-year residency requirement before qualified immigrants could access federal benefits. During debate over the bill, Rep. Nydia Velazquez (D-NY), the first Puerto Rican woman to serve in Congress, argued that "this bill . . . gives legal immigrants the shaft. Most of us here today descended from immigrant roots. Yet H.R. 3734 calls for an unprecedented denial of benefits for legal immigrants who, despite their contributions by working hard and paying taxes, fall on hard times" (*Congressional Record* 1996a). In the Senate, Sen. Al D'Amato (R-NY) defended the bill as a matter of fairness: "We did not design the system to say, 'Come here and get welfare benefits, and John Q. Public, hard-working middle-class families, are going to pay for it'" (*Congressional Record* 1996c).

PRWORA also redirected responsibility for immigrant health care from the federal government to state and local governments. This policy shift followed public opinion. In one 1995 Harvard/Kaiser poll, 52 percent of Americans favored welfare reform at the state level, while only 7 percent preferred the existing federal-oriented structure (Kaiser Family Foundation 1995). For immigrants, eligibility for public health benefits thus became contingent on state-level variation in public health benefit programs. By 2004, 23 states had extended coverage to immigrants who were otherwise ineligible for Medicaid or the Children's Health Insurance Program (CHIP) because of their immigration status. While some states extended prenatal care coverage regardless of immigration status, other states extended coverage to some or all immigrant pregnant women and children—providing the same benefits as Medicaid in some cases and reduced benefits in others. Some states elected to exercise CHIP funding to cover pregnant women, and others provided state funding. And yet other states extended coverage to other categories of qualified immigrants. Although noncitizens who lived in states with state-funded replacement programs were more likely to have insurance coverage, by 2003, over half of all recent immigrants living in the United States lacked insurance (Fremstad and Cox 2004).

The legacy of the 1996 welfare reform legislation has been and remains a focus of debate. Clinton remarked upon signing the bill into law that "welfare will no longer be a political issue" (Clines 1996), but that proved to be an overly optimistic prediction. After the 1997 Balanced Budget Act restored some benefits for some legal immigrants, namely Supplemental Security Income (SSI) benefits for disabled or elderly legal immigrants, one public opinion poll indicated that 56 percent of respondents disapproved of the restoration (Pew Research Center 1997). Five years later, a 2002 poll found that only 46 percent of Americans had a positive view of the 1996 reforms (Pew Research Center 2002). Supporters highlighted the decline in welfare enrollment, while critics argued that restrictive criteria impeded economic mobility for poor Americans and immigrants.

Data suggests that the 1996 welfare reform bill signed by Clinton adversely impacted the broader immigrant population in several ways. A 2004 analysis documented a decline in Medicaid enrollment among the larger group of qualified immigrants following welfare reform (Kandula et al. 2004). Similarly, a 2005 analysis recorded an increase in the proportion of uninsured among low-educated, foreign-born single women and their children (Kaushal and Kaestner 2005). Other researchers observed similar trends among older immigrants (Nam 2008). The Cato Institute's Michael Tanner later observed, "If welfare reform was not the disaster that its critics feared, neither was it the unalloyed success that its supporters claimed" (Tanner 2016).

In 2007, Sens. Hillary Clinton (D-NY) and Olympia Snowe (R-ME) introduced and sponsored the bipartisan Legal Immigrant Children's Health Improvement Act (ICHIA), which proposed restoring federal Medicaid and CHIP coverage to legal immigrant children and pregnant women within their first five years of legal residence in the United States. ICHIA was subsequently incorporated into the Children's Health Insurance Program Reauthorization Act of 2009 (CHIPRA). By 2011, 20 states and Washington, DC, had adopted the ICHIA option, accounting for an almost 25 percent increase in insurance coverage between 2007 and 2012 (Saloner, Koyawala, and Kenney 2014). As of January 2020, 34 states had exercised the ICHIA option to cover immigrant children and pregnant women within their first five years of legal residence.

During the Obama administration, several border states expanded local immigration enforcement measures. When Arizona's Gov. Jan Brewer (R) signed the Supporting Our Law Enforcement and Safe Neighborhoods Act in 2010, she defended her commitment to "protecting our state from crime associated with illegal immigration" (Brewer 2010). The act empowered law enforcement officials in the state to detain individuals who could not prove their citizenship upon request. Following enactment, however, Latino adolescent mothers reported a decline in utilization of preventive health care and public assistance programs—regardless of their citizenship status (Toomey et al. 2014). President Obama harshly criticized the law, asserting that it would "undermine basic notions of fairness that we cherish as Americans, as well as the trust between police and our communities that is so crucial to keeping us safe" (Archibold 2010).

Emboldened by passage of S.B. 1070, Arizona Republicans introduced a package of immigration bills in 2011, including S.B. 1405, which required hospitals to report uninsured patients who could not demonstrate their legal immigration status. Democrats questioned the administrative burden imposed on medical professionals by such proposals. As Democratic state senator Steve Gallardo argued, "Doctors that should be working to help treat ill patients are now turning into ICE agents" (CBS News 2011). Arizona state senator Steve Smith (R-AZ) countered that, "at emergency rooms, there is always a sign that says you will not be refused treatment. OK, good. Treat them, but there will be someone waiting there when they wake up" (InMaricopa 2011). Republican and Democratic state senators ultimately rejected the bills, in part due to the considerably negative press coverage of S.B. 1070.

In 2010, President Barack Obama signed into law his landmark health reform legislation, the Affordable Care Act (ACA), which had narrowly passed Congress despite receiving no Republican votes. The ACA's individual mandate applied to U.S. citizens and legal residents, but undocumented immigrants did not qualify for cost-sharing subsidies or premium tax credits. Undocumented immigrants were also disallowed from enrolling in health insurance exchanges. In July 2012, Obama announced the Deferred Action for Childhood Arrivals (DACA) program, a new policy to limit deportations of and grant work permits to undocumented immigrants who entered the United States as children. In November 2014, when Obama announced his intention to expand the program. 26 Republican-led states sued to prevent the executive action. The case eventually reached the U.S. Supreme Court, which ultimately blocked the expansion by rendering a 4–4 decision (the deadlock stemmed from the fact that the decision was handed down after the death of Justice Antonin Scalia but before his replacement, Neil Gorsuch, was sworn in). Although DACA protected certain undocumented immigrants from deportation, DACA-eligible immigrants were excluded from coverage through the ACA. In response, Democratic-led states expanded health care access to undocumented immigrants.

For example, California state law allowed DACA recipients to enroll in Medi-Cal, the state's Medicaid program, per S.B. 4, passed in 2015. Opinion polls indicated broad public support in California, where an estimated one-quarter of the nation's undocumented immigrant population resided at the time (Hayes and Hill 2017). In 2014, 54 percent of Californians supported expanding health insurance access to undocumented immigrants. Although the majority of Californians favored the proposal, partisan differences were clear: 70 percent of Democrats indicated support compared to 26 percent of Republicans (Metz and Strimple 2014).

Even as Republican-led states such as Arizona expanded local immigration enforcement measures, Democratic-led states and municipalities expanded health coverage to undocumented immigrants. Mayor Gavin Newsom (D) introduced one such initiative, Healthy San Francisco (HSF), in 2007. Designed to provide universal coverage for medical services provided within San Francisco, the program included an employer spending mandate. The program withstood legal challenges from the restaurant industry, which filed an appeal that the U.S.

Supreme Court subsequently declined to review (City Attorney of San Francisco 2010).

Following implementation of the ACA, many HSF enrollees gained coverage through the state's Medi-Cal expansion or through insurance subsidies on the Covered California marketplace exchange. This enrollment shift meant that undocumented immigrants constituted a sizeable proportion of HSF participants. In 2013, Tom Ammiano, a Democratic Assembly member who as city supervisor had helped establish HSF, touted the program as a clear success, declaring, "The denial of people's humanity and need is extremely unfortunate, but it doesn't fly here in San Francisco" (Knight 2013). In response to the Trump administration's later efforts to restrict immigration, John Coté, the communications director for City Attorney Dennis Herrera (D), affirmed in 2017 that the city would refuse to divulge medical records for undocumented immigrants to the federal government: "We can't envision a scenario where we would turn over those records, given medical privacy laws" (Arroyo 2017).

In 2014, New York City launched IDNYC, a municipal ID program that connected local residents, including undocumented immigrants, to the city's public facilities. The following year, the city launched ActionHealthNYC, a one-year pilot program funded through private philanthropy that extended public health system access to low-income adults who were ineligible for coverage through Medicaid or New York State of Health, the state's ACA marketplace exchange. Five years later, New York City Mayor Bill de Blasio (D) enacted the NYC Care program in May 2019. NYC Care extended access to primary care services offered by the city's public health clinics and hospital system, regardless of immigration status. As de Blasio argued, "Health care is a basic right and with NYC Care, we are ensuring that right for working people across our City and setting a nationwide model of what it means to provide low-cost, affordable health care" (City of New York 2019b).

Following de Blasio's unveiling, New York conservatives questioned how NYC Care would be funded. As Republican Assembly member Nicole Malliotakis tweeted, "Our citizens have [a] hard enough time covering their own healthcare costs. Now, [de Blasio] also wants them to pay for healthcare of 300,000 citizens of other countries. He must stop abusing the middle class and treating us like his personal ATM" (Malliotakis 2019). However, Democrats drew a direct connection between the program and broader progressive policy goals. As Assembly member Jeffrey Dinowitz (D) argued, "All New Yorkers should have access to high quality healthcare, regardless of their documentation status or ability to pay. The NYC Care program is a tremendous step forward towards the ultimate goal of universal healthcare" (City of New York 2019a).

California—which has voted for the Democratic presidential candidate since 1992—has continually expanded public health benefits to immigrants since 1996. In 2015, Gov. Jerry Brown (D) signed SB 4, the Health for All Act, which expanded

Medi-Cal eligibility to all low-income Californians regardless of immigration status. Republican state senator Andy Vidak, who voted in favor of the bill, explained that he did so because "taxpayers are already paying high health care costs for the undocumented Californians when they show up in our emergency rooms" (Koseff 2015). Vidak's observation reflected an unintended consequence of the Emergency Medical Treatment and Active Labor Act (EMTALA), signed by President Reagan in 1986, which required that any individual who came to an emergency room had to be treated regardless of insurance status or ability to pay—but because the law remains an unfunded mandate, taxpayers absorbed the cost of uncompensated care of undocumented immigrants seeking treatment in emergency rooms. Vidak's argument is also one traditionally put forward by Democrats: extending coverage to undocumented immigrants would be unlikely to lead to significant increases in overall health spending because immigrants could now obtain health care in settings other than (expensive) emergency rooms.

Although Republicans argued that extending public health benefits to immigrants would be fiscally irresponsible, peer-reviewed studies have indicated that immigrants' overall health care costs are less than those for U.S.-born individuals (Flavin et al. 2018). California's expansion of public health benefits to undocumented immigrants gained an increasingly positive reception from the electorate. In one 2015 public opinion poll, 54 percent of Californians supported extending Medi-Cal to cover undocumented immigrant children (Baldassare et al. 2015). The following year, SB 75 (Health for All Kids) extended full-scope Medi-Cal coverage to children under 19 regardless of immigration status. In 2019, another poll found that 64 percent of Californians favored extending Medi-Cal to cover undocumented immigrants (Baldassare et al. 2019). In January 2020, the state extended full-scope Medi-Cal to those 19–25 years of age regardless of immigration status (Mento 2020).

Nonetheless, the fact that a majority of Californians have reliably favored extending coverage to undocumented immigrants has obscured underlying political polarization within the state. For example, one 2015 poll indicated that 63 percent of Democrats favored "providing health care coverage for undocumented immigrants in California," while 87 percent of Republicans opposed doing so (Baldassare et al. 2015). In 2019, another survey found that 78 of identified Democrats favored state efforts to "protect the legal rights of undocumented immigrants in California," while the same proportion of Republicans disagreed (Baldassare et al. 2019).

In October 2019, Reps. Pramila Jayapal (D-WA) and Deb Haaland (D-NM) reintroduced the Health Equity and Access under the Law for Immigrant Women and Families Act (HEAL Act), which proposed removing the five-year waiting period for immigrants (Haaland 2019). As Haaland explained, "Under this administration, people in our country are denied access to health care because of where they come from—it's not what we stand for" (Turner 2019). Rep. Michelle Lujan

Grisham (D-NM) had previously introduced the HEAL Act in 2015 and again in 2017, arguing that the bill would "guarantee that lawfully present immigrants who work hard and contribute to our economy will be treated fairly by the health care system they support when they pay taxes" (Center for Reproductive Rights 2015). The 2019 version also proposed expanding ACA insurance exchange eligibility to undocumented immigrants.

Extending public health benefits to undocumented immigrants remained particularly polarizing. One 2019 CNN poll indicated that 66 percent of Democrats agreed that health coverage should be available to undocumented immigrants, while 88 percent of Republicans indicated that it should not (CNN 2019). As President Donald Trump put it during his third State of the Union address, "If forcing American taxpayers to provide free health care to illegal immigrants sounds fair to you, stand with the radical left. If you think we should defend patients and seniors, stand with me to pass legislation to prohibit free health care for illegal aliens" (Trump 2020).

Democrats on Immigrant Health Coverage

For Democrats, offering health coverage to noncitizens reflects a long-standing embrace of health care as a social right. Characterizing health care as a fundamental human right provides the foundation for many Democrats who support expanding access to health care services to all, regardless of immigration status. During one Democratic presidential primary debate in 2019, all Democratic candidates on the stage indicated that, if nominated, they would offer health insurance to undocumented immigrants (Bolton 2019).

Democrats argue that creating an inclusive health and social welfare care system is obligatory and that it is unfair to bar federal taxpayers from public benefits on the basis of their immigration status. As Sen. Claiborne Pell (D-RI) argued in 1996, "More often than not, legal immigrants are hard-working, tax paying individuals who deeply appreciate the freedom and opportunity of U.S. citizenship, which they hope to attain. To deny them so many of the benefits that they might legitimately need as they build a life here, seems unfair and unjustified" (*Congressional Record* 1996b). Almost two decades later, California state senator Ricardo Lara (D) emphasized the moral values behind this stance: "Ensuring that every child in California grows up healthy and with an opportunity to thrive and succeed is simply the right thing to do" (Koseff 2015). As Gov. Gavin Newsom (D) of California proclaimed in 2019, "Universal health care's a right, and we're delivering it—regardless of immigration status—to everyone up to the age of 26, and we're gonna get the rest of that done, mark my words" (Caiola 2019). Sen. Bernie Sanders (I-VT), an independent who has long caucused with Democrats and sponsored the Medicare for All Act of 2019, pledged that if Congress were to pass his bill, the

Immigrants Have Earned and Thus Deserve Public Benefits

On June 20, 2019, Rep. Barbara Lee (D-CA) addressed the U.S. House of Representatives to express her strong opposition to the Trump administration's proposal to add noncash benefits such as housing assistance and the Supplemental Nutrition Assistance Program (SNAP) to the criteria upon which the federal government makes "public charge" determinations.

> Let's get straight to the facts. This country was built and continues to stand on the strength of immigrants. We know that a little help for our hardworking immigrant families reaps exponential returns to our economy and society.
>
> Immigrants contribute in taxes, and they should be able to use social services when they need it, just like every other person in our Nation who pays taxes. Our immigrant community should not be seen as a drain on America but as an investment in our future. We are one Nation.
>
> In closing, I want to reiterate that it is the constitutional duty of Congress to write our immigration laws and ensure that they are equitable to all individuals, regardless of race, age, or socioeconomic status. That is why, last week, during the Homeland Security appropriations markup, I offered an amendment along with Congressmen Price, Pocan, and Aguilar that would make it clear that no Federal funds can be used to expand public charge. We must defeat this anti-immigrant and un-American public charge rule. I hope that all of my colleagues will stand up and demand that the administration abandon this plan once and for all.

Source

Congressional Record, vol. 165, no. 104 (June 20, 2019): H4923. Washington, DC: Government Printing Office. Accessed April 24, 2020. https://www.congress.gov/116/crec/2019/06/20/CREC-2019-06-20-pt1-PgH4923.pdf.

United States would "join the rest of the industrialized world and guarantee health care to all, including the undocumented" (Tin 2019).

How to achieve this progressive goal remains a point of disagreement. While progressive Democrats advocate for universal coverage, moderate Democrats favor extending unsubsidized coverage to undocumented immigrants. At the same time, moderates defend the ability of undocumented immigrants to obtain uncompensated emergency care. As former Vice President Joe Biden (D) offered in one interview, "How do you say, 'You're undocumented. I'm going to let you die, man'? What are you going to do?" (Brownstein 2019). When California's Democratic congressional delegation endorsed an innovation waiver to enable the state to offer unsubsidized coverage to undocumented immigrants through the state's marketplace exchange, Rep. Judy Chu (D-CA) stated, "We can begin getting all our residents the basic care they deserve, instead of having to wait for it to become an emergency. Being undocumented should not mean being unworthy" (Roybal-Allard 2016). Similarly, in 2016, Rep. Nydia Velazquez (D-NY) introduced the Mobile Medical

Immigrant Health Improvement Act, which proposed creating a federal partnership with hospitals and other health care facilities to develop and fund mobile medical services in immigrant communities. Velazquez emphasized how undocumented immigrants obtaining care from mobile medical facilities would be a more cost-effective use of limited government funds (U.S. Congress 2016).

As the Trump administration announced new immigration restrictions in the late 2010s, the health and welfare of detained migrants became another focus of attention for Democrats. After reports of inadequate sanitary conditions for detainees at U.S. Customs and Border Patrol facilities drew public attention, Democratic policy makers visited the facilities. Rep. Veronica Escobar (D-TX) expressed horror at what she saw, declaring that "our government's abuse of immigrant children is abhorrent and should be a wake-up call to our nation" (Valencia and Shoichet 2019). Rep. Ayanna Presley (D-MA), who called for an emergency hearing, claimed that "what's so troubling about this, beyond the cruelty of it, is the lack of transparency around the process" (Jordan and Dickerson 2019).

The health of the detainees emerged as one of the major sources of concern for Democrats. Rep. Lauren Underwood (D-IL) introduced the U.S. Border Patrol Medical Screening and Standards Act, which would require the Department of Homeland Security (DHS) to create and implement an electronic health record system to document migrants' medical screenings (Brufke 2019). The bill passed the House virtually along party lines, with 227 of 230 yea votes cast by Democrats. As of July 2020, the bill remained with the Senate Judiciary Committee.

While extending health coverage to undocumented immigrants has fostered considerable debate, so has extending coverage to legal immigrants and permanent residents. In particular, Democrats argue that the public charge rule, which requires immigrants to exhibit self-sufficiency to gain entry into the United States, discriminates against legal, taxpaying immigrants. When DHS proposed expanding the scope of the public charge rule in August 2019 to use an individual's history of public benefits to restrict visa eligibility, Democrats objected. As California Attorney General Xavier Becerra (D) insisted, "This Trump rule weaponizes nutrition, health care and housing" (Betz 2019). Michigan Attorney General Dana Nessel asserted that "Michigan is home to tens of thousands of legal immigrants who have every legal right to receive certain benefits to provide food, health care and shelter for their families" (Kovanis 2019). New York Attorney General Letitia James (D) declared that "under this rule, children will go hungry; families will go without medical care" (Alvarez, Sands and Luhby 2019).

In October 2019, federal judges from New York, California, and Washington issued injunctions to prevent the rule from taking effect (Wamsley, Fessler, and Gonzales 2019). In January 2020, however, the U.S. Supreme Court issued a 5–4 decision that allowed the Trump administration to enforce the rule while legal challenges proceeded (Luthi 2020). In April, the Supreme Court denied another motion to block implementation of the rule during the COVID-19 pandemic. In late July, though, a federal judge issued another temporary nationwide injunction, ruling that "adverse government action that targets immigrants . . . is particularly dangerous during a pandemic" (Weixel 2020).

In April 2020, Democrats across the country announced new local and state policies that extended health care benefits to undocumented immigrants during the COVID-19 pandemic. In Chicago, Mayor Lori Lightfoot (D) issued an executive order that all Chicago residents could access public health benefits and services regardless of immigration status. As Lightfoot stated, "We have been working around the clock to ensure that all our residents are secure and supported, including our immigrant and refugee communities, who are among the most vulnerable to the impact of this pandemic" (City of Chicago, Office of the Mayor 2020). When Gov. Gavin Newsom (D) announced a $125 million program to support undocumented families, he remarked, "Every Californian, including our undocumented neighbors and friends, should know that California is here to support them during this crisis" (Loiaconi 2020).

In early April 2020, five Democratic members of Congress introduced the Coronavirus Immigrant Families Protection Act to provide access to COVID-19 testing and treatment to vulnerable communities. Sen. Mazie Hirono (D-HI) defended the bill by arguing that "the coronavirus does not discriminate based on immigration status," and Rep. Raúl Grijalva (D-AZ) asserted that "COVID-19 does not care about your immigration status, so neither should our response" (Hirono 2020). Public opinion among Democratic voters echoed this sentiment. In one May 2020 poll, 85 percent of Democrats believed that the federal government had a responsibility to provide medical care to undocumented immigrants with COVID-19 (Krogstad and Lopez 2020). As of July 2020, the bill had yet to move to the House floor for a vote.

Republicans on Immigrant Health Coverage

For Republicans, long-standing conservative principles of personal responsibility and self-reliance guide their stances on immigration and social welfare policy reforms. Gov. John Kasich of Ohio, who introduced PRWORA as a congressman in 1996, later recalled that "these reforms, for the first time, introduced personal accountability into the welfare equation and began moving America down a better path" (Kasich 2016). These priorities have been reflected in such policy reforms as PRWORA and the Illegal Immigration Reform and Immigrant Responsibility Act of 1996, both of which received strong GOP support.

Generally speaking, Republicans have not strayed from this position in subsequent decades. When the Trump administration put forward more restrictive immigration reform proposals, such as limiting family chain migration and revising the public charge rule, Republicans defended such measures by arguing that it is unfair to provide health care to noncitizens when many American citizens are burdened with high health care costs. Rep. Glenn Grothman (R-WI) asked, "Can we really afford to be the healthcare provider for the entire Western Hemisphere?" (*Congressional Record* 2019). After Democratic candidates for the 2020 presidential nomination pledged to offer health insurance to undocumented immigrants if elected, Republican National Committee chair Ronna McDaniel tweeted that "millions of Americans struggle to pay their own health care bills. Now Democrats want us to pay illegal immigrants'? We can't afford their extreme agenda!" (McDaniel 2019).

The first three years of the Trump administration were punctuated by a series of controversial efforts to restrict immigration. In June 2019, news reports publicized inadequate sanitary conditions at several U.S. Customs and Border Patrol facilities that were holding unaccompanied migrant minors. Trump administration officials argued that government agencies lacked sufficient resources to manage the humanitarian crisis. As acting Customs and Border Protection Commissioner John Sanders explained, "The death of a child is always a terrible thing, but here is a situation where, because there is not enough funding . . . they can't move the people out of our custody" (Attanasio, Burke and Mendoza 2019). In August 2019, U.S. Citizenship and Immigration Services, without public comment, revoked a policy that had enabled immigrants to avoid deportation while undergoing life-saving medical treatment (Jordan and Dickerson 2019). Weeks later, the Trump administration reversed the policy.

As the Trump administration formulated increasingly restrictive immigration policy measures, public surveys demonstrated their early impact. In 2018, 45 percent of nonelderly undocumented immigrants were uninsured (Kaiser Family Foundation 2020). That same year, one in seven low-income adult immigrants reported that they or other family members did not participate in a public benefit program to avoid jeopardizing future green card applications (Bernstein et al. 2019). In 2019, nearly half of community health centers reported decreased rates of health care utilization among immigrant patients and their families (Tolbert, Artiga, and Pham 2019).

Republicans also argue that subsidizing care for undocumented immigrants would further incentivize illegal entry into the country and pose a significant financial burden to the nation. As Rep. Dana Rohrabacher (R-CA) argued in 2009, "If we provide the type of operations that we want for our own people—heart operations and various things that are very expensive operations for health care—to be granted to illegal aliens, you can expect that it will, number one, bankrupt the system; but, number two, we will have illegal aliens coming here from every part of the world. And, in fact, one of the problems right now is that we already provide too much health care for illegal immigrants" (*Congressional Record* 2009).

A decade later, Rep. Dan Crenshaw (R-TX) emphasized the disproportionate impact of illegal immigration on border states in particular. "Americans hospitals and schools are overwhelmed," he charged. "In Houston, which I represent, employees at one hospital designated for low-income Americans without insurance told me they spend 25 percent of their budget on illegal immigrants" (Crenshaw 2019). Former Arizona Gov. Jan Brewer (R) echoed these concerns, tweeting, "When I was Governor, illegal aliens cost [Arizona] taxpayers $1.6 billion/y[ea]r in education, health care and incarceration costs. So, why do we continue to bear these costs when sanctuary cities encourage illegal immigration?" (Gage 2019). In late 2018, Oklahoma state senator Paul Scott (R) introduced legislation to eliminate the state's benefits program for pregnant noncitizens: "Why would they go through the hassle of seeking citizenship or returning to their home country when we're providing them free services" (Oklahoma Senate 2018). Similarly, Rep. Doug LaMalfa (CA-R) insisted that Gov. Newsom's 2019 budget deal would "make California a magnet for illegal immigration" (LaMalfa 2019). In 2019, seven Republican senators and 28 Republican representatives introduced the Protect Medicaid Act in both chambers with the intention of preventing states from expanding Medicaid benefits to

Immigrants Should Not Take Advantage of Public Benefits

On February 27, 2020, Rep. Glenn Grothman (R-WI) addressed the U.S. House of Representatives to commend the Trump administration's proposed change to the public charge rule.

Ever since the 1800s in this country, we have tried to make it a point that people who come here from other countries not come here and wind up on public benefits or welfare or what have you.

Unfortunately, we weren't doing a very good job of enforcing this rule until President Trump stepped up and put a rule that went into effect last October, saying that if you are here as an immigrant, you are not eligible for food stamps; you are not eligible for low-income housing; you are not eligible for Medicaid; you are not eligible for other means-based benefits.

President Trump, having a soft heart, continues to allow immigrants, immigrant children, to receive free and reduced lunch, Medicaid, and even are eligible for student loans. Nevertheless, I think it was a very good thing for President Trump to do. Our immigrants are the future of America. Right now, in America, our immigrants are far more likely than the native-born to take advantage of public benefits.

The only reason we are trying to hold down the number of people who are here who are not citizens from getting benefits is President Trump. It could easily be true that by this time next year, we will go back to the days in which a high number of noncitizens are taking advantage of public benefits. Like I said, I think for some people, the generosity of the public benefits will encourage people to adapt a lifestyle in which they are eligible for them, which is a real crime.

Source

Congressional Record, vol. 166, no. 39 (February 27, 2020): H1244. Washington, DC: Government Printing Office. Accessed April 24, 2020. https://www.congress.gov/116/crec/2020/02/27/CREC-2020-02-27-pt1-PgH1244.pdf.

undocumented immigrants. As of November 2020, neither bill had received a vote in committee in the 116th Congress.

In October 2019, the Trump administration issued Presidential Proclamation 9945, which required applicants for immigrant visas to demonstrate the ability to obtain health insurance within one month. The proclamation noted that "while our healthcare system grapples with the challenges caused by uncompensated care, the United States Government is making the problem worse by admitting thousands of aliens who have not demonstrated any ability to pay for their healthcare costs" (White House 2019). After a district court in Oregon issued an injunction, the White House press secretary responded, "It is wrong and unfair for a single district court judge to thwart the policies that the President determined would best protect the United States healthcare system—and for the United States taxpayers to suffer the grave consequences of the immense strain inflicted on the healthcare system from subsidizing uncompensated care for those seeking admission" (Associated Press 2019). As of July 2020, the injunction remained in place following an appeals court's May 2020 denial of the federal government's request for a stay (American Immigration Lawyers Association 2020).

Republican claims that providing health care to immigrants would impose a significant financial burden expanded on the public charge doctrine, which has been a long-standing component of immigration policy in the United States. In August 2019, the Trump administration proposed changing the public charge rule to include non-cash-based public benefits, such as the Supplementary Nutrition Assistance Program (SNAP), Medicaid, and subsidies for Medicare Part D drug benefits (Tolbert, Artiga, and Pham 2019). When announcing the proposed change, Ken Cuccinelli, the acting director of the U.S. Citizenship and Immigration Services, argued, "We certainly expect people of any income to be able to stand on their own two feet" (Rodrigo 2019). In February 2020, the rule went into effect after the U.S. Supreme Court issued a 5–4 decision in which the conservative majority voted to allow implementation while legal challenges to the rule proceeded. In March 2021, the Biden administration rescinded the Trump-era policy (Kruzel 2021).

During the first months of 2020, Republicans criticized Democratic efforts to support undocumented immigrants and their families during the COVID-19 pandemic as political partisanship. California State Republican Leader Shannon Grove questioned Gov. Newsom's relief fund for undocumented immigrants, arguing that he "has chosen to irresponsibly pursue a left-wing path" at the expense of California citizens (Platt 2020). Rep. Jim Jordan (R-OH), meanwhile, stated, "We should not turn our back on the citizens and lawful immigrants of this great country to favor those that broke the law and came here illegally or overstayed their visas" (Committee on Oversight and Reform 2020). In March 2020, U.S. Citizenship and Immigration Services issued an alert stating that any individual with COVID-like symptoms should seek treatment and that such treatment would not impact any future public charge tests (U.S. Citizenship and Immigration Services 2020).

Public opinion among Republican voters echoed Jordan's sentiment, however, with polls regularly showing that a majority of self-identified Republicans believed that the federal government did not have a responsibility to provide medical care to undocumented immigrants with COVID-19 (Krogstad and Lopez 2020).

Todd M. Olszewski and Bethany Evans

Further Reading

An Act to Regulate Immigration. 1882. Public Law 47-376, *U.S. Statutes at Large* 214: 214–215. Accessed August 2, 2020. https://www.loc.gov/law/help/statutes-at-large/47th-congress/session-1/c47s1ch376.pdf.

Alvarez, Priscilla, Geneva Sands, and Tami Luhby. 2019. "Trump Admin Announces Rule That Could Limit Legal Immigration over Use of Public Benefits." CNN, August 13. Accessed May 19, 2020. https://www.cnn.com/2019/08/12/politics/legal-immigration-public-charge/index.html.

American Immigration Lawyers Association. 2020. "AILA Doc. No. 19103090." May 4. Accessed August 1, 2020. https://www.aila.org/infonet/complaint-filed-to-halt-implementation.

Archibold, Randal. 2010. "Arizona Enacts Stringent Law on Immigration." *New York Times*, April 23. Accessed May 18, 2020. https://www.nytimes.com/2010/04/24/us/politics/24immig.html.

Arroyo, Noah. 2017. "As Healthy S.F. Serves Mostly Spanish Speakers, City Vows to Shield Undocumented Clients." *San Francisco Public Press*, February 9. Accessed May 18, 2020. https://sfpublicpress.org/news/2017-02/as-healthy-sf-serves-mostly-spanish-speakers-city-vows-to-shield-undocumented-clients.

Associated Press. 2019. "US Judge Blocks Trump's Health Insurance Rule for Immigrants." November 3. Accessed March 7, 2021. https://apnews.com/article/59f973d6d02c46378ada739d129ab5f8.

Attanasio, Cedar, Garance Burke, and Martha Mendoza. 2019. "Attorneys: Texas Border Facility Is Neglecting Migrant Kids." Associated Press, June 21. Accessed May 19, 2020. https://apnews.com/46da2dbe04f54adbb875cfbc06bbc615.

Baldassare, Mark, Dean Bonner, Alyssa Dykman, and Rachel Ward. 2019. "PPIC Statewide Survey: Californians and Their Government." Public Policy Institute of California. Accessed May 18, 2020. https://www.ppic.org/wp-content/uploads/ppic-statewide-survey-californians-and-their-government-march-2019.pdf.

Baldassare, Mark, Dean Bonner, David Kordus, and Lunna Lopes. 2015. "PPIC Statewide Survey: Californians and Their Government." Public Policy Institute of California. Accessed May 18, 2020. https://www.ppic.org/content/pubs/survey/S_1215MBS.pdf.

Bernstein, Hamutal, Dulce Gonzalez, Michael Karpman, and Stephen Zuckerman. 2019. "One in Seven Adults in Immigrant Families Reported Avoiding Public Benefit Programs in 2018." Urban Institute. Accessed May 19, 2020. https://www.urban.org/sites/default/files/publication/100270/one_in_seven_adults_in_immigrant_families_reported_avoiding_publi_8.pdf.

Betz, Bradford. 2019. "California Leads Latest Lawsuit against Trump's 'Public Charge' Immigration Rule." Fox News, August 16. Accessed May 19, 2020. https://www.foxnews.com/us/california-lawsuit-against-trump-immigration-rule.

Bolton, Alexander. 2019. "All Candidates Raise Hands on Giving Health Care to Undocumented Immigrants." The Hill, June 27. Accessed August 1, 2020. https://thehill.com/homenews/campaign/450797-all-candidates-raise-hands-on-giving-health-care-to-undocumented-immigrants.

Brewer, Jan. 2010. "Statement by Governor Jan Brewer." April 23. Accessed July 10, 2020. http://i.cdn.turner.com/cnn/2010/images/04/23/brewer.statement.pdf.

Brownstein, Ronald. 2019. "The Democrats' Gamble on Health Care for the Undocumented." *The Atlantic*, July 11. Accessed May 19, 2020. https://www.theatlantic.com/politics/archive/2019/07/2020-democrats-undocumented-health-care/593761/.

Brufke, Juliegrace. 2019. "House Passes Bill to Revamp Medical Screenings for Migrants at Border." The Hill, September 26. Accessed May 19, 2020. https://thehill.com/latino/463303-house-passes-bill-to-revamp-medical-screenings-for-migrants-at-border.

Caiola, Sammy. 2019. "California Becomes First in Nation to Expand Medicaid to Undocumented Young Adults." Capital Public Radio, July 9. Accessed May 18, 2020. https://www.capradio.org/articles/2019/07/09/california-becomes-first-in-nation-to-expand-medicaid-to-undocumented-young-adults/.

CBS News. 2011. "Ariz. May Require Hospitals to Check Citizenship." February 14. Accessed May 18, 2020. https://www.cbsnews.com/news/ariz-may-require-hospitals-to-check-citizenship/.

Center for Reproductive Rights. 2015. "Congresswoman Lujan Grisham Introduces Federal Bill Restoring Vital Health Care Services to Immigrant Women and Families." April 22. Accessed May 19, 2020. https://reproductiverights.org/press-room/congresswoman-grisham-introduces-federal-bill-restoring-vital-health-care-services-to-immigrant-women-families.

City Attorney of San Francisco. 2010. "'Healthy San Francisco' Stands, as U.S. Supreme Court Denies Legal Challenge." June 28. Accessed May 18, 2020. https://www.sfcityattorney.org/2010/06/28/healthy-san-francisco-stands-as-u-s-supreme-court-denies-legal-challenge/.

City of Chicago, Office of the Mayor. 2020. "Mayor Lightfoot Signs Executive Order to Protect Immigrant and Refugee Communities during Covid-19." April 7. Accessed May 19, 2020. https://www.chicago.gov/city/en/depts/mayor/press_room/press_releases/2020/april/EOImmigrantRefugeeProtection.html.

City of New York. 2019a. "Mayor de Blasio Unveils NYC Care Card, Details Progress toward Launch of Guaranteed Health Care." May 7. Accessed May 18, 2020. https://www1.nyc.gov/office-of-the-mayor/news/239-19/mayor-de-blasio-nyc-care-card-details-progress-toward-launch-guaranteed-health-care#/0

City of New York. 2019b. "NYC Care: 5,000 New Yorkers Receiving Accessible and Affordable Health Care." October 4. Accessed May 18, 2020. https://www1.nyc.gov/office-of-the-mayor/news/463-19/nyc-care-5-000-new-yorkers-receiving-accessible-affordable-health-care.

Clines, Francis. 1996. "Clinton Signs Bill Cutting Welfare; States in New Role." *New York Times*, August 23. Accessed August 1, 2020. https://www.nytimes.com/1996/08/23/us/clinton-signs-bill-cutting-welfare-states-in-new-role.html.

CNN. 2019. "Democrats and Healthcare." July 1. Accessed July 11, 2020. http://cdn.cnn.com/cnn/2019/images/07/01/rel8a.-.democrats.and.healthcare.pdf.

Committee on Oversight and Reform. 2020. "Oversight Republicans Call Out Democrats for Using Coronavirus to Advance Their Radical Immigration Agenda." April 17. Accessed May 19, 2020. https://republicans-oversight.house.gov/release/oversight

-republicans-call-out-democrats-for-using-coronavirus-to-advance-their-radical-immigration-agenda/.

Congressional Record. 1996a. 104th Cong., 2nd sess., 142, no. 106: H 7792. Accessed July 10, 2020. https://www.congress.gov/104/crec/1996/07/18/CREC-1996-07-18-pt1-PgH7784-6.pdf.

Congressional Record. 1996b. 104th Cong., 2nd sess., 142, no. 116. Accessed July 10, 2020. https://www.congress.gov/104/crec/1996/08/01/CREC-1996-08-01-pt1-PgS9387.pdf.

Congressional Record. 1996c. 104th Cong., 2nd sess., 142, no. 106: S 8092. Accessed October 30, 2020. https://www.congress.gov/104/crec/1996/07/18/CREC-1996-07-18-pt1-PgS8076-2.pdf.

Congressional Record. 2009. 111th Cong., 1st sess., 155, no. 85. Accessed July 10, 2020. https://www.congress.gov/111/crec/2009/06/09/CREC-2009-06-09-pt1-PgH6400.pdf.

Congressional Record. 2019. 116th Congr., 1st sess., 165, no. 9. Accessed July 12, 2020. https://www.congress.gov/116/crec/2019/01/16/CREC-2019-01-16-pt1-PgH671-2.pdf.

Crenshaw, Dan. 2019. "Rep. Dan Crenshaw: Dems Are Doing Less Than Mexico to Solve Border Crisis." Fox News, June 20. Accessed May 19, 2020. https://www.foxnews.com/opinion/dan-crenshaw-democrats-mexico-border.

Dyck, Joshua, Gregg Johnson, and Jesse Wasson. 2012. "A Blue Tide in the Golden State: Ballot Initiatives, Population Change, and Party Identification in California." *American Politics Research* 40: 450–475.

Flavin, Lila, Leah Zallman, Danny McCormick, and J. Wesley Boyd. 2018. "Medical Expenditures on and by Immigrant Populations in the United States: A Systematic Review." *International Journal of Health Services: Planning, Administration, Evaluation* 48, no. 4: 601–621.

Fremstad, Shawn, and Laura Cox. 2004. "Covering New Americans: A Review of Federal and State Policies Related to Immigrants' Eligibility and Access to Publicly Funded Health Insurance." Kaiser Family Foundation. Accessed May 15, 2020. https://www.kff.org/wp-content/uploads/2013/01/covering-new-americans-a-review-of-federal-and-state-policies-related-to-immigrants-eligibility-and-access-to-publicly-funded-health-insurance-report.pdf.

Gage, John. 2019. "Ex-Arizona Governor: Trump Proposal to Dump Illegal Immigrants in Sanctuary Cities Is a 'Great Plan.'" *Washington Examiner*, April 16. Accessed May 19, 2020. https://www.washingtonexaminer.com/news/ex-arizona-governor-trumps-proposal-to-dump-illegal-immigrants-in-sanctuary-cities-a-great-plan.

Graham v. Richardson, 403 US 365 (1971).

Haaland, Deb. 2019. "Press Call on the Re-Introduction of the Health Equity and Access under the Law for Immigrant Women and Families Act (HEAL Act)." October 15. Accessed May 19, 2020. https://haaland.house.gov/media/press-releases/press-call-re-introduction-health-equity-and-access-under-law-immigrant-women.

Hayes, Joseph, and Laura Hill. 2017. "Just the Facts: Undocumented Immigrants in California." Public Policy Institute of California, March. Accessed August 2, 2020. https://www.ppic.org/publication/undocumented-immigrants-in-california/.

Hirono, Mazie. 2020. "Hirono, Harris, Chu, Grijalva, Correa Introduce Legislation to Provide Critical Assistance to Vulnerable Communities Impacted by COVID-19." April 3. Accessed May 19, 2020. https://www.hirono.senate.gov/news/press-releases/hirono-harris-chu-grijalva-correa-introduce-legislation-to-provide-critical-assistance-to-vulnerable-communities-impacted-by-covid-19-.

InMaricopa. 2011. "Maricopa's State Senator Pleased with Freshman Year's Success." April 27. Accessed May 18, 2020. https://www.inmaricopa.com/maricopas-state-senator-pleased-with-freshman-years-success/.

Jordan, Miriam, and Caitlin Dickerson. 2019. "Sick Migrants Undergoing Lifesaving Care Can Now Be Deported." *New York Times*, August 29. Accessed May 19, 2020. https://www.nytimes.com/2019/08/29/us/immigrant-medical-treatment-deferred-action.html.

Kaiser Family Foundation. 1995. "National Survey of Public Knowledge of Welfare Reform and the Federal Budget." January 12. Accessed August 2, 2020. https://www.kff.org/medicaid/poll-finding/national-survey-of-public-knowledge-of-welfare/.

Kaiser Family Foundation. 2020. "Health Coverage of Immigrants." March 18. Accessed May 19, 2020. https://www.kff.org/disparities-policy/fact-sheet/health-coverage-of-immigrants/.

Kandula, Namratha, Colleen Grogan, Paul Rathouz, and Diane Lauderdale. 2004. "The Unintended Impact of Welfare Reform on the Medicaid Enrollment of Eligible Immigrants." *HSR: Health Services Research* 39 (October): 1509–1526. Accessed August 2, 2020. https://www.ncbi.nlm.nih.gov/pmc/articles/PMC1361081/pdf/hesr_00301.pdf.

Kasich, John. 2016. "John Kasich: 20 Years after Reform, Welfare Is Still Broken." *New York Times*, August 22. Accessed August 2, 2020. https://www.nytimes.com/2016/08/22/opinion/john-kasich-20-years-after-reform-welfare-is-still-broken.html.

Kaushal, Neeraj, and Robert Kaestner. 2005. "Welfare Reform and Health Insurance of Immigrants." *HSR: Health Services Research* 40 (June): 697–721. Accessed August 1, 2020. https://www.ncbi.nlm.nih.gov/pmc/articles/PMC1361164/pdf/hesr_00381.pdf.

Knight, Heather. 2013. "Healthy S.F. Might Sicken Tea Partiers." *SFGATE*, October 26. Accessed May 18, 2020. https://www.sfgate.com/bayarea/article/Healthy-S-F-might-sicken-Tea-Partiers-4929116.php.

Koseff, Alexei. 2015. "California Senate Approves Health Care for Undocumented Immigrants." *Sacramento Bee*, June 2. Accessed July 10, 2020. https://www.sacbee.com/news/politics-government/capitol-alert/article22904433.html.

Kovanis, Georgea. 2019. "Michigan Attorney General Sues Federal Government for Violating Immigrants' Rights." *Detroit Free Press*, August 15. Accessed May 19, 2020. https://www.freep.com/story/news/local/michigan/detroit/2019/08/15/michigan-attorney-general-immigrant-rights-lawsuit/2009322001/.

Krogstad, Jens Manuel, and Mark Hugo Lopez. 2020. "Americans Favor Medical Care but Not Economic Aid for Undocumented Immigrants Affected by COVID-19." Pew Research Center, May 20. Accessed August 1, 2020. https://www.pewresearch.org/fact-tank/2020/05/20/americans-favor-medical-care-but-not-economic-aid-for-undocumented-immigrants-affected-by-covid-19/.

Kruzel, John. 2021. "Biden Rescinds Trump's 'Public Charge' Rule." The Hill, March 11. Accessed March 14, 2021. https://thehill.com/regulation/court-battles/542860-biden-rescinds-trumps-public-charge-rule

LaMalfa, Doug. 2019. "LaMalfa: California Providing Free Health Care to Illegal Immigrants Is Insane." June 12. Accessed May 19, 2020. https://lamalfa.house.gov/media-center/press-releases/lamalfa-california-providing-free-health-care-to-illegal-immigrants-is.

Loiaconi, Stephen. 2020. "Partisan Battle Lines Drawn over Aid to Undocumented amid Outbreak." ABC6, April 17. Accessed May 19, 2020. https://abc6onyourside.com/news/nation-world/partisan-battle-lines-drawn-over-aid-to-undocumented-amid-outbreak.

Luthi, Susannah. 2020. "Supreme Court Allows Trump to Enforce 'Public Charge' Immigration Rule." Politico, January 27. Accessed August 2, 2020. https://www.politico.com/news/2020/01/27/supreme-court-enforce-trump-immigration-rule-106520.

MacLeod, Laurie, Darrel Montero, and Alan Speer. 1999. "America's Changing Attitudes toward Welfare and Welfare Recipients, 1938–1995." *Journal of Sociology & Social Welfare* 26 (June): 175–186. Accessed August 1, 2020. https://scholarworks.wmich.edu/cgi/viewcontent.cgi?referer=&httpsredir=1&article=2574&context=jssw

Malliotakis, Nicole (@NMalliotakis). 2019. "Our Citizens Have Hard Enough Time Covering Their Own Healthcare Costs. Now, @nycmayor also Wants Them to Pay for Healthcare of 300,000 Citizens of Other Countries. He Must Stop Abusing the Middle Class and Treating Us Like His Personal ATM. #deBlasioCare." Twitter, January 8. https://twitter.com/NMalliotakis/status/1082674200245161984.

McDaniel, Ronna (@GOPChairwoman). 2019. "Millions of Americans Struggle to Pay Their Own Health Care Bills. Now Democrats Want Us to Pay Illegal Immigrants'? We Can't Afford Their Extreme Agenda!" Twitter, June 28. https://twitter.com/GOPChairwoman/status/1144611920953171968.

Mento, Tarryn. 2020. "Medi-Cal Expands Health Coverage for Young Adults Who Can't Prove Legal Residence." KPBS, January 2. Accessed May 19, 2020. https://www.kpbs.org/news/2020/jan/02/medi-cal-expansion-impact-estimated-10000-undocume/.

Metz, Dave, and Greg Strimple. 2014. "Findings of a Statewide Survey on Expanding Access to Health Coverage." Kaiser Family Foundation, September 30. Accessed August 2, 2020. https://www.kff.org/wp-content/uploads/sites/2/2014/10/fm3-gs_strat-final_memo.pdf.

Nam, Yunju. 2008. "Welfare Reform and Older Immigrants' Health Insurance Coverage." *American Journal of Public Health* 98, no. 11 (November): 2029–2034. Accessed August 2, 2020. https://www.ncbi.nlm.nih.gov/pmc/articles/PMC2636438/pdf/2029.pdf.

Noonan, Peggy. 2020. "New York Is the Epicenter of the World." *Wall Street Journal*, April 2. Accessed August 2, 2020. https://www.wsj.com/articles/new-york-is-the-epicenter-of-the-world-11585869852.

Nowrasteh, Alex. 2016. "Proposition 187 Turned California Blue." Cato Institute, July 20. Accessed August 2, 2020. https://www.cato.org/blog/proposition-187-turned-california-blue.

Oklahoma Senate. 2018. "Federal Government Forcing States to Pay for Pregnant Illegal Immigrants' Healthcare through CHIP." December 13. Accessed May 19, 2020. https://oksenate.gov/press-releases/federal-government-forcing-states-pay-pregnant-illegal-immigrants-healthcare-through.

Pew Research Center. 1997. "When Washington Works, Incumbents Proper." August 15. Accessed August 2, 2020. https://www.pewresearch.org/politics/1997/08/15/when-washington-works-incumbents-prosper/.

Pew Research Center. 2002. "Americans Struggle with Religion's Role at Home and Abroad." March 20. Accessed August 1, 2020. https://www.pewforum.org/2002/03/20/americans-struggle-with-religions-role-at-home-and-abroad/.

Platt, Jeff. 2020. "Grove Slams Newsom for Using Tax Dollars to Aid Undocumented Immigrants." KBAK, April 16. Accessed May 19, 2020. https://bakersfieldnow.com/news/local/grove-slams-newsom-for-using-tax-dollars-to-aid-undocumented-immigrants.

Rodrigo, Chris Mills. 2019. "Trump Administration Releases New 'Public Charge' Rule Making It Easier to Reject Immigrants." The Hill, August 12. Accessed May 19, 2020. https://thehill.com/homenews/administration/457077-trump-administration-releases-final-public-charge-rule.

Roybal-Allard, Lucille. 2016. "California Democratic Congressional Delegation Urges Approval of State Waiver to Allow Undocumented Immigrants to Buy into Obamacare." September 14. Accessed May 19, 2020. https://roybal-allard.house.gov/news/documentsingle.aspx?DocumentID=398116.

Saloner, Brendan, Neel Koyawala, and Genevieve M. Kenney. 2014. "Coverage for Low-Income Immigrant Children Increased 24.5 Percent in States That Expanded CHIPRA Eligibility." *Health Affairs* 33, no. 5: 832–839.

Tanner, Michael. 2016. "Twenty Years after Welfare Reform: The Welfare System Remains in Place." Cato Institute, May 2. Accessed August 2, 2020. https://www.cato.org/publications/commentary/twenty-years-after-welfare-reform-welfare-system-remains-place.

Tavernise, Sabrina. 2018. "U.S. Has Highest Share of Foreign-Born since 1910, with More Coming from Asia." *New York Times*, September 13. Accessed May 15, 2020. https://www.nytimes.com/2018/09/13/us/census-foreign-population.html.

Tin, Alexander. 2019. "Does Medicare for All Cover Undocumented Immigrants? Depends on Who You Ask." CBS News, June 13. Accessed May 19, 2020. https://www.cbsnews.com/news/does-medicare-for-all-cover-undocumented-immigrants-depends-on-who-you-ask/.

Tolbert, Jennifer, Samantha Artiga, and Olivia Pham. 2019. "Impact of Shifting Immigration Policy on Medicaid Enrollment and Utilization of Care among Health Center Patients." Kaiser Family Foundation, October 15. Accessed May 19, 2020. https://www.kff.org/report-section/impact-of-shifting-immigration-policy-on-medicaid-enrollment-and-utilization-of-care-among-health-center-patients-issue-brief/.

Toomey, Russell B., Adriana J. Umana-Taylor, David R. Williams, Elizabeth Harvey-Mendoza, Laudan B. Jahromi, and Kimberly A. Updegraff. 2014. "Impact of Arizona's SB 1070 Immigration Law on Utilization of Health Care and Public Assistance among Mexican-Origin Adolescent Mothers and Their Mother Figures." *American Journal of Public Health* 104 (Suppl. 1): S28–S34.

Trump, Donald. 2020. "State of the Union Address." February 4. Accessed July 12, 2020. https://www.govinfo.gov/content/pkg/DCPD-202000058/pdf/DCPD-202000058.pdf.

Turner, Scott. 2019. "Bill Would Ease Immigrants' Access to Health Care." *Albuquerque Journal*, October 20. Accessed May 19, 2020. https://www.abqjournal.com/1380989/bill-would-ease-immigrants-access-to-health-care.html.

U.S. Citizenship and Immigration Services. 2020. "USCIS Response to Coronavirus 2019 (COVID-19)." March 27. Accessed July 11, 2020. https://www.uscis.gov/green-card/green-card-processes-and-procedures/public-charge.

U.S. Congress, House. 2016. *Mobile Medical Immigrant Health Improvement Act of 2016*. H.R. 5981, 114th Cong., 2nd sess. Introduced in House September 9, 2016, https://www.govtrack.us/congress/bills/114/hr5981/text.

Valencia, Nick, and Catherine E. Shoichet. 2019. "Lack of Soap, Filthy Onesies and Too Few Beds Have Created a 'Heath Crisis' at Border Detention Facilities, Monitors Warn." CNN, June 21. Accessed May 19, 2020. https://www.cnn.com/2019/06/20/politics/border-detention-facilities-health/index.html.

Wamsley, Laurel, Pam Fessler, and Richard Gonzales. 2019. "Federal Judges in 3 States Block Trump's 'Public Charge' Rule for Green Cards." NPR, October 11. Accessed August 1, 2020. https://www.npr.org/2019/10/11/769376154/n-y-judge-blocks-trump-administrations-public-charge-rule.

Weixel, Nathaniel. 2020. "Federal Judge Blocks Immigration 'Public Charge' Rule due to Pandemic." The Hill, July 29. Accessed August 1, 2020. https://thehill.com/latino/509706-federal-judge-blocks-trump-immigration-public-charge-rule-due-to-pandemic.

White House. 2019. "Presidential Proclamation on the Suspension of Entry of Immigrants Who Will Financially Burden the United States Healthcare System." October 4. Accessed July 12, 2020. https://trumpwhitehouse.archives.gov/presidential-actions/presidential-proclamation-suspension-entry-immigrants-will-financially-burden-united-states-healthcare-system/.

Wills, Garry. 1997. "The Clinton Principle." *New York Times*, January 19. Accessed August 1, 2020. https://www.nytimes.com/1997/01/19/magazine/the-clinton-principle.html.

Individual Health Insurance Mandate

At a Glance

The Affordable Care Act (ACA), or Obamacare, which President Obama signed into law on March 23, 2010, includes a requirement that all individuals must provide proof of health insurance coverage or pay a penalty when filing their taxes. A health insurance mandate plays an essential role in reforming the health insurance marketplace by allowing insurers to spread the risk of illness among more subscribers. In the absence of an effective mandate, healthier individuals may opt out of the market, leaving fewer, and sicker, patients in the risk pool (Mach 2018). Over time, this drives premiums up, as only the sickest people opt to purchase increasingly expensive coverage.

The requirement to purchase health insurance was a key element of the ACA's "three-legged stool" of reforms—the others being premium subsidies and protections for persons with preexisting conditions—to the individual health insurance market (Brill 2015). Beginning in 2014, the ACA required individuals to maintain "minimum essential coverage" or pay a tax penalty (starting at $95 in 2014) and rising to either 2.5 percent of yearly household income or $695 (whichever is higher). Exemptions to the requirement are granted for religious reasons, financial hardship, and for individuals below the tax filing threshold, among others (Mach 2018).

On the same day Obama signed the ACA into law, 14 state attorneys general challenged the requirement to purchase health insurance in federal court (Klein 2012). Ultimately, 26 states—all with Republican governors or attorneys general—filed suit in federal court to challenge the constitutionality of the individual health insurance mandate. In 2012, the U.S. Supreme Court upheld the constitutionality of the individual mandate in *National Federation of Independent Business v. Sebelius*. Nevertheless, the mandate continued to be a lightning rod for public opposition to the ACA.

After the election of Donald Trump, congressional Republicans sought to fulfill their long-standing pledge to "repeal and replace" the ACA during the spring and summer of 2017. Despite several attempts, however, Republicans narrowly failed to cobble together a majority in the Senate to repeal the ACA.

Repealing "the Worst Parts of Obamacare"

Speaking on the floor of the House of Representatives on May 4, 2017, Rep. Diane Black (R-TN) urged her colleagues to repeal the Affordable Care Act by voting for H.R. 1628, the American Health Care Act.

Under ObamaCare, the situation is getting worse every day. . . . Throughout this process, our commitment to undoing the damage done by ObamaCare has remained steadfast. Day after day, my constituents call my office begging us to do something to save them from ObamaCare, and it is because ObamaCare is collapsing. In my State of Tennessee, families are suffering. Premiums have increased by 60 percent, while deductibles are so high that, even if someone has an insurance card, it doesn't mean they have guaranteed care.

There are parts of my State in Tennessee that don't have a single insurance provider in the marketplace, and two-thirds of the counties have only one provider. That is not competition. That is called a monopoly.

While no legislation is perfect, this bill makes some important changes to help American families get quality, affordable health insurance: It zeros out the mandates, it repeals the taxes, and it repeals the subsidies; it allows people to choose health insurance plans to meet the unique needs of their families instead of purchasing a one-size-fits-all plan mandated by a Washington bureaucrat; and it modernizes Medicaid, a once-in-a-lifetime entitlement reform.

Source

Congressional Record. House of Representatives. "The American Health Care Act of 2017." May 4. Accessed March 1, 2021. https://www.congress.gov/115/crec/2017/05/04/CREC-2017-05-04-pt1-PgH4149-2.pdf.

In late 2017, Republicans refocused their attention on repealing the individual mandate as part of a larger tax reform bill: the Tax Cuts and Jobs Act (TCJA). The TCJA ended the tax penalty for individuals without qualifying health coverage, effective January 1, 2019. However, the TCJA did not repeal the individual mandate itself.

By eliminating this shared responsibility payment, 20 Republican-led states—led by Texas—argued that Congress had removed the legal foundation for the mandate itself, which had previously been upheld by the U.S. Supreme Court as a tax. The lawsuit was filed in a federal district court, where Judge Reed O'Connor—a conservative judge appointed to the bench by President George W. Bush—heard the case. As Judge O'Connor wrote in his decision, "The Individual Mandate is no longer fairly readable as an exercise of Congress's Tax Power and continues to be unsustainable under Congress's Interstate Commerce Power. The Court therefore finds the Individual Mandate, unmoored from a tax, is unconstitutional" (O'Connor 2018, 34).

In December 2019, the Fifth Circuit Court of Appeals upheld O'Connor's assessment that the individual mandate was unconstitutional, although it sent the case back to Judge O'Connor for further review on whether this rendered the entire ACA unconstitutional. Judge Jennifer Elrod wrote for the 2–1 majority, "The individual mandate is unconstitutional because it can no longer be read as a tax, and there is no other constitutional provision that justifies this exercise of congressional power" (*Texas v. United States* 2019). In April 2020, the U.S. Supreme Court agreed to hear the case during its 2020–2021 term, leaving the future of the individual mandate in doubt.

Most Democrats regard the individual mandate as a cornerstone of the ACA. As such, the individual mandate is vital to sustaining functioning health insurance markets. Without an effective mandate, Democrats fear younger and healthier individuals will not purchase coverage. If only older and sicker individuals buy health insurance, premiums will increase sharply, raising the risk of a "death spiral" in the marketplace. As a result, Democrats warned that the repeal of the individual mandate will cause millions of Americans to lose their health insurance. In the end, Democrats believe that requiring individuals to purchase health insurance is necessary to pool the cost of illness among all citizens. While Democrats regarded the lawsuit as a frivolous challenge to the ACA, previous experience with *NFIB v. Sebelius* offered a cautionary tale, as federal courts had afforded a receptive audience for opponents of the ACA in the past.

Although many Republicans initially supported an individual mandate for the purchase of health insurance in the early 1990s, over the course of the 2010s, the party displayed near unanimous opposition to this feature of the ACA. Republicans described the ACA's individual mandate as an unwarranted intrusion into the health care marketplace. Because Republicans also viewed the mandate as the connective tissue linking the various components of the ACA together, they argued that repealing the individual mandate would cause the ACA to unravel. In addition, Republicans claimed that the individual mandate imposed a heavy financial burden on millions of Americans who did not qualify for premium subsidies. Thus, the mandate disproportionately affected families who were least able to afford the additional cost of purchasing health insurance. Furthermore, Republicans contended that the individual mandate coerced millions of Americans—particularly younger and healthier consumers—into buying more expensive insurance policies than they wanted or needed. From their perspective, Americans should be free to choose the insurance that is right for their own personal circumstances without interference from the government. The Trump administration refused to defend the constitutionality of the ACA during its journey through the federal courts and ultimately sided with opponents of the law who argued that the individual mandate—without a corresponding tax penalty—could no longer be upheld as a valid exercise of congressional power.

According to Many Democrats . . .

- The individual mandate is vital to the success of the Affordable Care Act by encouraging younger and healthier persons to sign up for insurance, offsetting the cost of older and sicker individuals.
- Eliminating the individual mandate will cause health insurance premiums to rise sharply.
- Repealing the individual mandate will cause millions of Americans to lose health insurance coverage.
- The individual mandate promotes shared responsibility for health that benefits all members of society.

According to Many Republicans . . .

- Repealing the individual mandate will cause the Affordable Care Act to collapse.
- The individual mandate imposes a heavy financial burden on millions of Americans who do not qualify for premium subsidies under the ACA.
- The individual mandate forces millions of Americans to buy more expensive insurance policies than they want or need.
- Americans should be free to choose the insurance that is right for their own personal circumstances without interference from the government.

Overview

An individual mandate to purchase health insurance has been hotly debated in the United States for over three decades. Other nations, such as the Netherlands, Singapore, and Switzerland, require individuals to purchase health insurance or pay a significant penalty. Each country enacted a strong mandate with significant penalties for noncompliance as a way to achieve universal coverage while preserving the role of private insurers. In Switzerland, for example, government garnishes the wages of individuals who do not comply with the mandate to recoup the cost of the premiums (Herzlinger, Richman, and Boxer 2017). Swiss cantons—the equivalent of U.S. states—can also impose a penalty, which ranges from 30 percent to 50 percent above the cost of insurance premiums for individuals who ignore the mandate; after three months, government can unilaterally enroll uninsured individuals in a health insurance plan (Zamosky 2016). Similarly, in the Netherlands, government may pick a health plan on a citizen's behalf and deduct the cost of the premium from his or her paycheck (Zamosky 2016). In other words, a strong mandate presents individuals with a choice of purchasing insurance or paying penalties that approximate, or exceed, the cost of insurance premiums.

In the United States, the individual health insurance mandate was originally the brainchild of a conservative think tank. The Heritage Foundation viewed such a requirement as a viable alternative to more sweeping proposals for national health care reform advanced by Democrats. In 1989, Stuart Butler, a research fellow at Heritage, observed that mandating individuals to "obtain adequate insurance" reflected "two important principles. First, that health care protection is a responsibility of individuals, not businesses. . . . Second, it assumes that there is an implicit contract between households and society" (Butler 1989). Butler's proposal on "Assuring Affordable Health Care for All Americans" envisioned a requirement for individuals to purchase inexpensive "catastrophic" coverage to protect against unexpected illnesses rather than a comprehensive health plan that covered routine health care services (Butler 2012). Butler argued that an individual mandate "certainly would force those with adequate means to obtain insurance protection, which would end the problem of middle-class 'free riders'" (Butler 1989). In addition, Butler noted that publicly funded premium subsidies could be introduced to help low-income individuals defray the cost of coverage.

During the debate over President Bill Clinton's comprehensive health care reform bill in 1993, Sen. John Chafee (R-RI) embraced an individual mandate as a Republican alternative to "Clinton Care." The Chafee bill, known as the Health Equity and Access Reform Today (HEART) Act, required all individuals to provide proof of health insurance coverage and included subsidies for low-income individuals to defray the cost of coverage (Kaiser Health News 2010). The individual mandate gained bipartisan traction in 2004 when Sen. John Edwards (D-NC) proposed an insurance mandate for children (not adults) during his unsuccessful campaign for the Democratic nomination (Cooper 2012). In 2007, Sen. Ron Wyden (D-OR) introduced the Healthy Americans Act, which required individuals not enrolled in a health plan to purchase coverage for themselves and their dependent children or pay a penalty. None of these federal initiatives received serious consideration in Congress.

At the state level, Gov. Mitt Romney of Massachusetts—a popular Republican—reached across the aisle in 2006 to enact the nation's first individual health insurance mandate. His proposal received support from Democratic legislators and the endorsement of leading liberals, such as Sen. Edward Kennedy (D-MA). The mandate offered policy makers a way to retain federal dollars from the state's existing Medicaid waiver, which paid hundreds of millions of dollars in additional payments annually to "disproportionate share hospitals" treating indigent patients. Kennedy and Romney argued that the state could increase coverage by subsidizing the cost of purchasing insurance rather than reimbursing providers for uncompensated care (McDonough 2011). However, the circumstances in the Bay State were unique. The expiration of the state's Medicaid waiver created a strong sense of urgency for policy makers. In effect, "Massachusetts put a financial gun to its head that made passage of universal coverage legislation a policy, political and financial necessity" (McDonough 2011).

Massachusetts's approach to health care reform is often compared to a "three-legged stool" (McDonough 2011). First, the state enacted insurance market reforms, such as protections for individuals with preexisting conditions, community-rated premiums, and a ban on health-based discrimination (a practice known as "medical redlining"). Second, the new law required individuals to purchase insurance or pay a fine of up to half of the cost of coverage. Third, Massachusetts incorporated generous public subsidies (funded by federal Medicaid waiver funds) alongside the new mandate to lower the cost of compliance. Massachusetts emerged as the principal model for the Affordable Care Act (ACA) after the election of Barack Obama in 2008 (McDonough 2011).

The individual mandate in the ACA was quite weak. Neither Democrats nor Republicans viewed strong penalties as a politically advantageous position. As a result, penalties for noncompliance were low compared to those instituted in other nations. The ACA also contained a wide range of exemptions that limited the scope of penalties for noncompliance, including hardship exemptions, affordability exemptions for low-income individuals, religious exemptions, and allowances for brief periods without insurance (Mach 2018). Furthermore, the individual mandate established by the ACA did not take effect until January 2014—nearly four years after President Obama signed it into law. Under pressure from Sens. Olympia Snowe (R-ME) and Chuck Schumer (D-NY), the ACA set the penalty for individuals who did not purchase health insurance that met the "minimum essential coverage" provisions established by the ACA at only $95 (or 1 percent of income, whichever was greater) during the first year (McDonough 2011). The penalties gradually increased over time, reaching $695 or 2.5 percent of income—whichever is greater—in 2017 (Mach 2018). The ACA penalties reflected a delicate political balance, as "the consequences needed to be enough to make you want to conform with the Act but not so onerous that Congress would be loathe to vote for it" (Erb 2015). As a result, the new mandate failed to provide a strong financial incentive for individuals to purchase coverage. Penalty and exemption data underscore the limits of the ACA mandate; more than twice as many individuals claimed exemptions than paid the mandate penalty (Mach 2018).

A stronger individual health insurance mandate (with penalties for noncompliance) was never popular with the American public. At the time of the congressional vote to approve the ACA in 2010, only 28 percent of the public favored an "individual mandate with penalties." When the subject of penalties was *not* included in questions, more than half of respondents expressed support for an "individual mandate with subsidies" (Blendon and Benson 2010). Notably, more than half (56 percent) of the public believed that the ACA would lead to too much government involvement in the health care system (Blendon and Benson 2010). As a new requirement that directly impacted individuals, the health insurance mandate embodied public fears of too much government. Public opposition to the mandate was not short-lived; the mandate remained one of most unpopular elements of the ACA. In 2017, only 35 percent of respondents favored "requiring nearly all Americans to have health insurance or else pay a fine" (Blendon and Benson 2017).

Public opinion displayed a sharp partisan divide. One poll found that only 21 percent of Republicans favored a mandate compared to 57 percent of Democrats (Blendon and Benson 2017). That same poll reported that 55 percent of Republicans favored "removing the requirement that people obtain health insurance or pay a penalty," but only 38 percent of Democrats supported its repeal (Blendon and Benson 2017). A 2017 poll by the Kaiser Family Foundation revealed an even wider partisan split on "no longer enforcing the requirement that all individuals have health insurance or pay a fine" (Kirzinger et al. 2017). While nearly all Democrats (94 percent) opposed this proposal, a solid majority (66 percent) of Republicans believed the Trump administration should no longer enforce the mandate. Public opinion polls also cast doubt about the significance and effectiveness of the mandate itself. In 2018, a Kaiser poll found that only one-third (34 percent) of individuals in the non–group insurance market cited the mandate as a "major reason" for purchasing health insurance (Kaiser Family Foundation 2018).

In 2017, a diverse coalition of health insurers, hospitals, and physician groups urged legislators "to maintain the individual mandate unless and until Congress can enact a package of reforms to adequately assure a balanced risk pool and prevent extraordinary premium increases" (America's Health Insurance Plans et al. 2017). Providers and insurers warned that "repealing the individual mandate without offering a workable alternative will reduce enrollment, further destabilizing an already fragile individual and small group health insurance market on which more than 10 million Americans rely" (America's Health Insurance Plans et al. 2017). As Sherry Glied (2008) noted, "Perhaps the most important benefit of mandates is symbolic. By mandating the purchase of health insurance, governments signal to their citizens that coverage is critical."

Substantial evidence exists that suggests the individual mandate contributed to a large reduction in the number of uninsured individuals. The uninsured rate fell sharply for individuals with incomes above 400 percent of the federal poverty line, who did not qualify for premium subsidies (Fiedler 2018). In addition, the proportion of young adults with insurance coverage also increased after the mandate took effect in 2014. Overall, the mandate reduced the number of uninsured by 4.6–8 million individuals in 2016 (Fiedler 2018). Without a mandate, the Congressional Budget Office (CBO) estimated that the number of uninsured Americans would increase by 13 million over a 10-year period, leading to significant increases in health insurance premiums as younger and healthier consumers dropped coverage (Sanger-Katz 2017). Despite these factors, the Republican-controlled Congress opted to repeal the financial penalty for not having health insurance as part of the Tax Cuts and Jobs Act (TCJA) passed in December 2017.

The individual health insurance mandate contained within the ACA led to numerous legal challenges as well. Opponents of the ACA—including 26 states

Individuals Need to Take Responsibility for Buying Health Insurance

On June 28, 2012, President Barack Obama underscored the significance of the Supreme Court's decision to uphold the Affordable Care Act's individual mandate in the case of National Federation of Independent Business v. Sebelius.

> Today, the Supreme Court also upheld the principle that people who can afford health insurance should take the responsibility to buy health insurance. This is important for two reasons. First, when uninsured people who can afford coverage get sick, and show up at the emergency room for care, the rest of us end up paying for their care in the form of higher premiums. And second, if you ask insurance companies to cover people with preexisting conditions, but don't require people who can afford it to buy their own insurance, some folks might wait until they're sick to buy the care they need—which would also drive up everybody else's premiums. That's why, even though I knew it wouldn't be politically popular, and resisted the idea when I ran for this office, we ultimately included a provision in the Affordable Care Act that people who can afford to buy health insurance should take the responsibility to do so. In fact, this idea has enjoyed support from members of both parties, including the current Republican nominee for President.

Source

Remarks by the President on Supreme Court Ruling on the Affordable Care Act. June 28. Accessed March 1, 2021. https://obamawhitehouse.archives.gov/the-press-office/2012/06/28/remarks-president-supreme-court-ruling-affordable-care-act.

with Republican governors or attorneys general—first challenged the validity of the individual mandate in the case of *National Federation of Independent Business (NFIB) v. Sebelius*. In a 5–4 decision in June 2012, the Supreme Court's five conservative justices held that the individual mandate was not a valid exercise of Congress' power to regulate commerce, as the Constitution does not empower Congress to compel individuals to participate in commercial activity. Instead, Chief Justice John Roberts sided with the court's four liberal justices to sustain the mandate as a valid exercise of Congress' well-established power to tax. As Roberts noted in his majority opinion for the court, "Congress's authority under the taxing power is limited to requiring an individual to pay money into the Federal Treasury, no more. . . . The Affordable Care Act's requirement that certain individuals pay a financial penalty for not obtaining health insurance may reasonably be characterized as a tax" (*National Federation of Independent Business v. Sebelius* 2012). However, the court's decision to uphold the ACA's individual mandate as a tax opened the door to a fresh legal challenge after Congress voted to repeal the tax penalty in 2017.

The passage of the TCJA in December 2017 removed the consequences for not having insurance, but it left the individual mandate untouched. Conservatives seized upon the new reality—a mandate to purchase insurance without an accompanying tax penalty—to mount a new legal challenge against Obamacare. Twenty states argued that Congress' decision to end the tax penalty for not having health insurance undermined the foundation of the ACA itself. In their brief for the Fifth Circuit, lawyers for the State of Texas noted, "The mandate now raises no revenue and therefore cannot by any conceivable definition be considered a tax. Stripped of its tax status, the individual mandate is nothing more than an unconstitutional congressional mandate to purchase health insurance" (Biskupic 2019).

In December 2018, federal district court Judge Reed O'Connor agreed: "In *NFIB*, the Supreme Court held the Individual Mandate was unconstitutional under the Interstate Commerce Clause but could fairly be read as an exercise of Congress's Tax Power because it triggered a tax. The TCJA eliminated that tax. The Supreme Court's reasoning in *NFIB*—buttressed by other binding precedent and plain text—thus compels the conclusion that the Individual Mandate may no longer be upheld under the Tax Power. And because the Individual Mandate continues to mandate the purchase of health insurance, it remains unsustainable under the Interstate Commerce Clause—as the Supreme Court already held" (O'Connor 2018). Judge O'Connor's ruling identified the individual mandate as a "signature provision" of ACA that was essential for the law's other insurance market reforms to operate.

Although Judge O'Connor's ruling invalidated the individual mandate—and with it the ACA in its entirety—this decision was stayed pending appellate review. In March 2019, the Trump administration declared its support for Judge O'Connor's ruling. In an unprecedented decision, the Justice Department declined to defend the ACA in court. It did not challenge the contentions of critics such as Texas Attorney General Ken Paxton, who declared that "Congress meant for the individual mandate to be the centerpiece of Obamacare. Without the constitutional justification for the centerpiece, the law must go down" (Paxton 2019).

In oral arguments before the Fifth Circuit Court of Appeals, Texas Solicitor General Kyle Hawkins charged that "the Affordable Care Act presents a standalone command to buy an insurance product that the federal government deems suitable, and it does so without raising a single dime of revenue" (Kendall 2019). In response, California's Deputy Solicitor General argued that "the individual mandate no longer requires anyone to do anything" (Kendall 2019). California officials supportive of the ACA also argued that upholding Judge O'Connor's decision "conflicts with the plain intent of Congress and could create chaos and harm tens of millions of Americans" (Biskupic 2019).

In December 2019, the U.S. Court of Appeals for the Fifth Circuit affirmed Judge O'Connor's ruling that the individual mandate, as amended by the TCJA, was unconstitutional because it could no longer be saved by Congress' power to tax since it no longer produced any revenue for the government (Musumeci 2020). The 2–1 decision was authored by two conservative judges, Jennifer Elrod and

Kurt Englehart, who were appointed to the appellate bench by Presidents George W. Bush and Donald Trump, respectively. The court's lone Democrat, Judge Carolyn King—filed a lengthy dissenting opinion (Keith 2019). But this decision is not the last legal word on the individual mandate or the ACA. The appellate court ruling will be reviewed once again by the U.S. Supreme Court during its 2020–2021 term. Thus, "10 years after its enactment, the only certainty for the ACA in the foreseeable future is that there is continuing uncertainty about its ultimate survival" (Musumeci 2020).

The most recent challenge underscores the sharp partisan divide over the individual mandate. "The case was brought by twenty states whose most distinct common quality is their redness. Maine and Wisconsin dropped out of the suit after the 2018 midterm elections when their Republican governors were replaced by Democrats. When the Trump administration declined to defend the law, a group of mostly blue states got permission from the district court to do so. They were joined by a lawyer for the Democratic-controlled House of Representatives" (Sorkin 2019).

In the wake of the TCJA and the recent court challenges to the constitutionality of the individual mandate—and by extension the ACA itself—several states took the lead in framing new mandates and penalties. As John McDonough, a health policy scholar at the Harvard School of Public Health, noted, "If future state and federal policymakers wish to surpass the high-water mark for insurance coverage attained under the ACA, restoring an individual mandate or something like it should be part of the policy conversation" (Fiedler 2018). In June 2019, the California State Legislature passed SB 78, a bill establishing a new state tax on individuals who do not purchase health insurance, effectively restoring the individual mandate repealed by Congress. The bill passed the California State Assembly by a 57–14 margin, with only one Democrat dissenting. The law imposed a $695 penalty on persons without qualifying health coverage, effective January 1, 2020. Undocumented individuals, incarcerated persons, and members of recognized American Indian tribes are exempt from the new mandate (East County Today 2019). Other states—including Massachusetts, New Jersey, and Vermont—also enacted state-level health insurance mandates (Young and Ibarra 2019).

Democrats and Republicans remain split about the consequences of repealing the individual health insurance mandate. Academic health policy experts are also divided. Some scholars warn that "without an individual mandate, the nongroup insurance pools will shrink, with healthy people being more likely to disenroll" (Blumberg and Holahan 2017). Others, however, argue that the repeal of the mandate is unlikely to have a significant impact because "the Obama administration, and subsequently the Trump administration, did not enforce it; and it's hard to have a powerful mandate if the administration is giving millions of exemptions and creating really broad exemption categories, which the Obama administration did for political reasons" (Lovelace 2018).

Despite the repeal of the individual mandate penalty in 2017, the number of Americans without health insurance did not increase significantly in 2018 (Keith 2018). As journalist Dylan Scott observed, "Obamacare, the imperfect product that it is, isn't going to collapse without the mandate. The law has proved rather resilient under Trump: Nearly as many people signed up for coverage for 2018 as did for 2017. The subsidies deserve the credit: For people with lower incomes, they help make insurance genuinely affordable or even free. That won't change when the mandate goes away. Even if insurers raise their premiums, the subsidies will protect the people who receive them from those hikes. So Obamacare is likely to keep its market of 10 million or so customers" (Scott 2018)

Democrats on the Individual Mandate

The Affordable Care Act (ACA) was the Obama administration's signature domestic policy achievement. The passage of the ACA, commonly known as Obamacare, represented the fulfillment of a decades-old promise by Democrats to move toward a health care system that provided coverage for all Americans. To preserve the role of private insurers in the U.S. health care system, the ACA incorporated an individual health insurance mandate along with fundamental reforms of the existing insurance market. The ACA limited the ability of insurers to "cherry pick" healthy subscribers, extended coverage for adult children, and introduced protections for individuals with preexisting conditions.

In exchange for complying with these new requirements, the ACA promised insurers millions of new paying customers. In particular, the Obama administration sought to bring millions of younger (and healthier) individuals into the insurance market. Because potential customers—also known as "young invincibles" in health policy circles—often opted to not purchase insurance, an individual mandate would bring them into the marketplace, significantly broadening the risk pool. As President Obama explained in 2009, "Unless everyone does their part, many of the insurance reforms we seek—especially requiring insurance companies to cover pre-existing conditions—just can't be achieved. That's why under my plan everyone will be required to carry basic health insurance, just as most states require you to carry auto insurance" (Obama 2009).

Democrats in Congress and the Obama administration defended the individual mandate as the only way to ensure that other elements of the ACA would work as designed. In 2016, Health and Human Services Secretary Sylvia Burwell compared the ACA to "a game of Jenga, where you have the puzzle pieces, and, if you pull one out, the thing will topple. And it's important to understand, when one has people with pre-existing conditions in the insurance pool, there are other things that you have to do. You have to make sure everybody is in the pool, so you spread that risk. That is what insurance is. It is about spreading risk. And that's why there is a mandate to have everyone in" (Woodruff 2016). In short, popular reforms to the insurance market were tightly interwoven with the less popular mandate to purchase health insurance or pay a penalty. Younger and healthier subscribers played a vital role in subsidizing the cost of coverage for older and sicker enrollees, as they contributed premiums while using, on average, fewer health care services. After the 2016 election, Democrats warned that Republican proposals to repeal the individual mandate would lead to the "destruction of the Affordable Care Act" and result in a "life-or-death struggle for millions of American families" (Miller 2017).

In addition, Democrats warned that repealing the individual health insurance mandate would raise health insurance premiums for millions of Americans. During the debate over the Tax Cuts and Jobs Act (TCJA) in 2017, House Minority Leader Nancy Pelosi (D-CA) argued that if the TCJA bill passed, "Those with private insurance will experience higher premiums and higher deductibles, with lower tax credits to help working families cover the costs, even as their plans might no longer cover pregnancy, mental health care, or expensive prescriptions. Discrimination based on pre-existing conditions could become the norm again. Millions of families will lose coverage entirely" (Newkirk 2017). Without a mandate, Democrats worried that younger and healthier subscribers would once again forego insurance coverage, creating an "adverse selection" problem for insurers in which predominantly older and sicker patients purchased coverage in the individual market. Over time, this would create a feedback loop—as premiums rose because only those with significant health risks or needs purchased coverage, more individuals would drop out, leading to a smaller and much more expensive market that catered to the sickest individuals. In this scenario, insurers would have no choice but to raise premiums. Senate Minority Leader Chuck Schumer (D-NY) warned, "The number of middle-class families who would lose money from this bill may be even higher now considering the 10 percent increase in premiums that will occur as a result of the Republican plan to repeal the individual mandate" (Miller 2017). This dire scenario, however, did not come to pass. Instead, average monthly premiums for the least expensive "silver" tier plan on health insurance marketplaces declined from $456 in 2018 to $442 in 2020 (Kaiser Family Foundation 2021).

Democrats painted a bleak picture of the consequences of repealing the individual mandate. In particular, Democrats seized on projections from the nonpartisan Congressional Budget Office (CBO) that repealing the individual mandate would result in millions of Americans losing coverage. Sen. Bernie Sanders (I-VT) described proposals to end the individual mandate as "a bad idea. This is going to throw 13 million Americans off the health insurance they currently have" (Miller 2017). After the failure of Republican efforts to repeal and replace the ACA in 2017, Sen. Kamala Harris (D-CA) echoed these concerns and attacked Republican proposals in the TCJA to eliminate the penalty for not having health insurance. She argued, "They're trying to turn this tax bill into a healthcare bill by repealing the individual mandate. So that means if you have health insurance, you could be one of 13 million people to become uninsured in the next decade or face premium increases of up to 10%" (Harris 2017). After the passage of the TCJA in December 2017, House Minority Leader Nancy Pelosi (D-CA) declared, "Republicans are fully responsible for this cruel decision and for the fear they have struck into millions of families across America who are now in danger of losing their health coverage" (Gray 2018). Democrats' fears about the erosion of coverage gains were partially borne out, but their dire projections did not materialize in the years following the passage of the TCJA. Despite a healthy—and growing—economy from 2017 to 2019, the number of uninsured Americans increased from 26.9 million (10 percent) in 2016 to 29.2 million (10.8 percent) in 2019 (Garfield and Tolbert 2020).

Aside from these concerns about rising costs and diminished coverage, Democrats defended the individual mandate on the grounds that it benefited society as a whole and emphasized the importance of shared responsibility in health care reform. President Barack Obama argued that young and healthy individuals who chose not to purchase coverage were engaging in "irresponsible behavior. . . . If there are affordable options and people still don't sign up for health insurance, it means we pay for those people's expensive emergency room visits" (Obama 2009). In other words, the individual mandate offered a solution to the problem of cost shifting. As Dr. Ezekiel Emanuel, one of President Obama's leading health policy advisers, wrote in 2013, "We need to make it clear as a society that buying insurance is part of individual responsibility. If you don't have insurance and you need to go to the emergency room or unexpectedly get diagnosed with cancer, you are free-riding on others. Insured Americans will have to pay more to hospitals and doctors to make up for your non-payment. The social norm of individual responsibility must be equated with purchasing health insurance" (Emanuel 2013).

Republicans on the Individual Mandate

The Affordable Care Act (ACA) passed Congress without a single Republican vote in 2010. Staunch opposition to the ACA was also seen by many political analysts as a factor in the Republican return to majority status in the House of Representatives in 2010 and their success in regaining control over the Senate in 2014. Repealing the ACA with a more market-oriented, competitive model became a top domestic policy priority for Republicans in Congress. No clear consensus emerged among congressional Republicans or the Trump administration over what a replacement for the ACA would look like. The Republican-controlled House voted to repeal, replace, or significantly modify the ACA more than fifty times between 2011 and 2016 (Berensen 2017). More than five years after President Obama signed the ACA into law, Rep. Tom Price (R-GA) complained that the "law violates the principles that every American holds dear when it comes to health care" (Woodruff 2016).

As a presidential candidate in 2016, Donald Trump also pledged to "end Obamacare" if elected. This view was shared by all of the 2016 contenders for the

Republican nomination. After taking office in 2017, he maintained that stance, endorsing efforts by Republicans in Congress to repeal and replace the ACA. Trump also issued numerous executive orders to weaken key elements of the law.

While Republicans were united in their opposition to Obamacare, the individual health insurance mandate drew particular ire. Like Democrats, Republicans regarded the mandate to purchase health insurance as the vital connective tissue that held the various parts of the ACA together. Unlike Democrats, their goal was to end, not amend, the ACA. Republicans saw excising the individual mandate as a way of making the carefully constructed framework of the entire Affordable Care Act collapse. As Sen. Orrin Hatch (R-UT) declared in December 2017, this "onerous and punitive individual mandate tax" was "a major pillar of what has proven to be an unworkable and unpopular law" (Hatch 2017). Repealing the individual mandate emerged as one of Republicans' principal arguments for passing the Tax Cuts and Jobs Act (TCJA) in December 2017. As Senate Majority Leader Mitch McConnell (R-KY) argued, "The repeal of the individual mandate takes the heart out of Obamacare" (Snell and Davis 2017). President Donald Trump proudly declared in his State of the Union address in January 2018 that with the passage of TCJA, "we repealed the core of the disastrous Obamacare. The individual mandate is now gone. Thank heaven" (CNN.com 2018).

Republicans characterized the individual mandate as an unfair, regressive tax for millions of Americans who did not qualify for premium subsidies. The Manhattan Institute—a conservative think tank—claimed that the main effect of the individual mandate "has been to concentrate more of the expense of covering the chronically ill on the relatively small cohort of working Americans who lack employer-sponsored coverage. By doing so, the mandate has served to obscure the total cost of the entitlement" (Pope 2017). The conservative Heritage Foundation concurred: "It is people buying health insurance without subsidies that most need relief from Obamacare's escalating premiums and the return of disappearing health plans" (Haislmaier 2017). Congressional leaders such as Sen. Orrin Hatch (R-UT) described the individual mandate as "regressive and punitive, disproportionately hurting low-income households. According to the IRS, nearly 80 percent of households that pay the penalty make less than $50,000 annually." Hatch noted that many "families were stuck paying up to $2,085 this year for simply not being able to afford health insurance. Obamacare premiums have unfortunately been so high that millions of Americans were forced to pay the Obamacare penalty because they could not afford the thousands of dollars for coverage that did not fit their needs. I am pleased that, moving forward [after the passage of TCJA], this penalty will no longer burden low-income Americans" (Hatch 2017).

This line of argument was a common one for the GOP. Indeed, Republicans repeatedly framed passage of TCJA in 2017 as a way to provide tax relief for hard-working American families. As President Trump noted in his 2018 State of the Union address, "We eliminated an especially cruel tax that fell mostly on Americans making less than $50,000 a year, forcing them to pay tremendous penalties simply because they couldn't afford government-ordered health plans" (CNN.com 2018). Seema Verma, the Trump administration's chief administrator for Medicare and Medicaid, described the individual mandate as "a perverse tax that charged people for not buying something they could not afford. Worse, the tax fell to lower income people—nearly 80 percent of the households paying the tax earned less than $50,000 annually" (Verma 2018). Republicans voiced similar concerns about state initiatives to establish individual mandates following the passage of the TCJA. David Wolfe, the legislative director of the Howard Jarvis Taxpayers' Association in California, decried Gov. Gavin Newsom's proposed tax penalty on Californians without health insurance as a "very costly and regressive tax on young people who can't afford it. They likely aren't going to get sick and they want to take that chance" (Young and Ibarra 2019).

Apart from concerns about the cost of health insurance, Republicans also objected to the individual mandate as a matter of principle. Republicans argued that the mandate forced millions of Americans to purchase more expensive insurance than they otherwise would and unnecessarily constrained consumer choice in the marketplace. This stance represented a marked shift from the 1990s, when Republicans in Congress supported an individual mandate as a market-oriented policy alternative to the Clinton administration's ambitious proposal to reinvent the American health care system. In 2006, Mitt Romney, the Republican governor of Massachusetts, gained national attention for embracing an individual mandate as part of the state's pathbreaking reform law. After the passage of the ACA in 2010, however, Republicans characterized a national mandate as an unwarranted imposition on individuals' ability to choose the health plan they felt best fit their needs. In 2013, for example, insurers canceled existing policies for millions of Americans because their current plans did not meet the "minimum essential coverage" requirements established by the ACA (*Wall Street Journal* 2013). In response, the Obama administration granted exemptions from the mandate for affected individuals. Critics, however, argued that this episode underscored how the law distorted the market by ignoring consumer preferences for less expensive "catastrophic" plans. As the *Wall Street Journal* editorialized, "Waiving ObamaCare rules for some citizens and continuing to squeeze the economic liberties of others by forcing them to buy what the White House now concedes is an unaffordable product is untenable" (*Wall Street Journal* 2013).

Republicans touted the importance of consumer choice in purchasing health insurance. As Sens. John McCain (R-AZ) and John Barrasso (R-WY) declared, "It is far past time for American families to once again have the freedom to make their own decisions about what is best for their families" (McCain and Barrasso 2015). At this point, Republicans contended that respecting consumer sovereignty meant empowering individuals to make their own choices about what type of health plan to purchase. As Sen. Orrin Hatch (R-UT) declared during the debate over the TCJA, "The individual mandate tax forces Americans to purchase health insurance they do not want or cannot afford and represents an excessive encroachment on Americans' ability to make their own health-care decisions" (Hatch 2017). Rather than a one-size-fits-all approach, Republicans argued that consumers should have the freedom to decide whether to purchase health insurance and, if so, to choose the type of policy that best fits their needs. As Sen. Lisa Murkowski (R-AK) stated, "I believe that the federal government should not force anyone to buy something they do not wish to buy, in order to avoid being taxed" (Paletta 2017).

Finally, Republicans defined their opposition to the individual mandate in terms of personal liberty. For Republicans, the mandate—and its tax for noncompliance—embodied unnecessary government intrusion into individuals' personal lives. Speaking on the campaign trail in 2014, future Texas governor Greg Abbott declared, "I have fought Obamacare from Day One and will continue to fight against this unworkable law, so our state remains a beacon of liberty" (Haberkorn 2015). In 2014, Sens. John McCain (R-AZ) and John Barrasso (R-WY) insisted that "health care should be based on the fundamental principle of freedom, and Americans should be able to have the ability to make their own health care decisions without fear that the government will extract onerous penalties from them." Republicans said that the Obamacare mandate established a dangerous precedent by forcing individuals to purchase a product that they otherwise would not choose to buy. Rep. Tom Price (R-GA)—later tapped by President Donald Trump to be his secretary of Health and Human Services—echoed this point on the campaign trail in 2016. Price promised that Republicans "will repeal things like the individual mandate and say, 'You should be free to pick whatever insurance plan meets your needs, not one Washington forces you to buy'" (Bacon 2016).

Republicans described the individual mandate to purchase health insurance—however well intended—as a fundamental threat to personal liberty and individual autonomy. As Sen. Orrin Hatch (R-UT) warned, "ObamaCare and its mandates put our nation on a fast-track to socialism. If the federal government can force you to buy health insurance, where does the government's power stop? Repealing the individual mandate tax restores liberty to the nation's health-care system. Once again, the American people will be back in charge of their health care—not Washington bureaucrats" (Hatch 2017).

Robert B. Hackey and Shannon McGonagle

Further Reading

America's Health Insurance Plans et al. 2017. Letter to Congressional Leaders. November 14. Accessed July 12, 2019. https://www.ahip.org/wp-content/uploads/2017/11/IM-Coalition-Letter-11_14_2017.pdf.

Bacon, Perry. 2016. "In Picking Rep. Price, Trump Signals Possible Aggressive Overhaul of Obamacare." NBC News, November 29. Accessed July 30, 2019. https://www.nbcnews.com/politics/white-house/picking-rep-price-trump-signals-aggressive-overhaul-obamacare-n689646.

Berensen, Tessa. 2017. "Reminder: The House Voted to Repeal ObamaCare More Than 50 Times." *Time*, March 24. Accessed August 7, 2019. https://time.com/4712725/ahca-house-repeal-votes-obamacare/.

Biskupic, Joan. 2019. "Affordable Care Act Gears Up for Momentous Test in Court." CNN, July 8. Accessed July 29, 2019. https://www.cnn.com/2019/07/08/politics/affordable-care-act-court/index.html.

Blendon, Robert, and John Benson. 2010. "Public Opinion at the Time of the Vote on Health Care Reform." *New England Journal of Medicine* 362 (April 22): e55. Accessed July 21, 2019. https://www.nejm.org/doi/full/10.1056/NEJMp1003844.

Blendon, Robert, and John Benson. 2017. "Public Opinion about the Future of the Affordable Care Act." *New England Journal of Medicine* 377 (August 31): e12. Accessed July 21, 2019. https://www.nejm.org/doi/full/10.1056/NEJMsr1710032.

Blumberg, Linda, and John Holahan. 2017. "Strengthening the ACA for the Long Term." *New England Journal of Medicine* 317, no. 22: 2105–2107. Accessed July 30, 2019. https://www.nejm.org/doi/full/10.1056/NEJMp1713247.

Brill, Steven. 2015. *America's Bitter Pill: Money, Politics, Backroom Deals, and the Fight to Fix Our Broken Healthcare System*. New York: Random House.

Butler, Stuart. 1989. "Assuring Affordable Health Care for All Americans." Heritage Foundation, October 1. Accessed July 12, 2019. https://www.heritage.org/social-security/report/assuring-affordable-health-care-all-americans.

Butler, Stuart. 2012. "Don't Blame Heritage for Obamacare Mandate." Heritage Foundation, February 6. Accessed March 19, 2019. https://www.heritage.org/health-care-reform/commentary/dont-blame-heritage-obamacare-mandate.

CNN.com. 2018. "State of the Union 2018." CNN.com. January 31. Accessed March 1, 2021. https://www.cnn.com/2018/01/30/politics/2018-state-of-the-union-transcript.

Cooper, Michael. 2012. "Conservatives Sowed Idea of Health Insurance Mandate, Only to Spurn It Later." *New York Times*, February 15. Accessed March 19, 2019. https://www.nytimes.com/2012/02/15/health/policy/health-care-mandate-was-first-backed-by-conservatives.html.

East County Today. 2019. "Insurance Mandate Is Back after California Legislator Approves SB-78." Accessed July 19, 2019. https://eastcountytoday.net/insurance-mandate-is-back-after-california-legislator-approves-sb-78/.

Emanuel, Ezekiel. 2013. "Health Care Exchanges Will Need the Young Invincibles." *Wall Street Journal*, May 6.Accessed March 1, 2021. https://www.wsj.com/articles/SB10001424127887324326504578467560106322692.

Erb, Kelly Phillips. 2015. "Opting Out of the Obamacare Tax: What Happens if You Don't Pay?" *Forbes*, April 28. Accessed August 15, 2019. https://www.forbes.com/sites/kellyphillipserb/2015/02/26/opting-out-of-the-obamacare-tax/#2e64ef6440a0.

Fiedler, Matthew. 2018. "Coverage Gains among Higher-Income People Suggest the ACA's Individual Mandate Had Big Effects on Coverage." Brookings Institution, May 31. Accessed March 19, 2019. https://www.brookings.edu/blog/usc-brookings-schaeffer-on-health-policy/2018/05/31/new-evidence-the-acas-individual-mandate-substantially-increased-insurance-coverage/.

Garfield, Rachel, and Jennifer Tolbert. 2020. "What We Do and Don't Know about Recent Trends in Health Insurance Coverage in the US." Kaiser Family Foundation, September 17. Accessed October 21, 2020. https://www.kff.org/policy-watch/what-we-do-and-dont-know-about-recent-trends-in-health-insurance-coverage-in-the-us/.

Glied, Sherry. 2008. "Universal Coverage One Head at a Time: The Risks and Benefits of Individual Health Insurance Mandates." *New England Journal of Medicine* 358, no. 15: 1540–1542. Accessed July 23, 2019. https://www.nejm.org/doi/full/10.1056/NEJMp0802027.

Gray, Sarah. 2018. "Democrats React with Fury after Federal Judge Rules That Obamacare Is Unconstitutional." *Business Insider*. December 14. Accessed March 1, 2021. https://www.businessinsider.com/reactions-to-judges-ruling-that-affordable-care-act-unconstitutional-2018-12.

Haberkorn, Jennifer. 2015. "Burwell Goes Deep in the Heart of Texas for Obamacare." Politico, February 15. Accessed July 15, 2019. https://www.politico.com/story/2015/02/sylvia-matthews-burwell-texas-obamacare-115205.

Haislmaier, Edmund. 2017. "How to Bring Real Stability to the Health Care Market." Heritage Foundation, September 5. Accessed August 19, 2019. https://www.heritage.org/node/699632/print-display.

Harris, Kamala. 2017. "At Budget Hearing, Harris Votes against GOP Tax Plan." Accessed March 1, 2021. https://www.legistorm.com/stormfeed/view_rss/1160933/member/3160.html. .

Hatch, Orrin. 2017. "Repealing the Individual Mandate Tax Is the Beginning of the End of the Obamacare Era." Fox News, December 20. Accessed July 17, 2019. https://www.foxnews.com/opinion/sen-orrin-hatch-repealing-the-individual-mandate-tax-is-the-beginning-of-the-end-of-the-obamacare-era.

Herzlinger, Regina, Barak Richman, and Richard Boxer. 2017. "Achieving Universal Coverage without Turning to a Single-Payer: Lessons from Three Other Countries." *JAMA* 317, no. 14: 1409–1410. Accessed August 19, 2019. https://jamanetwork.com/journals/jama/fullarticle/2607482.

Kaiser Family Foundation. 2018. "Poll: Survey of the Non-Group Market Finds Most Say the Individual Mandate Was Not a Major Reason They Got Coverage in 2018, and Most Plan to Continue Buying Insurance despite Recent Repeal of the Mandate Penalty" April 3. Accessed August 19, 2019. https://www.kff.org/health-reform/press-release/poll-most-non-group-enrollees-plan-to-buy-insurance-despite-repeal-of-individual-mandate-penalty/.

Kaiser Family Foundation. 2021. "Average Marketplace Premiums by Metal Tier: 2018–2021." Accessed February 13, 2021. https://www.kff.org/health-reform/state-indicator/average-marketplace-premiums-by-metal-tier/.

Kaiser Health News. 2010. "Summary of a 1993 Republican Health Reform Plan." Accessed March 19, 2019. https://khn.org/news/gop-1993-health-reform-bill/.

Keith, Katie. 2018. "Two New Federal Surveys Show Stable Uninsured Rate." *Health Affairs*, September 13. Accessed August 15, 2019. https://www.healthaffairs.org/do/10.1377/hblog20180913.896261/full/.

Keith, Katie. 2019. "Continued Uncertainty as Fifth Circuit Strikes Mandate, Remands on Rest of ACA." *Health Affairs*, December 19. Accessed October 21, 2020. https://www.healthaffairs.org/do/10.1377/hblog20191219.863104/full/.

Kendall, Brent. 2019. "Court Signals Peril for Health Law." *Wall Street Journal*, July 10: A6.

Kirzinger, Ashley, Bianca DiJulio, Bryan Wu, and Mollyann Brodie. 2017. "Kaiser Health Tracking Poll—August 2017: The Politics of ACA Repeal and Replace Efforts." Accessed March 19, 2019. https://www.kff.org/health-reform/poll-finding/kaiser-health-tracking-poll-august-2017-the-politics-of-aca-repeal-and-replace-efforts/.

Klein, Ezra. 2012. "Unpopular Mandate." *New Yorker*, June 25. Accessed July 18, 2019. https://www.newyorker.com/magazine/2012/06/25/unpopular-mandate.

Lovelace, Berkeley. 2018. "Obamacare Enrollment Sinks 11%—Historically Low Unemployment Is at Least Partly to Blame." CNBC, December 6. Accessed July 31, 2019. https://www.cnbc.com/2018/12/06/obamacare-enrollment-sinks-11percent-historically-low-unemployment-is-blamed.html.

Mach, Annie. 2018. *The Individual Mandate for Health Insurance Coverage: In Brief*. Washington, DC: Congressional Research Service. Accessed March 19, 2019. https://fas.org/sgp/crs/misc/R44438.pdf.

McCain, John, and John Barrasso. 2015. "ObamaCare Opt-Out Act: Let All Americans Make Their Own Health Care Decisions." Fox News, January 13. Accessed July 15, 2019. https://www.foxnews.com/opinion/obamacare-opt-out-act-let-all-americans-make-their-own-health-care-decisions.

McDonough, John. 2011. *Inside National Health Care Reform*. Berkeley: University of California Press.

Miller, Emily. 2017. "Democrats in Meltdown Mode as Obamacare Individual Mandate Moves toward Extinction." Daily Signal, November 20. Accessed July 16, 2019. https://www.dailysignal.com/2017/11/20/democrats-meltdown-mode-obamacare-individual-mandate-moves-toward-extinction/.

Musumeci, MaryBeth. 2020. "Explaining *Texas v. U.S.*: A Guide to the Case Challenging the ACA." Kaiser Family Foundation, March 10. Accessed May 28, 2020. https://www.kff.org/health-reform/issue-brief/explaining-texas-v-u-s-a-guide-to-the-case-challenging-the-aca/.

National Federation of Independent Business v. Sebelius. 2012. 567 U.S. __. Accessed August 15, 2019. https://www.oyez.org/cases/2011/11-393.

Newkirk, Vann. 2017. "Obama: 'This Bill Will Do You Harm.'" *The Atlantic*, June 22. Accessed July 15, 2019. https://www.theatlantic.com/politics/archive/2017/06/this-is-the-obamacare-speech-obama-never-gave/531330/.

Obama, Barack. 2009. "Obama's Health Care Speech to Congress." *New York Times*, September 9. Accessed July 16, 2019. https://www.nytimes.com/2009/09/10/us/politics/10obama.text.html.

O'Connor, Reed. 2018. "Memorandum Opinion and Order—*Texas, et al. v. United States of America, et al.* Civil Action No. 4:18-cv-00167-0. December 14. Accessed May 28, 2020. https://www.documentcloud.org/documents/5629711-Texas-v-US-Partial-Summary-Judgment.html.

Paletta, Damian. 2017. "Republican Sen. Lisa Murkowski Announces Support for Repealing Individual Mandate, a Potential Boost to Tax Overhaul." *Washington Post*, November 21. Accessed February 20, 2019. https://www.washingtonpost.com/news/business/wp/2017/11/21/republican-sen-lisa-murkowski-announces-support-for-repealing-individual-mandate-a-potential-boost-to-tax-overhaul/?utm_term=.d252ca572967.

Paxton, Ken. 2019. "AG Paxton Leads 18-State Brief Urging 5th Circuit to Declare Obamacare Unlawful." Press Release, May 1. Accessed August 15, 2019. https://www.texasattorneygeneral.gov/news/releases/ag-paxton-leads-18-state-brief-urging-5th-circuit-declare-obamacare-unlawful.

Pope, Chris. 2017. "The Individual Mandate Is Unnecessary and Unfair." Manhattan Institute, October 25. Accessed July 15, 2019. https://www.manhattan-institute.org/html/individual-mandate-unnecessary-and-unfair-10735.html.

Sanger-Katz, Margot. 2017. "Obamacare's Insurance Mandate Is Unpopular. Why Not Just Get Rid of It?" *New York Times*, November 14. Accessed July 12, 2019. https://www.nytimes.com/2017/11/14/upshot/obamacares-insurance-mandate-is-unpopular-so-why-not-just-get-rid-of-it.html.

Scott, Dylan. 2018. "A Requiem for the Individual Mandate." Vox, April 13. Accessed July 12, 2019. https://www.vox.com/policy-and-politics/2018/4/13/17226566/obamacare-penalty-2018-individual-mandate-still-in-effect.

Snell, Kelsey, and Susan Davis. 2017. "McConnell Ready to 'Move On' from Obamacare Repeal, Others in GOP Say Not So Fast." NPR, December 21. Accessed July 17, 2019. https://www.npr.org/2017/12/21/572588692/mcconnell-wants-bipartisanship-in-2018-on-entitlements-immigration-and-more.

Sorkin, Amy. 2019. "The Health Care Defense." *New Yorker*, July 22. Accessed July 29, 2019. https://www.newyorker.com/podcast/comment/the-health-care-defense.

Texas v. United States. 2019. U.S. Court of Appeals for the Fifth Circuit, Case No. 19-10011. Accessed May 28, 2020. http://www.ca5.uscourts.gov/opinions/pub/19/19-10011-CV0.pdf.

Verma, Seema. 2018. "Remarks by Administrator Seema Verma at the ALEC Policy Summit." Centers for Medicare and Medicaid Services, November 29. Accessed July 15, 2019. https://www.cms.gov/newsroom/press-releases/remarks-administrator-seema-verma-alec-policy-summit.

Wall Street Journal. 2013. "Obama Repeals ObamaCare." December 20. Accessed March 1, 2021. https://www.wsj.com/articles/SB10001424052702304367204579270252042143502.

Woodruff, Judy. 2016. "'Repeal and Replace'? More Like Repeal and Collapse, Warns HHS Secretary Burwell." *PBS News Hour*, December 12. Accessed July 30, 2019. https://www.pbs.org/newshour/show/repeal-replace-like-repeal-collapse-warns-hhs-secretary-burwell.

Young, Samantha, and Ana Ibarra. 2019. "California Gov. Newsom Proposes Penalty to Fund Health Insurance Subsidies." Kaiser Health News, June 4. Accessed July 23, 2019. https://khn.org/news/newsom-proposes-penalty-to-fund-health-insurance-subsidies/.

Zamosky, Lisa. 2016. "Do We Need a Stiffer Individual Mandate Penalty?" Healthinsurance.org, September 14. Accessed July 23, 2019. https://www.healthinsurance.org/blog/2016/09/14/do-we-need-a-stiffer-individual-mandate-penalty/.

Marijuana

At a Glance

After President Richard Nixon signed the Controlled Substances Act in 1970, marijuana reemerged as a touchpoint for partisan debates about how to categorize illicit drugs and reconcile public opinion with policy change. During the ensuing decades, Democrats and Republicans have disagreed about the criminal justice and public health implications of marijuana, fiercely debating the prospects and impact of decriminalization and legalization for medical and recreational use. Proponents of decriminalization argued in favor of eliminating criminal penalties for marijuana possession, leaving intact an unregulated marketplace, while proponents of legalization emphasized establishing regulatory frameworks that would include purchasing restrictions, licensing requirements, and taxation schemes.

As of March 2021, 36 states, the District of Columbia, Guam, Puerto Rico, and U.S. Virgin Islands have legalized marijuana for medical use. California became the first state to legalize medical marijuana with passage of Proposition 215 in 1996. Since Colorado and Washington first legalized marijuana for recreational use in 2012, 13 other states and three territories have followed suit. Public opinion polls indicate that since 2013, the majority of Americans have supported legalization; in 2018, one survey found that 66 percent of Americans favored legalizing marijuana for medical or recreational use (McCarthy 2018). Although marijuana has garnered bipartisan support over the past decade, rhetorical and policy differences between Democrats and Republicans still remain.

Democrats often frame decriminalizing marijuana as a restorative measure. In this view, decriminalizing marijuana will eliminate racist and wrongful marijuana enforcement practices and represent a significant advance in social justice reform. Democrats who advocate for legalizing medical marijuana defer to expert medical opinion, which has recently supported the therapeutic utilization of marijuana for pain management and symptom relief for certain medical conditions. Democrats also tend to view medical marijuana use as a decision to be made between patients and their physicians. They argue that states should remain free from federal interference and have the right to regulate marijuana for medical or recreational use for themselves. Public opinion polls indicate that the majority of Democratic voters have endorsed medical marijuana since 2008.

In contrast, Republicans present a less uniform front when it comes to marijuana policy. Historically, Republicans disapproved of state-level legalization efforts by reinforcing that marijuana remains illegal under federal law. Some Republican critics portray marijuana as a gateway drug with worrisome psychological effects. In this view, legalization and the broader social acceptance that would follow would lead to moral decline. More recently, however, a growing number of Republicans have expressed support for efforts to legalize marijuana for medical or recreational use. Republican advocates of legalization cite libertarian principles and emphasize the prioritization of individual freedom in private life and in medical practice. These advocates present marijuana as a safer alternative to prescription opioids. Although public opinion polls indicate that the majority of Republican voters have endorsed marijuana legalization since 2017, in 2018, the Trump administration announced its intention to strengthen enforcement of federal marijuana law.

According to Many Democrats . . .

- Current laws wrongfully punish marijuana users for minor offenses.
- Qualifying patients should have access to marijuana for medical use.
- The federal government should either not interfere with state legalization of marijuana for medical or recreational use or legalize it at the federal level.
- Marijuana can and should be regulated, much like alcohol and tobacco.

According to Many Republicans . . .

- Marijuana remains illegal under the Controlled Substances Act, which should be enforced as written.
- Allowing access to marijuana for medical use will lead to the broader social acceptance of marijuana for recreational use.
- Marijuana use endangers public health and public safety.

Overview

In 1971, Republican President Richard Nixon declared "a war on drugs," describing drug abuse as "public enemy number one" (Barber 2016). Nixon's initiative mobilized federal agencies to control the quantities of illicit drugs in the country and instituted severe punishment guidelines. The year before, the Democratic-led U.S. Congress passed the Controlled Substances Act, which deemed marijuana illegal and punishable by fines and prison time. Classified as a Schedule I drug—a drug with no recognized medical use and a high potential of abuse—marijuana joined a class that included heroin and psychedelics. Nixon also appointed the Shafer Commission to further study marijuana regulation. The commission produced a report that called for the decriminalization of marijuana possession and recommended clinical investigation into the medical benefits of marijuana (Nahas and Greenwood 1974). The Nixon administration did not implement the commission's major recommendations, however, and marijuana remained (and continues to remain) a Schedule I drug.

Since Nixon's "war on drugs" declaration, marijuana policy debates have not followed clearly partisan lines. Over the ensuing decades, nominal consensus regarding the illegality of marijuana morphed into partisan differences in rhetoric and policy reform. More recently, these partisan differences have given way to an emerging bipartisan consensus on legalization. Neither political party has enjoyed clear unanimity on the matter. Intraparty disagreement arose among Democrats in the 1990s and among Republicans in the 2010s. Between 1968 and 2018, Gallup polls indicated a marked increase in public support for marijuana legalization, from 12 percent in 1969 to 66 percent in 2018. According to Gallup, the majority of Americans have supported legalization since 2013 (McCarthy 2018). Legalization reached a particular milestone of support in 2017—the first year in which Gallup found that the majority of Republicans supported legalizing marijuana (McCarthy 2017). By 2019, several polls revealed that the majority of Americans supported legalizing marijuana for medical and recreational use. Although majorities of both parties now support legalization, Democrats remain much more supportive: 78 percent compared to 55 percent of Republicans, according to one 2019 poll (Daniller 2019).

Nixon's war on drugs brought federalism to the forefront of marijuana policy as legislators debated the scope of federal and state powers pertaining to drug policy. During the late 1970s and early 1980s, several states passed permissive marijuana-related legislation. States established therapeutic research programs, rescheduled marijuana at the state level, or declined to prosecute physicians for prescribing marijuana to patients. In one notable 1976 case, Robert Randall, a Washington, DC, resident with glaucoma, was arrested for growing marijuana to treat his affliction. A federal judge ruled in favor of Randall, accepting his argument that marijuana cultivation was medically necessary, and required the federal government to provide Randall with access to marijuana (Zielinski 2001).

In 1977, Democratic president Jimmy Carter announced his support for civil rather than criminal penalties for marijuana possession. In a message to Congress, Carter supported "leaving the States free to adopt whatever laws they wish concerning marijuana," but he also acknowledged that "decriminalization is not legalization" (Carter 1977). The federal government reached a settlement in the Randall case, which led to the establishment of the FDA's Compassionate Investigational New Drug (IND) Program to provide medical marijuana to a small group of qualified patients. By 1979, eleven states had enacted legislation that decriminalized the possession of small amounts of marijuana (Pacula, Chriqui, and King 2003).

Republicans upheld Nixon's war on drugs, however, and the GOP often equated marijuana use with crime throughout the 1980s and 1990s. The Reagan administration renewed attention to illicit drug use, particularly marijuana, throughout Reagan's two terms in office. Reagan sponsored "Just Say No" and Drug Abuse Resistance Education (D.A.R.E.), nationwide campaigns that warned of the dangers of drug use and abuse. Bipartisan passage of the Anti-Drug Abuse Act of 1986 set mandatory criminal punishments for simple possession of any controlled substance and imposed prison sentences on marijuana users who possessed small amounts of marijuana.

Drug-related incarceration rates rose during the Reagan administration. In 1980, the national drug incarceration rate had been 15 people per 100,000; by 1990, it had risen to just under 100 people per 100,000 (Travis and Western 2014). Republican president George H. W. Bush, who served as vice president under Reagan, retained and expanded the Reagan administration's drug enforcement initiatives. In 1989, the Bush administration mobilized DEA raids on marijuana-growing

Medical Marijuana Policy Requires Clarity

On March 10, 2015, Sen. Cory Booker (D-NJ) offered the following remarks when introducing the Compassionate Access, Research Expansion, and Respect States Act (CARES Act). The bill, which did not come up for a vote, would have moved marijuana from Schedule I to Schedule II status and allowed states to set medical marijuana policy without federal interference.

> Individual users of medical marijuana in States with legalized medical marijuana continue to be targeted by the Drug Enforcement Agency. That is unacceptable and must change. Individuals who use medical marijuana in States where it is legal should not fear prosecution simply based on prosecutorial discretion. We can do better.
>
> I am encouraged that the winds of change are blowing at the Federal level on whether to prosecute medical marijuana, but confusion remains. While the 2013 guidance likely trumps the prior two memorandum, what message do these documents send? Is medical marijuana legal or not? Is it right that the law can be changed at a moment's notice by an unelected Federal prosecutor? And what protection does State law afford medical marijuana users when State and Federal law collide, especially when marijuana is classified by the Federal Government as a schedule I drug? This legislation brings certainty and uniformity to these issues.

Source

Congressional Record, vol. 161, no. 40 (March 10, 2015): S1385. Washington, DC: Government Printing Office. Accessed March 13, 2021. https://www.congress.gov/114/crec/2015/03/10/CREC-2015-03-10-pt1-PgS1385.pdf.

operations across forty-six states, leading to over one hundred arrests and the confiscation of six thousand marijuana plants (Carmichael 1989). In 1992, Bush also closed the window for new medical marijuana applicants to the Compassionate IND Program (Congressional Research Service 2010).

During the 1990s, Democrats presented a less unified front on marijuana policy than Republicans. Early in his presidential tenure, President Bill Clinton acknowledged experimenting with marijuana but famously remarked that he "didn't inhale it." Although U.S. Surgeon General Joycelyn Elders voiced public support for medical marijuana (one of several controversial statements that ultimately led her to resign under pressure), U.S. Secretary of Health and Human Services Donna Shalala criticized legalization efforts occurring during the Clinton administration. In his 1996 State of the Union address, Clinton affirmed his predecessors' drug awareness programs, calling on "Congress not to cut our support for drug-free schools" (Clinton 1996). That same year, however, California voters approved Proposition 215, the nation's first ballot initiative that legalized the cultivation or possession of marijuana for medical use (Matthews 1996). The Clinton administration denounced the initiative, and in September 1998, the Republican-led U.S. House of Representatives voted 310–93 to oppose subsequent state efforts to legalize marijuana for medical use (H.J. Res. 117 1998). Rep. Henry Waxman (D-CA) argued that the bill, which received bipartisan support, was nonetheless driven by GOP political considerations: "[Republicans] want to deprive seriously ill patients of potential therapies because they have a political agenda. They think we should just say no to sick and dying patients because it looks like we are getting tough on illegal drugs" (Congressional Record 1998).

During the following decade, debates continued about legalizing marijuana for medical use at both the state and federal levels. Several major U.S. cities and states decriminalized marijuana during the 2000s, and states that included Colorado, Hawaii, Montana, Maine, and Nevada legalized medical marijuana via ballot initiative or new legislation. As a presidential candidate, George W. Bush opposed medical marijuana but supported states' rights to legalize or prohibit the substance (Hsu 1999). After he assumed the presidency, the U.S. Supreme Court issued two significant rulings pertaining to medical marijuana. The first case, *U.S. v. Oakland Cannabis Buyers' Cooperative* (2001), followed court challenges after the U.S. Department of Justice sought to close marijuana distribution centers operating under California state law that allowed for local cultivation and distribution. The court issued an 8–0 decision that "a medical necessity exception for marijuana is at odds with the terms of the Controlled Substances Act." In 2005, the Supreme Court issued a 6–3 decision in *Gonzales v. Raich* that Congress could criminalize marijuana use even if allowed under state law for medical use, as congressional power to regulate commerce extended to intrastate "activities that have a substantial effect on interstate commerce."

Medical marijuana policy during the Obama administration marked both a continuation of and a departure from the Clinton and George W. Bush administrations. By 2008, more than a dozen states had legalized medical marijuana, and in 2009, Deputy Attorney General David Ogden issued a memorandum (later referred to as the "Ogden memo") that directed federal prosecutors to focus on illegal drug manufacturing and trafficking rather than individuals who were in compliance with state laws allowing medical marijuana (Ogden 2009). As Attorney General Eric Holder indicated, "It will not be a priority to use federal resources to prosecute patients with serious illnesses or their caregivers who are complying with state laws on medical marijuana" (Stout and Moore 2009). While the Obama administration de-emphasized marijuana as a prosecutorial priority, public opinion polls in 2010 indicated that a plurality of conservative Republicans continued to oppose efforts to legalize marijuana for medical use (Pew Research Center 2010). As Rep. Lamar Smith (R-TX) argued, "If we want to win the war on drugs, federal prosecutors have a responsibility to investigate and prosecute all medical marijuana dispensaries and not just those that are merely fronts for illegal marijuana distribution" (Stout and Moore 2009). In a series of subsequent memos in 2011 and 2013, Deputy Attorney General James Cole—Ogden's successor—further clarified that commercial operations were not shielded from federal prosecution and that federal enforcement priorities would focus on preventing marijuana sales by criminal enterprises, preventing access to minors, and preventing diversion across state lines (Cole 2013). The Cole memos spurred federal prosecution of state-approved medical marijuana dispensaries, as the George W. Bush administration had done. In 2016, President Obama suggested that "I do believe that treating this as a public-health issue, the same way we do with cigarettes or alcohol, is the much smarter way to deal with it" (Wenner 2016).

The 2016 presidential election reinforced how Democrats and Republicans prioritized marijuana policy in different ways. The Republican Party's 2016 platform included no mention of medical marijuana. The Democratic Party's platform, on the other hand, supported reclassifying marijuana to acknowledge its potential medical utility and establishing a "pathway for future legalization" (Weigel 2016). Democratic nominee Hillary Clinton remarked that "there's some great evidence about what marijuana can do for people who are in cancer treatment, who have other kind of chronic diseases, who are suffering from intense pain. . . . There's great, great anecdotal evidence but I want us to start doing the research" (Berke 2016). While the 2016 presidential candidates debated broader health policy issues—namely the future of the Affordable Care Act and how to control rising health care costs—one 2016 peer-reviewed study determined that Medicare Part D prescription drug spending decreased in states that had legalized medical marijuana for certain medical conditions, suggesting that legalization could become a source of public health cost savings (Bradford and Bradford 2016).

Marijuana policy reform gained bipartisan appeal during the Obama and Trump administrations, however. For example, Democratic and Republican lawmakers collaborated on several efforts to clarify the separation of federal and state powers in terms of marijuana regulation. In 2014, Reps. Dana Rohrabacher (R-CA) and Sam Farr (D-CA) reintroduced an amendment to prohibit federal interference with state medical marijuana laws. Previous efforts to pass the amendment had failed multiple times over the preceding decade, but the Rohrabacher-Farr amendment—now the Rohrabacher-Blumenauer amendment—passed the U.S. House and was inserted into spending bills signed by President Obama in 2014 and 2015 and by President Trump in 2017, 2018, and 2019 (Abreu 2018). In 2017, Democratic Reps. Jared Polis (CO) and Earl Blumenauer (OR) and Republican Reps. Dana Rohrabacher (CA) and Don Young (AK) launched the bipartisan Cannabis Caucus. The Cannabis Caucus formed to address conflicts between state and federal regulation of marijuana. As Rohrabacher noted, "Not only have incalculable amounts of taxpayers' dollars been wasted, but countless lives have been unnecessarily disrupted and even ruined by misguided law enforcement" (Ingraham 2017). On the House floor, Polis emphasized how "states like Colorado, and now dozens of other states, have proven that allowing responsible adults to legally purchase marijuana, gives money to classrooms, not cartels; creates jobs, not addicts; and boosts our economy, not our prison population" (Congressional Record 2017). Bipartisan support for medical marijuana blended the Democratic embrace of traditionally conservative support for states' rights and the Republican acknowledgment of traditionally liberal critiques of the law enforcement system.

Although Democrats and Republicans expressed recent bipartisan support for revamping marijuana policy, the Trump administration indicated its commitment to federal marijuana enforcement under the Controlled Substances Act. In 2018, White House press secretary Sarah Huckabee Sanders noted that Trump "believes in enforcing federal law. That would be his top priority, and that is regardless of what the topic is" (Hulse 2018). These remarks marked a departure from Trump's 2016 presidential campaign, when he advocated for states' rights with respect to marijuana regulation. As a candidate, Trump declared, "I think it should be up to the states, absolutely" (Krane 2018).

In January 2018, Attorney General Jeff Sessions promised a "return to the rule of law" and reversed the Ogden and Cole memos released by the Obama administration. In his own memo, Sessions directed the U.S. Department of Justice "to use previously established prosecutorial principles that provide them all the necessary tools to disrupt criminal organizations, tackle the growing drug crisis, and thwart violent crime across our country" (Sessions 2018). In April 2019, Sessions's successor, Bill Barr, stated that "I would still favor one uniform federal rule against marijuana" (Godlewski 2019). In August 2019, U.S. Surgeon General Jerome Adams and U.S. Health and Human Services Secretary Alex Azar issued a health advisory cautioning Americans that legalization dampened public perceptions of the dangers associated with marijuana use. As Azar noted, "This ain't your mother's marijuana" (Fearnow 2019). That same year, President Trump donated his second-quarter salary to a public awareness campaign about the negative effects of marijuana use (Cha 2019).

Democrats on Marijuana

During the 2020 presidential primaries, almost every Democratic candidate supported legalization (Politico 2020). Candidates who were sitting members of Congress, including Sens. Cory Booker, Amy Klobuchar, Bernie Sanders, and Elizabeth Warren, had either cosponsored or signaled support for legislation that would legalize marijuana or introduce other criminal justice reform measures related to past marijuana-related convictions. Notably, former Vice President Joe Biden and former New York City mayor Mike Bloomberg had long championed criminal penalties for marijuana possession throughout their political careers. During the primaries, however, both candidates signaled support for letting states decide how to regulate marijuana. One health journalist even contended that support for marijuana legalization had become "the new Democratic litmus test" (Demko 2019).

Democrats now often frame support for marijuana decriminalization as a matter of social justice. Rep. Donna Shalala (D-FL) exemplifies that shift in attitude among many Democrats. Shalala opposed legalizing medical marijuana when she served as the secretary of health and human services under President Bill Clinton, but in 2018, she tweeted that "decriminalizing marijuana shouldn't just be a policy priority—but a moral imperative" (Shalala 2018). Democrats contended that many Americans have been wrongfully punished for minor marijuana possession charges and that minority groups in the United States had been most heavily affected. As Sen. Cory Booker (D-NJ) argued in 2018, "There's no difference in America between blacks or whites for using or selling marijuana, but African-Americans are almost 3.7 times more likely to be arrested for that" (Bowden 2018). With Democratic Senate colleagues, Booker cosponsored the Marijuana Justice Act, which called for removing marijuana from the federal list of controlled substances and expunging marijuana convictions. Rep. Tim Ryan (D-OH) applauded the bill, which he said "could save $7.7 billion in averted enforcement costs and add $6 billion in additional tax revenue—a $13.7 billion net savings" (Ryan 2018).

When Booker reintroduced the Marijuana Justice Act in 2019, he tweeted that "it's not enough to legalize marijuana at the federal level—we should also help those who have suffered due to its prohibition" (Booker 2019). Thirty Democratic representatives, led by Rep. Barbara Lee (D-CA), cosponsored the U.S. House version of the bill. In October 2018, Rep. Earl Blumenauer (D-OR) released a "Blueprint to Legalize Marijuana," which laid out a schedule of legislative priorities that included legalizing marijuana at the federal level and extending access to medical marijuana for veterans with PTSD or pain management needs (Blumenauer 2018). In November 2019, the Democratic-led House Judiciary Committee approved a bill to decriminalize marijuana. The Marijuana Opportunity Reinvestment and Expungement (MORE) Act of 2019, introduced by Rep. Jerrold Nadler (D-NY), proposed removing marijuana as a Schedule I drug. As Nadler emphasized, "For far too long, we have treated marijuana as a criminal justice problem instead of a matter of personal choice and public health" (Gehlen 2019). House Majority Leader Steny Hoyer (D-MD) announced that the House would vote on the MORE Act in September 2020, but the vote was eventually delayed to focus on COVID-19 relief legislation.

Democrats assert that states should be able to determine how to regulate marijuana for medical or recreational use. In 2015, during the 114th Congress, Rep. Jared Polis (D-CO) introduced the Regulate Marijuana Like Alcohol Act, which proposed allowing states to make that regulatory decision. When no further action was taken on that bill, Polis reintroduced the measure during the 115th Congress (to the same effect), and Rep. Earl Blumenauer (D-OR) reintroduced the measure yet again during the 116th Congress. After Attorney General Jeff Sessions indicated that the Trump administration would enforce federal marijuana law under the Controlled Substances Act in 2018, House Minority Leader Nancy Pelosi (D-CA) tweeted that "your unjust war against Americans who legally use marijuana is shameful & insults the democratic processes that played out in states across the country" (Pelosi 2018). Sen. Chuck Schumer (D-NY) contended that "the States should continue to be the labs of democracy when it comes to recreational & medical marijuana. . . . This is one place where states' rights works. Let each state decide" (Schumer 2018).

For Democrats, a regulated, legal marketplace ensures patient access to a safer, potentially standardized product. In May 2019, Gov. Steve Bullock of Montana signed into law Senate Bill 265, sponsored by state senator Tom Jacobson (D). By "untethering" patients from a single provider and giving patients the freedom of choice, the bill clarified how patients would register and gain access to marijuana and how providers would undergo licensing and product monitoring. As Montana state representative Zach Brown (D) argued, "The state has an obligation to provide a regulatory framework that provides certainty for cancer patients and other types of patients, so that they know that their medicine is safe and effective, and they know where it came from" (Ambarian 2019).

In July 2019, New Jersey's Gov. Phil Murphy (D) signed the Jake Honig Compassionate Use Medical Cannabis Act, which enabled physician assistants and advanced practice nurses to authorize medical marijuana, raised the monthly consumption limit, introduced employment protections for medical marijuana patients, and established a new regulatory commission. As New Jersey state senator Joseph Vitale (D), who sponsored the bill, proclaimed, "We will treat patients with the dignity they deserve, recognize the full benefits of cannabis and ensure that compassion is a mainstay in New Jersey's medical marijuana program" (Murphy 2019). Moreover, Murphy argued that the act would "break down barriers to ensure this life-changing medical treatment is affordable and accessible for those who need it most" (Murphy 2019). This patient-centered sentiment resonates with Democrats who endorse expanding access to medical marijuana. As Texas state senator Jose Menendez (D) remarked in March 2019, "I don't understand why politicians are trying to get between the doctor and the patient on something that doesn't do anything but help the patient" (Samuels 2019). In August 2019, Gov. J. B. Pritzker (D) of Illinois signed legislation that allows school nurses to administer cannabis products. One month later, Washington, DC, Mayor Muriel Bowser (D) also approved emergency legislation that allows students participating in the District's medical marijuana program to be treated at school (Yu 2019).

The Democratic consensus around medical marijuana remains stronger than that regarding recreational marijuana. In some blue states that allow medical marijuana, legalizing marijuana for recreational use has proven challenging. For example, the Hawaii State Legislature approved medical marijuana in 2000. Since then—and despite Democratic control of the executive and legislative branches of state government—multiple recreational marijuana bills have failed in the state, most recently in 2019 (McAvoy 2019). In June 2019, New York lawmakers decriminalized the possession of small amounts of marijuana but failed to legalize marijuana despite public support from Gov. Andrew Cuomo (D) (McKinley and Wang 2019). In New Jersey, legislative efforts to legalize marijuana failed under Gov. Chris Christie (R) and Gov. Phil Murphy (D) despite overwhelming public support. One 2019 Monmouth University poll indicated that 62 percent of New Jersey adults supported legalizing marijuana, including 72 percent of Democrats (Monmouth University Poll 2019). In November 2020, New Jersey voters approved a ballot measure to amend the New Jersey Constitution to legalize marijuana for recreational use.

Republicans on Marijuana

Until the mid-2010s, Republicans reliably opposed legalizing marijuana for medical or recreational use. However, during that decade, public opinion polls across the country indicated a gradual warming to the idea among self-identified Republicans, and 2017 marked the first year that Gallup recorded that the majority of Republican voters supported legalizing marijuana (McCarthy 2017). Even in traditionally conservative states, polling indicated that Republicans are increasingly receptive to marijuana. For example, a 2018 Ball State University poll indicated that 76 percent of Indiana Republicans supported legalizing marijuana for medical or recreational use (Ball State University 2018). In Kentucky—which has voted for every Republican presidential candidate since 2000—a February 2020 poll indicated that 90 percent of Kentucky Republicans supported legalizing marijuana for medical use (Foundation for a Healthy Kentucky 2020). Another early 2020 poll recorded that 81 percent of Iowans supported expanding the state's medical marijuana program and that the majority of Iowans, for the first time, supported legalizing marijuana for recreational use (Coltrain 2020). In light of these shifts in public sentiment, even among Republican voters, Republican lawmakers have not taken a uniform approach to marijuana policy. Republican detractors of marijuana are increasingly at odds with a voter base that is amenable to legalization. Intraparty debates revolve around three distinct themes: marijuana's health impact, its association with individual liberty, and its regulatory status.

Republicans interpret marijuana's impact on health in different ways. While some Republicans endorse marijuana's medical benefits, others highlight its public health dangers. When the Texas State Senate subsequently passed a legalization bill unanimously in May 2019, state senator Brian Birdwell (R) indicated that "I will not allow it to become a road to perdition for Texas that has manifested in Colorado" (Allen 2019). Birdwell's "road to perdition" echoed claims from anti-marijuana advocates that legalization in Colorado (and elsewhere) spurred increases

Unanswered Questions about Marijuana Remain

On October 10, 2019, Sen. John Cornyn (R-TX) questioned the emerging consensus for legalizing marijuana.

> I am looking forward to our second hearing tomorrow, which I will talk about briefly, where we will have experts testifying on the public health effects of the most commonly used illicit drug—marijuana.
>
> A 2018 report found that an estimated 43.5 million Americans used marijuana in the last year. That is the highest percentage since 2002. While marijuana is still a prohibited drug under Federal law, we know that more than half of the States have legalized it in some form, making the rise in usage not all that surprising.
>
> Now, there is no shortage of people who claim that marijuana has endless health benefits and can help patients struggling with everything from epilepsy to anxiety to cancer treatments. This reminds me of some of the advertising we saw from the tobacco industry years ago where they actually claimed public health benefits from smoking tobacco, which we know, as a matter of fact, were false and that tobacco contains nicotine, an addictive drug, and is implicated with cancers of different kinds.
>
> We are hearing a lot of the same happy talk with regard to marijuana and none of the facts that we need to understand about the public health impact of marijuana use. We have heard from folks here in Congress, as well as a number of our Democratic colleagues who are running for President, about their desire to legalize marijuana at the Federal level. But for the number of voices in support of legalization, there are even more unanswered questions about both the short-term and long-term public health effects.

Source

Congressional Record, vol. 165, no. 167 (October 22, 2019): S5935. Washington, DC: Government Printing Office. Accessed June 27, 2020. https://www.congress.gov/116/crec/2019/10/22/CREC-2019-10-22-pt1-PgS5932-3.pdf.

in opioid deaths and marijuana use among youth. In 2020, Gov. Pete Ricketts (R) argued that impaired driving and psychological damage would follow if marijuana were legalized in Nebraska. As Ricketts argued, legalization "communicates that a dangerous drug is nothing to worry about" (Office of Governor Pete Ricketts 2020). Indiana's Gov. Eric Holcomb (R) argued that "if you want young people to do more of something, legalize it. And we simply cannot afford that for any age group for that matter" (Segall 2020).

On the other hand, Republicans who support medical marijuana offer it as an alternative to prescription opioids, particularly in areas most affected by the opioid crisis. In 2016, Gov. Bruce Rauner (R) of Illinois signed legislation that established the Opioid Alternative Pilot Program, which granted patients access to medical marijuana in place of opioid prescriptions. "We've got to do everything we can to stop this vicious epidemic," said Rauner, "and today, I'm proud to sign a bill that helps us stop this epidemic" (Schuba 2019). In February 2019, the Kentucky Legislature considered Senate Bill 170, sponsored by state senator Stephen West (R), and House Bill 136 to legalize medical marijuana. West justified his bill as a way to combat opioid misuse: "You clearly are going to have a reduction in addiction, and as you well know Kentucky is one of the worst in the United States when it comes to the opioid crisis" (Gillespie 2019). When the Georgia General Assembly considered marijuana bills in 2019, state representative David Clark (R) emphasized his belief that the patients who would benefit "are parents. These are kids. These are veterans who are begging for it, can't get access and get it legally" (Gazaway 2019).

Some Republicans perceive marijuana legalization as leading to social and moral decay. When Wisconsin legislators considered a legalization bill in early 2019, Speaker Robin Vos (R) posited that the bill could lead to "pot on every corner" (Associated Press 2019). In November 2019, South Dakota's Gov. Kristi Noem (R) opposed two ballot initiatives to establish a medical marijuana program and legalize marijuana in the state. As Noem argued, "I believe the social experiment our nation is conducting with highly potent legal weed will end poorly" (Noem 2019). Kayleigh McEnany, before becoming White House press secretary, insisted that "the legalization of marijuana is a proxy war, setting the stage for legalization of a variety of these other vice crimes" (McEnany 2014).

On the other hand, Republicans who advocate marijuana legalization draw upon libertarianism to emphasize freedom of choice. As Gov. Phil Scott (R) of Vermont stated in 2018, "I personally believe that what adults do behind closed doors and on private property is their choice. So long as it does not negatively impact the health and safety of others" (Office of Governor Phil Scott 2018). In December 2019, Wisconsin state representative Mary Felzkowski sponsored a proposal to create a state licensing program for medical marijuana dispensaries. As she argued, "There's being conservative but there's being libertarian too. . . . Having been through what I've gone through [as a cancer survivor], I don't think the government should tell me what I could take" (DuPont 2019). Kentucky state representative Jason Nemes made a similar argument in support of his own proposed legalization bill: "If a physician thinks [marijuana] will help his or her patient, the legislators need to get out of the way and let the doctors do their job" (Latek 2019). For some Republicans, legalization would advance the causes of individual freedom for patients and professional autonomy for physicians.

Republicans also differ on the regulatory status of marijuana. Some advocate for federal uniformity, while others argue that states should be able to regulate marijuana free from federal interference. During his 2018 U.S. Senate campaign, Mitt Romney (R-UT) argued for an agency-based approach to achieve uniformity. He stated, "Let's take this [marijuana] off the category one designation and let it be evaluated through a normal FDA-type process" (Wood 2018). In April 2019, Attorney General Bill Barr indicated that "I would still favor one uniform federal rule against marijuana" (Godlewski 2019). Elsewhere, other Republicans argued that because of lingering unanswered questions about marijuana's public health impact, state governments remain insufficiently equipped to make an informed judgment about loosening marijuana regulation. In 2019, for example, Lt. Gov. Dan Patrick (R) of Texas claimed that he "remains wary of the various medicinal use proposals that could become a vehicle for expanding access to this drug" (Samuels 2019). In 2018, South Carolina's Gov. Henry McMaster (R) argued, "We are not in a position to appropriately regulate medical marijuana" (Shain 2018). In December 2019, the Trump administration announced that it would enforce federal drug law despite bipartisan congressional efforts to protect citizens who complied with state medical marijuana laws from federal prosecution (Angell 2019).

While the Trump administration preferred a universal federal rule, as Barr indicated, several Republican members of Congress followed the example set by the bipartisan Cannabis Caucus and introduced bipartisan bills that promote states' rights to set marijuana policy. In 2018, Sen. Cory Gardner (R-CO) collaborated with Sen. Elizabeth Warren (D-MA) to introduce the Strengthening the Tenth Amendment through Entrusting States (STATES) Act. The STATES Act protected states that legalized marijuana from federal intervention. As Gardner argued, the "bipartisan, commonsense bill ensures the federal government will respect the will of the voters—whether that is legalization or prohibition—and not interfere in any states' legal marijuana industry" (Aiello 2018). In 2019, Rep. Matt Gaetz (R-FL) collaborated with Rep. Donna Shalala (D-FL) to introduce the Expanding Cannabis Research and Information Act. Intended to further biomedical and public health research on marijuana—and to address certain concerns raised by Republican colleagues wary of the public health impact of marijuana—Gaetz said that the bill would "help unlock cures for America's most vulnerable populations" (Shalala 2019).

Other Republican operatives envision marijuana policy as a potentially promising wedge issue as public perception shifts in favor of marijuana. In April 2020, one Republican polling firm concluded from a survey of Pennsylvania voters that Republican legislative candidates could gain electoral support among both

Republican and Democratic voters by supporting marijuana use (Harper Polling 2020). In October 2020, Vermont legalized recreational marijuana sales by an act of the Democratic-led state legislature after Gov. Phil Scott (R) allowed the bill to become law without his signature (Wilson 2020). As a growing proportion of Republican voters support legalization, many political analysts expect Republican officeholders to follow suit—and for the partisan gap on marijuana policy between Democrats and Republicans to further diminish.

Todd M. Olszewski and Keith Vieira Jr.

Further Reading

Abreu, Danielle. 2018. "Spending Plan Protects Medical Marijuana Laws from Feds." NBC Connecticut, March 23. Accessed July 28, 2020. https://www.nbcconnecticut.com/news/national-international/spending-bill-includes-medical-marijuana-protections-from-doj-sessions/2006580/.

Aiello, Chloe. 2018. "Senators Gardner and Warren Release Bipartisan Marijuana Bill That Prioritizes States' Rights." CNBC, June 7. Accessed December 17, 2018. https://www.cnbc.com/2018/06/07/senators-gardner-and-warren-release-bipartisan-marijuana-bill.html.

Allen, Rebekah. 2019. "Bill to Expand Medical Marijuana in Texas Heads to Governor's Desk." *Dallas News*, May 24. Accessed July 7, 2020. https://www.dallasnews.com/news/politics/2019/05/24/bill-to-expand-medical-marijuana-in-texas-heads-to-governor-s-desk/.

Ambarian, Jonathan. 2019. "Montana House Endorses Medical Marijuana Reform Bill, Including 'Untethering' Patients." KPAX, April 15. Accessed July 8, 2020. https://www.kpax.com/news/montana-legislature/2019/04/15/montana-house-endorses-medical-marijuana-reform-bill-including-untethering-patients/.

Angell, Tom. 2019. "Trump Says He Can Ignore Medical Marijuana Protections Passed by Congress." *Forbes*, December 21. Accessed July 24, 2020. https://www.forbes.com/sites/tomangell/2019/12/21/trump-says-he-can-ignore-medical-marijuana-protections-passed-by-congress/#2a9f16e4256f.

Associated Press. 2019. "Vos Fears Evers' Plan to OK Medical Marijuana Is 'Slippery Slope.'" WPR, January 22. Accessed July 3, 2020. https://www.wpr.org/vos-fears-evers-plan-ok-medical-marijuana-slippery-slope.

Ball State University. 2018. "Hoosier Survey." Accessed July 10, 2020. http://bowencenterforpublicaffairs.org/wp-content/uploads/2018/11/ONB-BSU-2018-Hoosier-Survey.pdf.

Barber, Chris. 2016. "Public Enemy Number One: A Pragmatic Approach to America's Drug Problem." Richard Nixon Foundation, June 29. Accessed July 10, 2020. https://www.nixonfoundation.org/2016/06/26404/.

Berke, Jeremy. 2016. "Here's Where Donald Trump and Hillary Clinton Stand on Marijuana Legalization." Business Insider, November 5. Accessed December 17, 2018. https://www.businessinsider.com/trump-and-clinton-on-weed-legalization-2016-11/.

Blumenauer, Earl. 2018. "Blueprint to Legalize Marijuana in the 116th Congress." Accessed July 10, 2020. https://assets.documentcloud.org/documents/5017819/2018-Fall-Blumenauer-Cannabis-Memo-for-116th.pdf.

Booker, Cory (@CoryBooker). 2019. "It's not Enough to Legalize Marijuana at the Federal Level—We Should also Help Those Who Have Suffered Due to Its Prohibition." Twitter, March 5. Accessed July 10, 2020. https://twitter.com/CoryBooker/status/1103119742599131136.

Bowden, John. 2018. "Cory Booker Slams Marijuana Convictions Ahead of 4/20." The Hill, April 20. Accessed December 17, 2018. https://thehill.com/homenews/senate/384188-cory-booker-slams-marijuana-convictions-ahead-of-4-20.

Bradford, Ashley, and W. David Bradford. 2016. "Medical Marijuana Laws Reduce Prescription Medication Use in Medicare Part D." *Health Affairs* 35, no. 7: 1230–1236. Accessed July 8, 2020. https://www.healthaffairs.org/doi/pdf/10.1377/hlthaff.2015.1661.

Carmichael, Dan. 1989. "Operation 'Green Merchant.'" UPI, October 26. Accessed December 17, 2018. https://www.upi.com/Archives/1989/10/26/Operation-Green-Merchant/5761625377600/.

Carter, Jimmy. 1977. "Drug Abuse Remarks on Transmitting a Message to Congress." Online by Gerhard Peters and John T. Woolley, the American Presidency Project. Accessed July 10, 2020. https://www.presidency.ucsb.edu/node/243649.

Cha, Ariana Eunjung. 2019. "'A Dangerous Drug': Surgeon General Warns against Marijuana Use by Pregnant Women, Youths." *Washington Post*, August 29. Accessed July 10, 2020. https://www.washingtonpost.com/health/2019/08/29/dangerous-drug-surgeon-general-warns-against-marijuana-use-by-pregnant-women-youth/.

Clinton, William J. 1996. "State of the Union Address." January 23. Accessed July 10, 2020. https://clintonwhitehouse2.archives.gov/WH/New/other/sotu.html.

Cole, James. 2013. "Guidance Regarding Marijuana Enforcement." U.S. Department of Justice, Office of the Deputy Attorney General, August 29. Accessed July 5, 2020. https://www.justice.gov/iso/opa/resources/3052013829132756857467.pdf.

Coltrain, Nick. 2020. "Iowa Poll: Most Iowans Support Expanding Medicinal Cannabis and Legalizing Recreational Marijuana." *Des Moines Register*, March 15. Accessed July 5, 2020. https://www.desmoinesregister.com/story/news/politics/2020/03/15/iowa-poll-iowans-support-legal-recreational-expanded-medical-marijuana/5026342002/.

Congressional Record, 105th Cong., 2nd sess., 1998, 144, no. 22. Accessed on July 10, 2020. https://www.congress.gov/crec/1998/09/15/CREC-1998-09-15-pt1-PgH7719.pdf.

Congressional Record, 115th Cong., 1st sess., 2017, 163, no. 80. Accessed on July 10, 2020. https://www.congress.gov/115/crec/2017/11/06/CREC-2017-11-06-pt1-PgE1516-2.pdf.

Congressional Research Service. 2010. "Medical Marijuana: Review and Analysis of Federal and State Policies." April 2. Accessed July 10, 2020. https://www.everycrsreport.com/files/20100402_RL33211_081e74fb2f48cc27b945f5c649493cb60d013658.pdf.

Daniller, Andrew. 2019. "Two-Thirds of Americans Support Marijuana Legalization." Pew Research Center, November 14. Accessed July 10, 2020. https://www.pewresearch.org/fact-tank/2019/11/14/americans-support-marijuana-legalization/.

Demko, Paul. 2019. "Legalizing Pot Is the New Democratic Litmus Test." Politico, April 3. Accessed July 9, 2020. https://www.politico.com/story/2019/04/03/democrats-presidential-candidates-marijuana-1312878.

DuPont, Amy. 2019. "'People Are Asking for Medical Marijuana': GOP Support Grows with Unveiling of 1st Bill." FOX6, December 11. Accessed July 10, 2020. https://fox6now.com/2019/12/11/gop-support-grows-to-legalize-medical-marijuana-in-wisconsin/.

Fearnow, Benjamin. 2019. "Top Trump Health Officials Warn against Marijuana Legalization: 'This Ain't Your Mother's Marijuana.'" *Newsweek*, August 29. Accessed July 2, 2020.

https://www.newsweek.com/marijuana-trump-administration-advisory-legalization-surgeon-general-warning-adolescents-pregnancy-1456836.

Foundation for a Healthy Kentucky. 2020. "Kentucky Health Issues Poll: Support for Medical Marijuana in Kentucky Jumps to 90 Percent." February 5. Accessed July 1, 2020. https://www.healthy-ky.org/newsroom/news-releases/article/415/kentucky-health-issues-poll-support-for-medical-marijuana-in-kentucky-jumps-to-90-percent.

Gazaway, Wright. 2019. "GA Senate Passes Bill Legalizing Cultivation, Distribution of Medical Marijuana." WTOC, March 29. Accessed July 5, 2020. https://www.wtoc.com/2019/03/29/ga-senate-passes-medical-marijuana-measure/.

Gehlen, Bobby. 2019. "Landmark Bill Legalizing Marijuana at the Federal Level Passes House Committee." ABC News, November 20. Accessed July 6, 2020. https://abcnews.go.com/Politics/house-judiciary-passes-bill-legalize-marijuana-federal-level/story?id=67174950.

Gillespie, Lisa. 2019. "Another Kentucky Republican Introduces Medical Marijuana Legislation." WKMS, February 12. Accessed July 7, 2020. https://www.wkms.org/post/another-kentucky-republican-introduces-medical-marijuana-legislation#stream/0.

Godlewski, Nina. 2019. "Attorney General Barr Says He Would Favor Making Marijuana Illegal across the United States." *Newsweek*, April 10. Accessed July 10, 2020. https://www.newsweek.com/attorney-general-barr-marijuana-law-1392561.

Gonzales v. Raich, 545 US 1 (2005). Oyez. Accessed June 25, 2020. https://www.oyez.org/cases/2004/03-1454.

Harper Polling. 2020. "Key Findings—Survey of PA Voters on Adult Use Cannabis." April 27. Accessed July 6, 2020. https://drive.google.com/file/d/18rM2UjQGvrqL0FHk64TR_dA-LzelHCgA/view.

H.J. Res. 117, 105th Cong. (1997–1998). Accessed July 28, 2020. https://www.congress.gov/bill/105th-congress/house-joint-resolution/117/all-actions.

Hsu, Spencer. 1999. "Bush: Marijuana Laws up to States." *Washington Post*, October 22. Accessed July 10, 2020. https://www.washingtonpost.com/wp-srv/politics/campaigns/wh2000/stories/bush102299.htm.

Hulse, Carl. 2018. "New Pot Policy by Trump Administration Draws Bipartisan Fire." *New York Times*, January 5. Accessed December 17, 2018. https://www.nytimes.com/2018/01/05/us/politics/trump-marijuana-policy-bipartisan-fire.html.

Ifill, Gwen. 1992. "The 1992 Campaign: New York; Clinton Admits Experiment with Marijuana in 1960s." *New York Times*, March 30. Accessed July 10, 2020. https://www.nytimes.com/1992/03/30/us/the-1992-campaign-new-york-clinton-admits-experiment-with-marijuana-in-1960-s.html.

Ingraham, Christopher. 2017. "Just How Mainstream Is Marijuana? There's Now a 'Congressional Cannabis Caucus.'" *Washington Post*, February 17. Accessed on July 7, 2020. https://www.washingtonpost.com/news/wonk/wp/2017/02/17/just-how-mainstream-is-marijuana-theres-now-a-congressional-cannabis-caucus/.

Krane, Kris. 2018. "Why President Trump Is Positioned to Be Marijuana's Great Savior & How the Democrats Blew It." *Forbes*, July 11. Accessed December 17, 2018. https://www.forbes.com/sites/kriskrane/2018/07/11/why-president-trump-could-be-marijuanas-savior/#99dbb8820a0d.

Latek, Tom. 2019. "Ky. Republican Lawmaker Proposing Bill to Legalize Medical Marijuana." Kentucky Today, November 1. Accessed July 3, 2020. https://www.kentuckytoday.com/stories/ky-republican-lawmaker-proposing-bill-to-make-medical-marijuana-legal,22447.

Matthews, Jon. 1996. "Supporters of Medical Marijuana Rejoice—Possession Still against U.S. Law, Opponents Note." *Sacramento Bee*, November 7, A4.

McAvoy, Audrey. 2019. "Liberal Hawaii Decides Again Not to Legalize Marijuana." Associated Press, March 1. Accessed July 9, 2020. https://apnews.com/008c88116a3c4aa38cc229404faeb5c0.

McCarthy, Justin. 2017. "Record-High Support for Legalizing Marijuana Use in U.S." Gallup, October 25. Accessed July 1, 2020. https://news.gallup.com/poll/221018/record-high-support-legalizing-marijuana.aspx.

McCarthy, Justin. 2018. "Two in Three Americans Now Support Legalizing Marijuana." Gallup, October 22. Accessed July 1, 2020. https://news.gallup.com/poll/243908/two-three-americans-support-legalizing-marijuana.aspx.

McEnany, Kayleigh. 2014. "Perverse Liberty and the Danger of Pot Legalization." Daily Caller, October 9. Accessed July 24, 2020. https://dailycaller.com/2014/10/09/perverse-liberty-and-the-danger-of-pot-legalization/.

McKinley, Jesse, and Vivian Wang. 2019. "Marijuana Decriminalization Is Expanded in N.Y., but Full Legalization Fails." *New York Times*, June 20. Accessed October 31, 2020. https://www.nytimes.com/2019/06/20/nyregion/marijuana-laws-ny.html.

Monmouth University Poll. 2019. "New Jersey: Support for Legal Weed Stays High." February 18. Accessed July 8, 2020. https://www.monmouth.edu/polling-institute/documents/monmouthpoll_nj_021819.pdf/.

Murphy, Phil. 2019. "Governor Murphy Signs Legislation to Dramatically Reform New Jersey's Medical Marijuana Program, Expand Patient Access." July 2. Accessed July 8, 2020. https://www.nj.gov/governor/news/news/562019/approved/20190702d.shtml.

Nahas, Gabriel, and Albert Greenwood. 1974. "The First Report of the National Commission on Marihuana (1972): Signal of Misunderstanding of Exercise in Ambiguity." *Bulletin of the New York Academy of Medicine* 50: 55–75. Accessed July 10, 2020. https://www.ncbi.nlm.nih.gov/pmc/articles/PMC1749335/pdf/bullnyacadmed00168-0058.pdf.

Noem, Kristi. 2019. "Why I Won't Support Legalizing Hemp." *Wall Street Journal*, September 9. Accessed July 7, 2020. https://www.wsj.com/articles/why-i-wont-support-legalizing-hemp-11568068697.

Office of Governor Pete Ricketts. 2020. "An Honest Look at Marijuana." January 27. Accessed July 24, 2020. https://governor.nebraska.gov/press/honest-look-marijuana.

Office of Governor Phil Scott. 2018. "Governor Phil Scott Signs H. 511." January 22. Accessed July 28, 2020. https://governor.vermont.gov/press-release/governor-phil-scott-signs-h-511.

Ogden, David. 2009. "Investigations and Prosecutions in States Authorizing the Medical Use of Marijuana." U.S. Department of Justice, Office of the Deputy Attorney General, October 19. Accessed July 5, 2020. https://www.justice.gov/sites/default/files/opa/legacy/2009/10/19/medical-marijuana.pdf.

Pacula, Rosalie Liccardo, Jamie Chriqui, and Joanna King. 2003. "Marijuana Decriminalization: What Does It Mean in the United States?" NBER Working Paper No. 9690. National Bureau of Economic Research. Accessed July 8, 2020. https://www.nber.org/papers/w9690.pdf.

Pelosi, Nancy (@SpeakerPelosi). 2018. "Attorney General Sessions, Your Unjust War against Americans Who Legally Use #marijuana Is Shameful & Insults the Democratic Processes That Played Out in States across the Country." Twitter, January 4. Accessed July 10, 2020. https://twitter.com/SpeakerPelosi/status/948975525850222593.

Pew Research Center. 2010. "Public Support for Legalizing Medical Marijuana." April 1. Accessed July 3, 2020. https://www.pewresearch.org/politics/2010/04/01/public-support-for-legalizing-medical-marijuana/.

Politico. 2020. "Legalizing Marijuana." February 19. Accessed July 8, 2020. https://www.politico.com/2020-election/candidates-views-on-the-issues/marijuana-cannabis-legalization/legalizing-marijuana/.

Ryan, Tim. 2018. "Rep. Tim Ryan: Marijuana Should Be Legal in All 50 States." CNN, July 20. Accessed December 17, 2018. https://www.cnn.com/2018/07/20/opinions/legalize-marijuana-all-50-states-ryan/index.html.

Samuels, Alex. 2019. "Medical Cannabis Expansion Has High Support in the Texas Legislature. But Dan Patrick Might Stand in the Way." *Texas Tribune*, March 19. Accessed July 3, 2020. https://www.texastribune.org/2019/03/19/texas-medical-cannabis-dan-patrick-senate-hurdle/.

Schuba, Tom. 2019. "Pritzker Makes Medical Marijuana Program Permanent, Adds List of New Conditions." *Chicago Sun-Times*, August 12. Accessed July 7, 2020. https://chicago.suntimes.com/cannabis/2019/8/12/20802391/pritzker-makes-medical-marijuana-program-permanent-adds-list-new-conditions.

Schumer, Chuck (@SenSchumer). 2018. "I Believe That the States Should Continue to Be the Labs of Democracy When It Comes to Recreational & Medical Marijuana. Jeff, This Is One Place Where States' Rights Works. Let Each State Decide." Twitter, January 6. Accessed July 10, 2020. https://twitter.com/SenSchumer/status/949739211938201600.

Segall, Bob. 2020. "Don't Look Now, Indiana Lawmakers, but Your Republican Neighbors Are All Legalizing Marijuana." WTHR, February 25. Accessed July 7, 2020. https://www.wthr.com/article/news/investigations/13-investigates/dont-look-now-indiana-lawmakers-your-republican-neighbors-are-all-legalizing-marijuana/531-f551ebd2-6f1e-480f-9a92-45fcb6a9be99.

Sessions, Jefferson. 2018. "Marijuana Enforcement." U.S. Department of Justice, Office of the Attorney General, January 4. Accessed July 7, 2020. https://www.justice.gov/opa/press-release/file/1022196/download.

Shain, Andy. 2018. "We Gave SC Governor Candidates 10 Questions. Here's Where They Stand on Top Issues." *Post and Courier*, October 14. Accessed July 24, 2020. https://www.postandcourier.com/politics/we-gave-sc-governor-candidates-questions-here-s-where-they/article_f1c9d7d6-ce3c-11e8-8e5b-5fb0725a8c4f.html.

Shalala, Donna E. (@DonnaShalala). 2018. "Minorities and People of Lower-income Are 10 Times More Likely to Be Arrested for Nonviolent Marijuana Offenses. Decriminalizing Marijuana Shouldn't Just Be a Policy Priority—But a Moral Imperative. Stand with Me in This Fight for Progressive Justice: https://donnashalala.com/marijuana/." Twitter, April 20. Accessed July 8, 2020. https://twitter.com/DonnaShalala/status/987463473125838848.

Shalala, Donna E. 2019. "Representatives Donna Shalala and Matt Gaetz Introduce the Expanding Cannabis Research and Information Act." September 12. Accessed on July 7, 2020. https://shalala.house.gov/news/documentsingle.aspx?DocumentID=2035.

Stout, David, and Solomon Moore. 2009. "U.S. Won't Prosecute in States That Allow Medical Marijuana." *New York Times*, October 19. Accessed July 5, 2020. https://www.nytimes.com/2009/10/20/us/20cannabis.html.

Travis, Jeremy, and Bruce Western. 2014. *The Growth of Incarceration in the United States: Exploring Causes and Consequences*. Washington, DC: National Academies Press.

United States v. Oakland Cannabis Buyers' Coop, 532 US 483 (2001). Oyez. Accessed June 25, 2020. https://www.oyez.org/cases/2000/00-151.

Weigel, David. 2016. "Democrats Call for 'Pathway' to Marijuana Legalization." *Washington Post*, July 9. Accessed on July 1, 2020. https://www.washingtonpost.com/news/post-politics/wp/2016/07/09/democrats-call-for-pathway-to-marijuana-legalization/.

Wenner, Jann. 2016. "The Day After: Obama on His Legacy, Trump's Win and the Path Forward." *Rolling Stone*, November 29. Accessed on July 1, 2020 https://www.rollingstone.com/politics/politics-features/the-day-after-obama-on-his-legacy-trumps-win-and-the-path-forward-113422/.

Wilson, Reid. 2020. "Vermont to Legalize Recreational Marijuana." The Hill, October 9. Accessed October 31, 2020. https://thehill.com/homenews/state-watch/520373-vermont-to-legalize-recreational-marijuana.

Wood, Benjamin. 2018. "Romney and Wilson Split on Utah's Medical Marijuana Initiative, Medicaid Expansion and the Future of U.S. Health Care." *Salt Lake Tribune*, September 24. Accessed December 17, 2018. https://www.sltrib.com/news/politics/2018/09/24/romney-wilson-split-utahs/.

Yu, Elly. 2019. "Medical Marijuana Patients Will Be Able to Get Treatment in D.C. Schools under Emergency Legislation." WAMU, September 18. Accessed July 9, 2020. https://wamu.org/story/19/09/18/medical-marijuana-patients-will-be-able-to-get-treatment-in-d-c-schools-under-emergency-legislation/.

Zielinski, Graeme. 2001. "Activist Robert C. Randall Dies." *Washington Post*, June 8. Accessed July 28, 2020. https://www.washingtonpost.com/archive/local/2001/06/08/activist-robert-c-randall-dies/c6e832a4-55e2-47fc-a3c8-5e011da66e04/.

Medicaid Expansion

At a Glance

A decade after its passage in 2010, the Medicaid expansion introduced by the Affordable Care Act (ACA) remains "one of the most consequential policy decisions of the law" (McDonough 2011, 141). Prior to 2010, eligibility for Medicaid varied widely among states. The ACA, also known as Obamacare, required states to expand eligibility for Medicaid up to 133 percent of the federal poverty line (FPL). Medicaid expansion offered federal policy makers a practical tool to expand health insurance coverage through a well-established and familiar program. The federal government covered 100 percent of the cost of newly eligible beneficiaries; beginning in 2020, states would be responsible for 10 percent of the cost of Medicaid expansion. States had a compelling rationale to expand eligibility, as any state that did not comply with the new coverage requirements risked losing *all* federal Medicaid funds (not merely the additional funding to expand coverage).

In response, 26 Republican-led states filed suit in federal court in March 2010, arguing that Congress exceeded its authority by threatening noncompliant states with the loss of all Medicaid funding. In June 2012, the U.S. Supreme Court concurred. The court's decision in *National Federation of Independent Business v. Sebelius* struck down the new Medicaid coverage requirement. Writing for a 7–2 majority, Chief Justice John Roberts compared the threatened loss of all Medicaid funds to "a gun to the head" for state policy makers. In the wake of the court's decision, decisions about Medicaid expansion fell to state governors and legislatures. A majority of the states declined to expand their Medicaid programs in 2014. By 2019, however, 36 states and the District of Columbia had voted to expand Medicaid eligibility. In some cases, such as Maine, a switch in party control of the governor's office led states to embrace Medicaid expansion. In 2014, Gov. John Kasich (R) of Ohio defied legislators in his own party who opposed the ACA by expanding Medicaid eligibility for more than 600,000 Ohioans. Kasich argued that the state could not pass up the opportunity to secure more than $13 billion in federal funding for low-income residents (Kasler 2018). Several states with Republican governors and Republican-controlled legislatures have also opted

Expansion of Medicaid Provides Hope to Citizens in Maine

In January 2019, Maine's newly elected Democratic governor, Janet Mills, reversed her Republican predecessor's long-standing opposition to Medicaid expansion. Medicaid expansion was a cornerstone of her 2018 campaign, and on her first day in office, Mills fulfilled her promise to voters by making Medicaid accessible to all eligible residents.

> Medicaid expansion is the law of the land in Maine, and that is why on my first day in office I issued Executive Order Number One which directs the Department of Health and Human Services to implement Medicaid expansion as swiftly and aggressively as possible. That was just over a week ago. Since then already we've enrolled 529 Mainers in health care coverage under the Medicaid expansion program. For many of these people, this has the power to change their lives for the better and even save their lives. Now they can see a doctor, receive preventive care, afford critical prescription medications, and much more. Now they can stay healthy, work, and care for their families. And we're just getting started. My Administration will review the applications that were previously denied to ensure that every eligible Mainer is able to access the health care coverage they need. We will team up with health care providers, advocates, patients, the business community and others to help enroll more eligible Mainers. And, my Administration will work with the Legislature to craft a biennial budget that ensures that Maine people can receive appropriate health care coverage.

Source

Mills, Janet. 2019. "Radio Address: Governor Mills: 'Health Care Is a Human Right.'" January 11, 2019. Accessed February 20, 2021. https://www.maine.gov/governor/mills/news/radio-address-governor-mills-health-care-human-right-2019-01-11.

to expand Medicaid in recent years. Republican support for expanding Medicaid in Kentucky and Virginia, for example, was linked to the introduction of work requirements for new enrollees (Armour 2018).

Democrats assert that the infusion of federal funding for Medicaid expansion allows states to address other important policy priorities. Democrats also argue that expanding Medicaid will significantly reduce the number of uninsured adults, relieving the burden of uncompensated care for hospitals and other health providers. Furthermore, with more paying patients covered under Medicaid, Democrats contend Medicaid expansion will create jobs in the health care industry and improve the financial well-being of hospitals. Financially vulnerable rural hospitals, in particular, stand to reap significant benefits from Medicaid expansion. Democrats also believe that expanding eligibility for Medicaid will improve health outcomes. Since insured individuals are more likely to receive preventative care and ongoing care for chronic conditions, Democrats contend that improved coverage will reduce unnecessary emergency visits and improve overall population health.

Medicaid Expansion Yields "Deplorable Results"

In March 2015, Sen. Mike Lee (R-UT) challenged the assumption underlying Medicaid expansion and highlighted the pitfalls of Medicaid for providers and patients.

> The rollout of the Affordable Care Act (ACA) has been so calamitous in so many ways that it can be easy to overlook the problems created by the law's Medicaid expansion. Historically, Medicaid has been a program with admirable intentions, but deplorable results. Prior to the ACA, Medicaid's objective was to provide health care and insurance to our most vulnerable populations, such as individuals with disabilities, as well as low-income children, pregnant women, and seniors. But Medicaid is notorious for trapping its beneficiaries in third-rate care. Matters have only gotten worse under the ACA, which fails to improve the quality of care for our society's most vulnerable, while expanding Medicaid's eligibility to include anyone up to 138 percent of the federal poverty level. Many states, including Utah, are trying to succeed where the ACA has failed, by agreeing to the new, expanded Medicaid eligibility requirements, but only on their own terms.

Source

Lee, Mike. 2015. "Medicaid Expansion." March 27, 2015. Accessed February 20, 2021. https://www.lee.senate.gov/public/index.cfm/2015/3/medicaid-expansion.

Republicans, on the other hand, assert that Medicaid expansion poses a significant threat to state budgets. If Congress reduces the generous federal funding for Medicaid expansion in the future, Republicans warn that states will face difficult choices. Cash-strapped states will be forced to either increase state funding to preserve eligibility—likely requiring significant tax increases—or limit eligibility and remove thousands of individuals from the Medicaid rolls. Republicans also believe Medicaid expansion leads many individuals to substitute public coverage for existing private health insurance. This, they argue, promotes dependency on government. Finally, Republicans argue that Medicaid expansion offers "second-rate" coverage compared to private insurance, as many state Medicaid programs restrict patients' choice of providers through "narrow networks" and low reimbursement rates that discourage many providers from accepting Medicaid.

According to Many Democrats . . .

- Medicaid expansion relieves states of the burden of caring for the uninsured.
- Medicaid expansion provides a much-needed infusion of funds for hospitals.
- Medicaid expansion increases the use of primary care and preventive services and improves health outcomes.

- Medicaid expansion brings millions of working families into the mainstream of American health care.

According to Many Republicans . . .

- Medicaid expansion is unaffordable and places a growing burden on state budgets over time.
- Medicaid expansion promotes dependency by encouraging individuals to substitute public coverage for private health insurance plans.
- Medicaid expansion reinforces the existing two-tiered health care system. Medicaid offers fewer participating providers, narrow networks, and low reimbursement for participating providers compared to private insurers.

Overview

Each state Medicaid program is unique, even though the federal government establishes basic eligibility criteria and a core set of services. States determine eligibility, certify participating providers, and reimburse providers for covered services. On several occasions over the past four decades, Republicans in Congress (joined by President Ronald Reagan) proposed to devolve responsibility for Medicaid to the states by transforming the program into a block grant that would expand state discretion but also cap federal funding (Thompson 1998). None of these proposals won widespread support. After Republicans regained control over the House of Representatives for the first time in four decades in 1994, Speaker Newt Gingrich (R-GA) revived the idea of a block grant. President George W. Bush also supported transforming Medicaid into a block grant in 2003. After the passage of the Affordable Care Act (ACA), many prominent Republicans in Congress, including House Speaker Paul Ryan (R-WI) and Rep. Tom Price (R-GA), continued to press for a Medicaid block grant, which they described as a way to foster state innovation and increase program efficiency (Luthra 2017).

As a result, Medicaid remains a classic case of shared governance in the federal system. Financing is shared between states and the federal government, the latter of which provides 50–77 percent of program funding in every state. The federal government's share of Medicaid costs, known as the Federal Medical Assistance Percentage (FMAP), varies widely. Thirteen states with higher levels of per capita income shouldered 50 percent of the cost of their state Medicaid programs, while in Mississippi—with the nation's lowest per capita income—the federal government funded 77 percent of program costs (*Federal Register* 2018). States may request waivers from the federal requirements, but the Centers for Medicare and Medicaid Services (CMS) must approve all waiver requests. Waivers can include eligibility for coverage, the type of covered services, provider payment, and reporting, among others.

Eligibility for Medicaid varied widely before the passage of the ACA. Congress expanded eligibility for pregnant women and children during the 1980s, but non-disabled adults without children were largely excluded from coverage. In FY 2007, the year before the beginning of the Great Recession, the total federal and state expenditures on Medicaid was $333.3 billion. However, Medicaid spending is cyclical. Both enrollment and expenditures rise when the economy enters a recession, as more individuals qualify for benefits (Scott 2019).

This presents a difficult fiscal challenge for states because Medicaid spending increases at the same time state revenues decline. Unlike the federal government, every state except Vermont has a legal obligation to balance its budget (National Conference of State Legislatures 1999). While Medicaid expansion is popular when the economy is growing, the threat of an economic downturn worries state policy makers. Medicaid is one of the largest line items in state budgets, and its share of spending from state general funds has steadily increased over the past three decades, from less than 10 percent in 1990 to nearly 20 percent in 2016 (MACPAC 2019b).

The ACA sought to nationalize Medicaid coverage in all states by establishing a common floor for eligibility. Many Republican governors, however, saw Medicaid expansion as coercive, for "if a state refused to accept this 'new' Medicaid expansion, the federal government could 'penalize' the state by terminating its participation in—and all federal funding for—the 'old' Medicaid program" (Mariner, Glantz, and Annas 2012). In the 2012 case of *National Federation of Independent Business v. Sebelius*, the U.S. Supreme Court considered whether Congress exceeded its authority by forcing states to expand Medicaid to all individuals under the age of 65 with incomes below 133 percent of the federal poverty line (FPL). By a 7–2 majority—including two of the court's liberal members—Stephen Breyer and Elena Kagan, the justices rejected this requirement. As Chief Justice John Roberts noted in his majority opinion for the court, "The threatened loss of over 10 percent of a State's overall budget . . . is economic dragooning that leaves the States with no real option but to acquiesce in the Medicaid expansion" (*National Federation of Independent Business v. Sebelius* 2012). With this ruling, "the Court today limits the financial pressure the Secretary may apply to induce States to accept the terms of the Medicaid expansion. As a practical matter, that means States may now choose to reject the expansion; that is the whole point. But that does not mean all or even any will" (*National Federation of Independent Business v. Sebelius* 2012).

The court's decision transformed the politics of Medicaid expansion. The ruling exposed a major rift over the implantation of the ACA between Democratic- and Republican-controlled states. More than half of the states rejected Medicaid expansion when the program was implemented in 2014. No states with unified Republican government chose to expand eligibility, while all states with unified Democratic control opted for expansion (Beland, Rocco, and Waddan 2016, 95). As of 2019, 36 states and the District of Columbia had expanded Medicaid eligibility. Total Medicaid enrollment reached 65 million in 2014 (nearly double its level in 2007).

Medicaid enrollment peaked at 74.6 million in December 2017 before falling to 73 million in December 2018 (Kaiser Family Foundation 2019a). After the coronavirus pandemic battered the U.S. economy in 2020, Medicaid enrollment rebounded to 74.6 million in June 2020. Medicaid enrollment increased during the economic shutdown in early 2020, as millions of Americans who lost jobs—and thus met the income eligibility criteria for enrollment—qualified for benefits. In addition, the Families First Coronavirus Response Act (FFCRA) requires states to maintain coverage for current Medicaid enrollees (Corallo and Rudowitz 2020).

States followed different pathways to expand Medicaid eligibility. The Obama administration encouraged states to expand Medicaid by applying for Section 1115 waivers. Waivers provide states with greater flexibility to experiment with new approaches to enhance coverage or improve services. Obama administration officials carefully reviewed waiver proposals to ensure they would increase coverage and conform to the minimum essential coverage requirements established by the ACA. Arkansas, for example, became the first state to adopt a "private option" in which Medicaid funds would be used to purchase private health insurance for beneficiaries through the state's health insurance marketplace rather than enrolling eligible individuals in "traditional" Medicaid. Federal officials approved the state's proposal in 2013; soon afterward, New Hampshire followed suit with a similar Medicaid expansion plan in 2014.

The Trump administration adopted a different approach to Medicaid waivers. While CMS officials continued to approve state waiver applications, Trump administration officials welcomed Medicaid expansions that imposed new conditions on beneficiaries favored by conservative lawmakers (e.g., work requirements). As of 2019, 9 states were operating their Medicaid expansion under a 1115 waiver, and 14 other Republican-led states continued to reject Medicaid expansion (Kaiser Family Foundation 2019b).

The range of state experiences with Medicaid expansion is diverse. The experiences of an early adopter (California), a Section 1115 waiver applicant (Arkansas), a ballot initiative state (Utah), and a steadfast opponent (Texas) illustrate the choices faced by state officials in deciding whether to expand Medicaid eligibility. The positions of key policy makers and interest groups, state ideology, and public opinion all shaped state responses.

California

California is a deep blue state that strongly supported President Obama in both the 2008 and 2012 presidential elections. In 2013, Democrats held strong majorities in both the Assembly and the Senate and also controlled the governor's office. Gov. Jerry Brown (D) signed the state's Medicaid expansion into law in 2013. His successor, Gavin Newsom (D), also embraced Medicaid expansion as a cornerstone of the state's progressive health care agenda. California's Medicaid program (known as Medi-Cal) covers 13 million people; 3.8 million individuals became eligible for Medicaid as a result of the state's Medicaid expansion in 2014 (Norris 2018). Thanks in large part to this expansion, the uninsured rate in California fell 58 percent from 2013 to 2017 (Norris 2018). By 2017, Medi-Cal insured nearly one in three (29 percent) Californians (California Health Care Almanac 2019).

Medicaid expansion remains popular in California. In 2016, voters approved two ballot measures to increase funding for Medi-Cal. Proposition 52, which extended hospital fees to fund Medi-Cal health care services and care for uninsured patients, passed with 70 percent of the vote. Two-thirds of voters (64 percent) also endorsed Proposition 56, which raised the tax on cigarettes to support Medi-Cal and other public health programs (Norris 2018). Public opinion polls underscore the popularity of Medicaid expansion in California. In 2018, 70 percent of Californians held a "very favorable" or "somewhat favorable" view of Medicaid (California Health Care Almanac 2019). While Democrats are most supportive of Medicaid in California, it is notable that a majority of Republicans living in the state also held either very favorable or somewhat favorable views of the program. In addition, 76 percent of Californians in one 2019 survey of the state's population rated Medi-Cal as "very important" to the state, and another 15 percent regarded it as "somewhat important" (California Health Care Almanac 2019). Overall, an overwhelming proportion of both Democrats (89 percent) and Republicans (71 percent) regarded Medi-Cal as "very important" to California.

Arkansas

In 2013, Gov. Mike Beebe (D) signed Arkansas's nontraditional "private option" into law after the Republican-controlled state legislature balked at approving a traditional Medicaid expansion. In response, policy makers developed a proposal to use Medicaid funds to purchase private health insurance through the state's ACA health insurance marketplace. Despite its unconventional approach, officials in the Obama administration were eager to accommodate the state's interest in pursuing expansion and approved the scheme. By expanding Medicaid in this manner, Arkansas reduced its uninsured rate by 51 percent from 2013 to 2017. More than 321,000 individuals gained coverage as a result of the expansion (Norris 2019a).

Asa Hutchinson (R) replaced Beebe as governor in 2015, giving Republicans unified control over the legislature and the governorship. When the state's Section 1115 waiver came up for renewal, Hutchinson proposed a new approach known as Arkansas Works, which established community engagement as a requirement of eligibility of receiving benefits for nondisabled adults. In June 2018, the Trump administration approved Arkansas's proposed work requirement for Medicaid beneficiaries. Under this new rule, eligible individuals must work or participate in approved community engagement activities (e.g., job training) for 80 hours per month and report their work hours to the state. After the implementation of the new requirements, more than 18,000 individuals lost Medicaid benefits for failure to meet the work and reporting requirements (Froelich 2019).

In March 2019, a federal judge overturned the state's new rules, arguing the new policy was inconsistent with the goal of the Medicaid program to expand access to coverage for low-income individuals. The Trump administration appealed this ruling, but in February 2020, the U.S. Court of Appeals for the D.C. Circuit rejected the use of mandatory work requirements in Arkansas in a unanimous decision (Pradhan and Luthi 2020). In February 2020, the D.C. Circuit Court of Appeals reaffirmed this decision, invalidating the use of work requirements as a condition of Medicaid eligibility (Schneider 2020).

Public support for Medicaid expansion in Arkansas was sharply divided along party lines, but over time, the program gained popularity among Arkansans. In 2012, one poll found that 64 percent of Republican voters opposed Medicaid expansion, and only 21 percent supported expansion (Barth 2018). By 2016, however, after Gov. Hutchinson (R) expressed support for Medicaid expansion and rebranded the program as Arkansas Works, Republican opposition fell to 34 percent (Barth 2018). Notably, 70 percent of Democrats also endorsed the new Arkansas Works program (Brock 2018). Even after the introduction of the new work requirement, support for Medicaid expansion across the state remained essentially bipartisan (Barth 2018).

Utah

The state of Utah, where Republicans have maintained a firm grip on both houses of the legislature and the governor's office since 1992, was one of the original litigants in the legal challenge against the ACA in March 2010. Nevertheless, Utah's Gov. Gary Herbert developed a Medicaid expansion proposal in 2014, but this plan failed to win the endorsement of key legislators (Advisory Board 2020). In 2018, voters approved Proposition 3, a ballot measure to fully expand Medicaid eligibility to 150,000 Utahns, by a margin of 53 percent to 47 percent. Proposition 3 "earned majority support in 17 out of 29 state Senate districts and 44 out of 75 state House districts" (Wood 2019b). Utah legislators, however, continued to favor a more limited Medicaid expansion, delaying implementation until January 1, 2020.

In 2019, the Utah State Legislature passed, and Governor Herbert signed, a bill authorizing a partial Medicaid expansion (Advisory Board 2020).

Although supporters of Proposition 3 were outraged by this action, newly elected Utah Senator Mitt Romney (R-UT) claimed that the "state's plan is better than the ballot measure" (Weixel 2018). Federal officials in the Trump administration approved Utah's partial Medicaid expansion in March 2019, allowing the state to impose work requirements and cap enrollment if the state lacked sufficient funds (Advisory Board 2020). Utah's Medicaid expansion was implemented on January 1, 2020, opening up eligibility to individuals earning up to 138 percent of the FPL after the Trump administration approved the state's "Fallback Plan" waiver request (Kaiser Family Foundation 2021). The state's waiver proposal initially incorporated a work requirement for newly eligible adult enrollees, but federal courts blocked the implementation of work requirements in 2020 as an "arbitrary and capricious" action by the secretary of Health and Human Services (Schneider 2020).

Support for Medicaid expansion in Utah displayed a wide partisan divide. While 94 percent of Democrats and 71 percent of independents supported the expansion, 43 percent of Republicans opposed it according to one public survey (Lockhart 2018). Utah's Medicaid expansion underscores the role of state officials in coverage decisions, as legislators and the governor both continued to harbor concerns about the fiscal implications of expansion.

Texas

Texas is a solid red state. Since George W. Bush won the governor's office in 1995, Republicans have held the governorship in each successive election (Legislative Reference Library of Texas 2019a). Republicans have also maintained control of both houses of the state legislature since 2003 (Legislative Reference Library of Texas 2019a). Texas staunchly opposed the Medicaid expansion proposed by the ACA and became one of the original litigants in the *National Federation of Independent Business v. Sebelius* lawsuit filed in March 2010. Ironically, Texas took the lead in the fight against Medicaid expansion despite the fact that it had led the nation in the percentage of uninsured residents for more than a decade; in 2018, its uninsured rate was 19.6 percent, more than twice as high as the average for expansion states (Kaiser Family Foundation 2018).

For Texas Republicans, Medicaid expansion is a nonstarter because of the threat it could pose to their political reputation. Republican officeholders in Texas never approved of Obamacare and continued to challenge the law in court in the case of *Texas v. United States*—a legal challenge filed after Congress repealed the individual mandate penalty in December 2017. This case, which was filed in a federal district court in North Texas, was heard by the U.S. Supreme Court in November 2020. Advocates for Medicaid expansion in Texas, including hospitals and other health providers, face significant obstacles because Texas passed a bill that requires the state legislature to approve any future Medicaid expansion decisions (Norris 2019b). Both former and present Texas governors, Rick Perry (Republican 2000–2015) and Greg Abbott (Republican 2015–present), have said that the 10 percent share of Medicaid costs that Texas would have to cover in 2020 if they chose to expand would be too burdensome on the state budget (Norris 2019b).

Although Texas Democrats file legislation to expand Medicaid during each legislative session, their efforts consistently fail to gain traction in the Republican-dominated legislature (Waller 2018). As a result, every Dallas County property owner paid $535 on average to Parkland Health and Hospital System in 2018 to compensate it for providing $1 billion in uncompensated care to uninsured patients (Schutze 2019).

Not surprisingly, public opinion data reveals a stark partisan divide on Medicaid expansion within the state. In a poll conducted by the Commonwealth Foundation in 2013, 70 percent of voters agreed that Medicaid should not be expanded until "waste, fraud, and abuse" is cleaned up (Commonwealth Foundation 2013). In addition, 60 percent of voters and 84 percent of Republicans said the argument that "we can't count on the federal government to keep its funding commitment" was convincing (Commonwealth Foundation 2013).

A 2018 poll conducted by the Kaiser Family Foundation found that 82 percent of Texas Democrats and 71 percent of independents supported Medicaid expansion. Republican opposition remained strong, however, with 59 percent of Republicans expressing a desire to keep the state's current Medicaid program and reject expansion (Kaiser Family Foundation and Episcopal Health Foundation 2018). The same poll also found that nearly half (46 percent) of Texans believe expanding Medicaid to low-income Texans should be a top priority (Kaiser Family Foundation and Episcopal Health Foundation 2018).

Across the nation, about 16 million people gained coverage as a result of states expanding Medicaid under the ACA. An additional 5 million individuals could be insured if every state expanded eligibility to 133 percent of the FPL. In 2020, the federal government will pick up 90 percent of the cost of Medicaid, leaving participating states to foot the bill for the remaining 10 percent.

The health impacts of Medicaid expansion are well documented in the medical literature (Antonisse et al. 2018). For example, Benjamin Sommers and his coauthors compared the experience of states that expanded Medicaid (Arkansas and Kentucky) with states that refused to expand eligibility (Texas). In states that expanded Medicaid, more individuals reported having a personal physician, fewer individuals skipped taking medications because of cost concerns, and fewer individuals relied on hospital emergency rooms for primary care (Sommers et al. 2016). Proponents of Medicaid expansion also point out that expanding insurance coverage more than doubled the use of preventative services such as mammography and annual physicals (Sommers et al. 2016). In addition, states that expanded Medicaid eligibility also reported lower age-adjusted cardiovascular mortality rates among residents aged 45 to 64 years after expansion compared to nonexpansion states (Khatana, Bhatla and Nathan 2019).

Democrats on Medicaid Expansion

Democrats contend that Medicaid expansion offered states a win-win proposition. Democrats note that the initial cost of expansion would be fully financed by the federal government. Furthermore, since the funding formula was much more generous than for individuals who qualified under "traditional" Medicaid, Democrats felt that most, if not all, states would embrace the opportunity to expand eligibility. After the Supreme Court's decision in the case of *National Federation of Independent Business v. Sebelius*, House Speaker Nancy Pelosi (D-CA) declared, "Once this bill is rolling and people experience benefits of it, it's very hard for a state to say [no]"

(Khimm 2012). Kentucky's Gov. Steve Beshear echoed this sentiment: "Not only can states afford to expand Medicaid, but they also really can't afford not to do it" (Beshear 2015). The reality, as Democrats soon discovered, was far different; a majority of Republican-led states rejected the financial carrot offered by the Obama administration and refused to expand Medicaid eligibility in 2014.

Democrats argued that increased access to health insurance paid substantial dividends for hospitals and other health providers. Speaking on behalf of Medicaid expansion in 2019, Gov. Laura Kelly argued, "It's long past time to expand Medicaid so that more Kansans have access to affordable healthcare, our rural hospitals can stay open, and the tax dollars we send to Washington can come back home to Kansas to help our families. This bill meets the unique needs of Kansas patients, hospitals, providers" (Shorman 2019). Medicaid funds provided a vital infusion for cash-strapped hospitals serving vulnerable populations. As Gov. Tom Wolf Pennsylvania noted, "We've been able to keep hospitals that are and were on the financial edge open because now they're getting reimbursed for treatments that they weren't getting reimbursed for before" (Wolf 2017). Before Medicaid expansion, hospitals treated a higher proportion of uninsured patients, many of whom delayed seeking care because of financial concerns.

Democratic legislators thus repeatedly emphasized the benefits of expansion for health providers. Rep. Peter Schweyer (PA) noted that Medicaid expansion "saved hundreds of jobs in downtown Allentown by increasing the number of patients actually seeing the doctor and by reducing uncompensated care which in turn strengthened the bottom line of our hospitals and clinics" (Wolf 2018). By providing more patients with comprehensive insurance coverage, Medicaid expansion offered hospitals two concrete benefits. On the one hand, hospitals needed to provide less uncompensated care to indigent patients. On the other, hospitals saw the demand for their services increase, as formerly uninsured patients were able to access care outside of emergency settings for the first time.

Democratic governors touted the benefits of expanding Medicaid eligibility. As Gov. Jay Inslee of Washington declared, "It is absolutely nuts not to accept free money to help this effort when people need health care" (Miller 2018. Conversely, Democrats in states that refused to expand Medicaid displayed growing frustration over time, for their states left millions—if not billions—of dollars on the table. One Democratic state senator in Mississippi complained, "As a result of us not taking advantage of the Affordable Care Act we lost about $9 billion that could have benefited so many Mississippians. And when I say Mississippians, I'm not talking about just those people who are the recipients of Medicaid. I'm talking about those health care providers, those doctors, those nurses, those community hospitals that are closing" (Campbell 2018).

In addition, Democrats noted that Medicaid expansion provided a lifeline for struggling rural hospitals. In fact, the rate of hospital closures for rural hospitals in nonexpansion states is six times greater than in expansion states (Bullock 2019).

As Gov. Laura Kelly declared, "It's long past time to expand Medicaid so that more Kansans have access to affordable healthcare, our rural hospitals can stay open, and the tax dollars we send to Washington can come back home to Kansas to help our families" (Shorman, 2019).

Democrats also touted Medicaid expansion as a way to increase the use of primary care and preventive services and improve health outcomes. States that expanded Medicaid reported reduced infant mortality, increases in cancer diagnosis, and better adherence to prescription medications for treating opioid disorders (Antonisse et al. 2018. Furthermore, individuals with Medicaid coverage used hospital emergency departments at the same rate as people with private insurance (Perkins and McDonald 2017). Medicaid expansion also took on renewed importance in light of the opioid epidemic. In Pennsylvania, Gov. Tom Wolf noted, "We were able to provide access to critical drug and alcohol treatment to 124,170 newly eligible Pennsylvanians, which is helping to battle the opioid and heroin public health crisis" (Wolf 2017).

Finally, Democrats believe that Medicaid expansion moves millions of working families from the margins into the mainstream of American health care. Gov. Mike Beebe of Arkansas argued in 2012 that Medicaid expansion is "good for our people because it's helping folks that don't have insurance now that are working their tails off. They're not sitting on a couch somewhere asking for something" (Brantley 2012). In 2014, President Barack Obama declared, "Because of [the ACA], millions of our fellow citizens know the economic security of health insurance who didn't just a few years ago—and that's something to be proud of" (Obama 2014). For President Obama, increased access to health insurance meant better health care—and better health—for millions of Americans. He argued, "That's what the Affordable Care Act, or Obamacare, is all about—making sure that all of us, and all our fellow citizens, can count on the security of health care when we get sick; that the work and dignity of every person is acknowledged and affirmed" (Obama 2014).

Republicans on Medicaid Expansion

Some Republicans, including Gov. Terry Branstad (Iowa), Gov. John Kasich (Ohio), Gov. Brian Sandoval (Nevada), and Gov. Rick Snyder (Michigan), embraced ACA-sponsored Medicaid expansion as a means of leveraging additional federal funding to address their states' health care needs. As Gov. Kasich argued, "If other people don't want to take the money, that's up to them, but I got money I can bring home to Ohio. It's my money. There's no money in Washington. It's my money. It's the money of the people who live in my state" (Montanaro 2015). Two-thirds of the nation's Republican governors, however, opposed Medicaid expansion, arguing that it is unaffordable in the long run and will place a growing burden on state budgets. Texas's Gov. Greg Abbott captured the sentiments of a majority of his fellow Republican governors in 2019. He declared that he was opposed to expanding Medicaid "because the eventual 10 percent of the cost that the state would pay by 2020 would be too much for the budget" (Norris 2019b). In Louisiana, a conservative think tank called the Pelican Institute argued that "Washington is spending billions annually funding Medicaid for people with prior health coverage" (Jacobs 2019). A 2019 study by the National Bureau of Economic Research (NBER) of health insurance changes in nine states that expanded Medicaid found that 800,000 individuals obtained Medicaid coverage even though they did not meet the income criteria for enrollment. As a result, conservative health policy scholars argued that "ObamaCare has turned out to be a giant welfare program, with millions of working- and middle-class Americans improperly receiving Medicaid" (Blase and Yelowitz 2019).

Republican legislators echoed these concerns. As Utah state senator Dan Hemmert warned in 2018, "Obamacare Medicaid expansion includes no cost or enrollment circuit breakers, and once we are in, we will never get out. The payment is undetermined and 'term of the loan' is indefinite. Our decision will determine our future ability to fund vital state needs such as education, transportation and public safety" (Hemmert 2018). Hemmert challenged supporters of Utah's Medicaid expansion ballot initiative in 2018, noting that "Medicaid currently absorbs 18.7 percent of Utah's General Fund budget. How much more can we afford without more tax hikes or major cuts in services? That is happening in other states. So what are we willing to cut, or which taxes are we willing to raise, to pay for it?" Medicaid expansion, in this view, presents policy makers with a choice. As states must balance their budgets, legislators cannot spend more on Medicaid without either raising taxes or cutting other important programs. In 2013, Sen. Ted Cruz (R-TX) told Texas voters, "If you want state funds to provide for our prisons and law enforcement to incarcerate violent criminals and keep them off the streets, you should be glad we're not signing up for this Medicaid expansion, because every state that does so is going to be regretting it mightily because the pressure is going to crowd out just about every other priority in the budget" (Johnson 2013).

Republicans contend that expanding Medicaid will inevitably push state budgets into the red. Republican legislators in Kansas worried that "the feds may pull the rug out from under them and argue the state would face a heavy burden if Washington stops funding the expansion, as has happened with other government programs" (Patton 2019). Many Republicans cite this alleged uncertainty about future costs as a major deterrent to adopting Medicaid expansion. In Utah, Sen. Dan Hemmert (2018) argued that "in every expansion state, enrollment and cost estimates have been way off; reality has sometimes doubled projections, thus doubling the costs." In this context, Republicans see Medicaid expansion as a fiscally risky proposition.

Since the end of the Great Recession, Medicaid's share of state budgets has continued to grow—an unexpected development in an economic recovery (Scott 2019). Republican opponents emphasize that if federal policy makers ever decide to reduce or eliminate enhanced reimbursement for newly eligible individuals, states will be responsible for millions (if not billions) of dollars they do not have. Republican leaders in the Kansas Senate maintained "the state can't afford to take on the costs of expanding Medicaid, despite the promise from Washington that the federal government will pick up 90 percent of the tab" (Greenblat 2019). Gov. Greg Abbott of Texas claimed "that he is opposed to expanding Medicaid because the eventual 10 percent of the cost that the state would pay by 2020 would be too much for the budget" (Norris 2019b). In Utah, Sen. Dan Hemmert warned that the state's share of Medicaid expenditures would increase steadily over time. "In 2000," Hemmert noted, "Utah spent $774 million on Medicaid; $127 million of that was Utah's share, or 11.8 percent of Utah's budget. In 2016, the most recent year for which we have complete data, Utah's total Medicaid expenditure was $2.5 billion, a whopping 229 percent increase in Medicaid alone. Utah's share increased to $893 million, a 603 percent increase since 2000. And that was without Medicaid expansion under Obamacare" (Hemmert 2018).

In addition to voicing fiscal concerns about Medicaid expansion, Republicans worry that increasing the number of publicly insured individuals encourages dependency on government. Republicans believe that many Medicaid beneficiaries can, and should, obtain private insurance rather than relying on public coverage. As Arthur Brooks noted in the *Conservative Heart*, "We have seen how the number of Americans on federal nutritional assistance ('food stamps') has skyrocketed in recent years. Some look at those figures and see great success. They say, 'Hey, look! We helped all these people! Isn't that fantastic?' But conservatives in touch with their hearts will reply with incredulity: 'We have sixty-some percent more people on food stamps five years after the end of the recession than we had at the beginning? That isn't success. It is failure'" (Brooks 2016).

Conservative critics of the ACA also often cite concerns about Medicaid "crowding out" private coverage. Given the choice between subsidized (or free) public insurance and private coverage, many Republicans argue that individuals will cancel their existing private policies. In this view, crowding out not only increases the cost of Medicaid but also promotes dependency. As the Pelican Institute noted, "Thousands of Louisiana residents dropped their private coverage to enroll in Medicaid under the expansion." As a result, "the number of people covered by private health insurance declined by tens of thousands, even as Medicaid enrollment skyrocketed by more than 141,000" (Jacobs 2019).

Republicans draw a distinction between deserving and undeserving beneficiaries of public funds. In many Republican-controlled states, winning support for Medicaid expansion hinges on convincing legislators and voters that recipients are "deserving." Arkansas gained national attention for instituting work requirements for newly eligible Medicaid beneficiaries; such requirements address concerns that expansion promotes dependency. Gov. Asa Hutchinson of Arkansas asserted, "We are simply saying if you are able-bodied and able to work, and you don't have dependent children at home you ought to either be working or you ought to be in school or you ought to be volunteering or contributing" (Froelich 2019). Sen. Orrin Hatch (R-UT) worried that Medicaid expansion could change individuals' relationship with government. "The public," Hatch argued, "wants every dime they can be given. . . . Let's face it, once you get them on the dole, they'll take every dime they can. We've got to find some way of getting things under control or this country and your future is going to be gone" (May 2017).

Finally, Republicans argue that Medicaid expansion reinforces the existing two-tiered health care system. As Medicaid programs often offer individuals narrow provider networks and lower reimbursement for participating providers, Republicans describe Medicaid as "second-rate" health care coverage. On April 1, 2013, Gov. Rick Perry made it clear that Texas would not expand Medicaid eligibility. Perry quipped, "The first day of April. Seems to me an appropriate April Fool's Day—makes it perfect to discuss something as foolish as Medicaid expansion and to remind everyone that Texas will not be held hostage by the Obama administration's attempt to force us into this fool's errand of adding more than a million Texans to a broken system" (Goodwyn 2015). For former House Speaker Paul Ryan (R-WI), the issue was simple: "What good is your coverage if you can't get a doctor?" (Kodjak 2017). Even if patients can find a participating provider, conservative critics argued that waiting for appointments can take months. "Expanding Medicaid, as prescribed in Obamacare, will crowd out the most vulnerable in our state who are already using Medicaid while pushing tens of thousands off of their private insurance onto taxpayer-funded government-run healthcare" (Marso and Shorman 2019).

Robert B. Hackey and Anne Capozzoli

Further Reading

Advisory Board. 2020. "Where the States Stand on Medicaid Expansion." October 8. Accessed March 9, 2021.https://www.advisory.com/daily-briefing/resources/primers/medicaidmap.

Antonisse, Larisa, Rachel Garfield, Robin Rudowitz, and Samantha Artiga. 2018. "The Effects of Medicaid Expansion under the ACA: Updated Findings from a Literature Review." Kaiser Family Foundation, March. Accessed October 30, 2020. http://files.kff.org/attachment/Issue-Brief-The-Effects-of-Medicaid-Expansion-Under-the-ACA-Updated-Findings-from-a-Literature-Review.

Armour, Stephanie. 2018. "Medicaid Expansion Gains Popularity in Red States." *Wall Street Journal*, June 14. Accessed October 30, 2020. https://www.wsj.com/articles/medicaid-expansion-gains-popularity-in-red-states-1528974001.

Barth, Jay. 2018. "Medicaid Favor." *Arkansas Times*, April 26. Accessed October 30, 2020. https://arktimes.com/columns/jay-barth/2018/04/26/medicaid-favor.

Beland, Daniel, Philip Rocco, and Alex Waddan. 2016. *ObamaCare Wars: Federalism, Politics and the Affordable Care Act*. Lawrence: University Press of Kansas.

Beshear, Steve. 2015. "Medicaid Expansion: Kentucky Governor Explains His State's Success." *Richmond Times-Dispatch*, August 17. Accessed June 26, 2019. https://www.richmond.com/opinion/their-opinion/guest-columnists/medicaid-expansion-kentucky-governor-explains-his-state-s-success/article_23612d66-b0f8-5956-92fe-7b895c630e58.html.

Blase, Brian, and Aaron Yelowitz. 2019. "ObamaCare's Medicaid Deception." *Wall Street Journal*, August 15. Accessed October 30, 2020. https://www.wsj.com/articles/obamacares-medicaid-deception-11565822360.

Brantley, Max. 2012. "It's Official: Gov. Beebe Supports Medicaid Expansion." *Arkansas Times*, September 11. Accessed June 25, 2019. https://arktimes.com/arkansas-blog/2012/09/11/its-official-gov-beebe-supports-medicaid-expansion.

Brock, Roby. 2018. "Poll: 2nd District Democrats Show Strong Support for Arkansas Works, Gun Regulation." Talk Business & Politics, May 10. Accessed October 30, 2020. https://talkbusiness.net/2018/05/poll-2nd-district-democrats-show-strong-support-for-arkansas-works-gun-regulation/.

Brooks, Arthur. 2016. *The Conservative Heart*. New York: Harper Collins/Broadside Books.

Bullock, Steve. 2019. "Governor Steve Bullock's 2019 State of the State Address." State of Montana Newsroom, January 31. Accessed March 9, 2021. https://news.mt.gov/governor-steve-bullocks-2019-state-of-the-state-address.

California Health Care Foundation. 2019. *California Health Care Almanac: Medi-Cal Facts and Figures: Crucial Coverage for Low-Income Californians*. Oakland: California Health Care Foundation. Accessed February 14, 2021. https://www.chcf.org/wp-content/uploads/2019/02/MediCalFactsFiguresAlmanac2019.pdf.

Campbell, Larrison. 2018. "Democrats Futilely Push for Medicaid Expansion in Tech Bill." *Mississippi Today*, February 7. Accessed February 14, 2021. https://mississippitoday.org/2018/02/06/democrats-futilely-push-medicaid-expansion-tech-bill/.

City Wire. 2013. "Beebe Defends Arkansas' Medicaid Expansion." Talkbusiness.com, June 26. Accessed June 25, 2019. https://talkbusiness.net/2013/06/beebe-defends-arkansas-medicaid-expansion/.

Commonwealth Foundation. 2013. "Public Opinion of Medicaid Expansion." Accessed October 30, 2020. https://www.commonwealthfoundation.org/docLib/20130812_PublicOpinionofExpansion.pdf.

Corallo, Bradley, and Robin Rudowitz. 2020. "Analysis of Recent National Trends in Medicaid and CHIP Enrollment." Kaiser Family Foundation, October 15. Accessed October 30, 2020. https://www.kff.org/coronavirus-covid-19/issue-brief/analysis-of-recent-national-trends-in-medicaid-and-chip-enrollment/.

Federal Register. Department of Health and Human Services. 2018. "Federal Financial Participation in State Assistance Expenditures; Federal Matching Shares for Medicaid, the Children's Health Insurance Program, and Aid to Needy Aged, Blind, or Disabled Persons for October 1, 2019 through September 30, 2020." Vol. 83. No. 229: 61159. (November 28, 2018). Accessed March 9, 2021. https://www.govinfo.gov/content/pkg/FR-2018-11-28/pdf/2018-25944.pdf.

Froelich, Jacqueline. 2019. "In Arkansas, Thousands of People Have Lost Medicaid Coverage over New Work Rule." NPR, February 18. Accessed June 25, 2019. https://www.npr.org/sections/health-shots/2019/02/18/694504586/in-arkansas-thousands-of-people-have-lost-medicaid-coverage-over-new-work-rule.

Goodwyn, Wade. 2015. "Texas Politicians and Businesses Feud over Medicaid Expansion." NPR, May 29. Accessed June 25, 2019. https://www.npr.org/sections/health-shots/2015/05/29/410520561/texas-politicians-and-businesses-feud-over-medicaid-expansion.

Hemmert, Dan. 2018. "Proposition 3 Is Not Right for Utah." *Deseret News*, September 22. Accessed February 14, 2021. https://www.deseretnews.com/article/900032994/guest-opinion-proposition-3-is-not-right-for-utah.html.

Jacobs, Chris. 2019. "Medicaid Expansion Has Louisianans Dropping Plans." *Wall Street Journal*, June 8–9: A13.

Johnson, Luke. 2013. "Ted Cruz: Medicaid Expansion Will Worsen Health Care for the Poor." HuffPost, April 2. Accessed June 25, 2019. https://www.huffpost.com/entry/ted-cruz-medicaid_n_2998105.

Kaiser Family Foundation. 2018. "Key Facts about the Uninsured Population." Accessed July 3, 2019. https://www.kff.org/uninsured/fact-sheet/key-facts-about-the-uninsured-population/.

Kaiser Family Foundation. 2019a. "Analysis of Recent Declines in Medicaid and CHIP Enrollment." Accessed June 18, 2019. https://www.kff.org/medicaid/fact-sheet/analysis-of-recent-declines-in-medicaid-and-chip-enrollment/.

Kaiser Family Foundation. 2019b. "Status of State Action on the Medicaid Expansion Decision." https://www.kff.org/health-reform/state-indicator/state-activity-around-expanding-medicaid-under-the-affordable-care-act/.

Kaiser Family Foundation. 2021. "Status of State Medicaid Expansion Decisions." March 8. Accessed March 9, 2021. https://www.kff.org/medicaid/issue-brief/status-of-state-medicaid-expansion-decisions-interactive-map/.

Kaiser Family Foundation and Episcopal Health Foundation. 2018. "Poll: Texans' Top State Health Priorities Include Lowering Out-of-Pocket Costs and Reducing Maternal Mortality." https://www.kff.org/health-reform/press-release/poll-texans-health-priorities-costs-maternal-mortality-medicaid/.

Kasler, Karen. 2018. "Ohio Gov. Kasich Stumps Again in Support of Medicaid Expansion." NPR, August 21. Accessed October 30, 2020. https://www.npr.org/sections/health-shots/2018/08/21/640636316/ohio-gov-kasich-stumps-again-in-support-of-medicaid-expansion.

Khatana, Sameed, Angali Bhatla, and Ashwin Nathan. 2019. "Association of Medicaid Expansion with Cardiovascular Mortality." *JAMA Cardiology*, June 5. Accessed June 25, 2019. https://jamanetwork.com/journals/jamacardiology/fullarticle/2734704.

Khimm, Suzy. 2012. "Pelosi: No, Governors Won't Opt Out of the Medicaid Expansion." *Washington Post*, June 28. Accessed July 2, 2019. https://www.washingtonpost.com/news/wonk/wp/2012/06/28/pelosi-no-governors-wont-opt-out-of-the-medicaid-expansion/.

Kodjak, Alison. 2017. "Survey Says: Medicaid Recipients Really Like Their Coverage and Care." NPR, July 10. Accessed October 30, 2020. https://www.npr.org/sections/health-shots/2017/07/10/536448362/survey-says-medicaid-recipients-like-their-coverage-and-care.

Legislative Reference Library of Texas. 2019a. "Governors of Texas 1846 to the Present." Accessed June 23, 2019. https://lrl.texas.gov/legeLeaders/governors/govBrowse.cfm.

Legislative Reference Library of Texas. 2019b. "Party Affiliation on the First Day of the Legislative Session." Accessed June 23, 2019. https://lrl.texas.gov/legeLeaders/members/partyList.cfm.

Lockhart, Ben. 2018. "Strong Majority of Utah Voters Favor Medicaid Expansion Ballot Measure, New Poll Says." *Deseret News*, June 18. Accessed October 30, 2020. https://www.deseretnews.com/article/900022085/strong-majority-of-utah-voters-favor-medicaid-expansion-ballot-measure-new-poll-says.html.

Luthra, Shefali. 2017. "Everything You Need to Know about Block Grants—The Heart of GOP's Medicaid Plans." Kaiser Health News, January 24. Accessed October 30, 2020. https://khn.org/news/block-grants-medicaid-faq/.

Mariner, Wendy, Leonard Glantz, and George Annas. 2012. "Reframing Federalism—The Affordable Care Act (and Broccoli) in the Supreme Court." *New England Journal of Medicine* 367, no. 12: 1154–1158. Accessed October 30, 2020. https://www.nejm.org/doi/full/10.1056/NEJMhle1208437.

Marso, Andy, and Jonathan Shorman. 2019. "JoCo Senator's 'pass' Vote Was Key as Kansas Medicaid Expansion Attempt Fails." *Kansas City Star*, May 1. Accessed March 10, 2021. https://www.kansascity.com/news/politics-government/article229895904.html.

May, Charlie. 2017. "Orrin Hatch Makes Clear the Conservative Case against Obamacare: Once the Public 'Is on the Dole, They'll Take Every Dime They Can.'" Salon, May 10. Accessed June 25, 2019. https://www.salon.com/2017/05/09/orrin-hatch-makes-clear-the-conservative-case-against-obamacare-once-the-public-is-on-the-dole-theyll-take-every-dime-they-can/.

McDonough, John. 2011. *Inside National Health Care Reform.* Berkeley: Milbank/University of California Press.

Medicaid and CHIP Payment and Access Commission (MACPAC). 2019a. "Medicaid Enrollment Changes Following the ACA." Accessed June 25, 2019. https://www.macpac.gov/subtopic/medicaid-enrollment-changes-following-the-aca/.

Medicaid and CHIP Payment and Access Commission (MACPAC). 2019b. "Medicaid's Share of State Budgets." Accessed June 21, 2019. https://www.macpac.gov/subtopic/medicaids-share-of-state-budgets/.

Miller, Kevin. 2018. "LePage Says He'll Go to Jail before He Lets Maine Expand Medicaid without Funding." *Portland Press-Herald*, July 18. Accessed October 30, 2020. https://www.pressherald.com/2018/07/12/paul-lepage-says-hed-go-to-jail-before-he-expands-medicaid/.

Montanaro, Domenico. 2015. "Ohio Republican Gov. Kasich on Expanding Medicaid: 'It's My Money.'" NPR, May 1. Accessed October 30, 2020. https://www.npr.org/sections/itsallpolitics/2015/05/01/403610372/ohio-republican-gov-kasich-on-expanding-medicaid-its-my-money.

National Conference of State Legislatures 1999. "State Balanced Budget Requirements." Accessed June 21, 2019. http://www.ncsl.org/research/fiscal-policy/state-balanced-budget-requirements.aspx.

National Federation of Independent Business v. Sebelius. 2012. 567 U.S. 519. https://supreme.justia.com/cases/federal/us/567/519/#tab-opinion-1970522.

Norris, Louise. 2018. "California and the ACA's Medicaid Expansion: Eligibility, Enrollment and Benefits." Healthinsurance.org, November 29. Accessed July 2, 2019. https://www.healthinsurance.org/california-medicaid/.

Norris, Louise. 2019a. Arkansas and the ACA's Medicaid Expansion: Eligibility, Enrollment and Benefits." Healthinsurance.org, May 7. Accessed July 2, 2019. https://www.healthinsurance.org/arkansas-medicaid/.

Norris, Louise. 2019b. Texas and the ACA's Medicaid Expansion: Eligibility, Enrollment and Benefits." Healthinsurance.org, January 10. Accessed July 2, 2019. https://www.healthinsurance.org/texas-medicaid/.

Obama, Barack. 2014. "Remarks by the President on the Affordable Care Act." April 1. Accessed July 2, 2019. https://obamawhitehouse.archives.gov/the-press-office/2014/04/01/remarks-president-affordable-care-act.

Obama, Barack. 2016. "Remarks by the President on the Affordable Care Act." October 20. Accessed July 2, 2019. https://obamawhitehouse.archives.gov/the-press-office/2016/10/20/remarks-president-affordable-care-act.

Patton, Zach. 2019. "The Governor, House and Most Senators in Kansas Want to Expand Medicaid. So Why Did It Just Fail?" *Governing*, May 1. Accessed October 30, 2020. https://www.governing.com/topics/health-human-services/gov-kansas-medicaid-expansion-vote-fails.html.

Perkins, Jane, and Ian McDonald. 2017. "50 Reasons Medicaid Expansion Is Good for Your State." National Health Law Program, January 31. Accessed March 9, 2021. https://9kqpw4dcaw91s37kozm5jx17-wpengine.netdna-ssl.com/wp-content/uploads/2017/01/Why-Medicaid-Expansion-is-Good-for-States.pdf.

Pradhan, Rachana. 2019. "Utah Officials Moved Fast to Shrink Voter-Approved Medicaid Expansion; Documents Show." Politico, February 22. Accessed October 30, 2020. https://www.politico.com/story/2019/02/22/utah-medicaid-expansion-trump-administration-1202200.

Pradhan, Rachana, and Susannah Luthi. 2020. "Appeals Court Rejects Trump-Approved Medicaid Work Requirements." Politico, February 14. Accessed May 18, 2020. https://www.politico.com/news/2020/02/14/appeals-court-rejects-trump-approved-medicaid-work-requirements-115221.

Schneider, Andy. 2020. "Medicaid Work Requirements: News from the Litigation Front." Georgetown University Health Policy Institute Center for Children and Families, May 27. Accessed March 9, 2021. https://ccf.georgetown.edu/2020/05/27/medicaid-work-requirements-news-from-the-litigation-front/.

Schutze, Jim. 2019. "In Mayoral, City Council Runoff Election, Morning News Goes Full Cold War." *Dallas Observer*, June 3. Accessed October 30, 2020. https://www.dallasobserver.com/news/morning-news-reverts-to-cold-war-name-baiting-in-runoff-11675904.

Scott, Dylan. 2019. "Can Medicaid Handle Another Recession?" Vox, June 3. Accessed July 3, 2019. https://www.vox.com/policy-and-politics/2019/6/3/18650609/health-care-medicaid-expansion-recession.

Shorman, Jonathan. 2019. "Gov. Laura Kelly Sends Medicaid Expansion Plan to Lawmakers. It Faces GOP Opposition." *Wichita Eagle*, January 29. Accessed October 30, 2020. https://www.kansas.com/news/politics-government/article225228705.html.

Shorman, Jonathan, and Chance Swaim. 2019. "Medicaid Expansion Supporters Block Kansas Budget to Pressure Republican Leaders." *Kansas City Star*, May 3. Accessed October 30, 2020. https://www.kansascity.com/news/politics-government/article229984989.html.

Sommers, Benjamin D., Robert Blendon, E. John Orav, and Arnold Epstein. 2016. "Changes in Utilization and Health among Low-Income Adults after Medicaid Expansion or Expanded Private Insurance." *JAMA Internal Medicine* 176 (October): 1501–1509. Accessed October 30, 2020. https://jamanetwork.com/journals/jamainternalmedicine/fullarticle/2542420.

Thompson, Frank J. 1998. *Medicaid and Devolution*. Washington, DC: Brookings.

Waller, Allyson. 2018. "Texas Still Hasn't Expanded Medicaid. That's Leaving a Gap in Coverage for Hundreds of Thousands." *Texas Tribune*, December 17. Accessed October 30, 2020. https://www.texastribune.org/2018/12/17/what-medicaid-coverage-gap-means-texans-without-health-insurance/.

Weixel, Nathaniel. 2018. "Romney Opposes Utah's Medicaid Expansion Ballot Measure." The Hill, September 25. Accessed October 30, 2020. https://thehill.com/policy/healthcare/408319-romney-opposes-utahs-medicaid-expansion-ballot-measure.

Wolf, Tom. 2017. "Over 700,000 Enrolled in Gov. Wolf's Medicaid Expansion." February 2. Accessed July 3, 2019. https://www.governor.pa.gov/over-700000-additional-pennsylvanians-enrolled-in-governor-wolfs-medicaid-expansion-plan/.

Wolf, Tom. 2018. "Governor Wolf: Medicaid Expansion Has Helped Local Economies, Hospitals." April 27. Accessed July 3, 2019. https://www.governor.pa.gov/newsroom/governor-wolf-medicaid-expansion-helped-local-economies-hospitals/.

Wood, Benjamin. 2019a. "Prop 3 Was More Popular with Utah Voters Than 9 of the Republican Lawmakers Who Voted to Repeal and Replace It." *Salt Lake Tribune,* Accessed February 19, 2021. https://www.sltrib.com/news/politics/2019/02/20/prop-was-more-popular/.

Wood, Benjamin. 2019b. "Vote Analysis Says Utah's Prop 3 Expanding Medicaid Not Only Passed Statewide, but in Most Legislative Districts." *Salt Lake Tribune*, January 25. Accessed February 19, 2021. https://www.sltrib.com/news/politics/2019/01/25/vote-analysis-says-utahs/.

Medicaid Work Requirements

At a Glance

Medicaid is the nation's major public health insurance program for low-income and disabled individuals. Established in 1965, Medicaid is now the nation's largest insurer, providing coverage for more than 27 million nondisabled adults in 2020. Beginning in 2018, 16 states sought waivers to establish work requirements for nondisabled adults insured by Medicaid. This flurry of activity reflected new guidance from the Trump administration that encouraged states to explore the option of instituting "work and community engagement" requirements as a condition of program participation. However, the new work requirement applied only to "able-bodied" adults and included exemptions for the elderly, children, pregnant women, and the disabled. Proponents argued the new requirements would improve enrollees' health and well-being by helping "individuals and families rise out of poverty and attain independence . . . in furtherance of Medicaid program objectives" (Sarlin 2018). As of December 2019, the Trump administration had approved 10 state waiver applications to establish work requirements for Medicaid beneficiaries (Campo-Flores 2019). Arkansas was the first state to implement work requirements in 2018.

Opponents of the new work requirements mounted legal challenges in federal court; in 2019, District Court Judge James Boasberg set aside the Trump administration's approved waivers in Arkansas, Kentucky, and New Hampshire. In February 2020, a federal appellate court unanimously rejected the Trump administration's appeal (Pradhan and Luthi 2020). As a result, the future of work requirements for Medicaid remains uncertain. In addition, two states that received approval to institute work requirements, Maine and Kentucky, ended their participation after electing Democratic governors. Utah, which implemented its community engagement program for Medicaid beneficiaries in January 2020, suspended its work and reporting requirements in April 2020 in response to the COVID-19 pandemic (Utah Department of Health 2020).

Democrats favor expanding, not restricting, access to Medicaid coverage. Thus, they regard work requirements as unlawful and punitive because they undermine Medicaid's principal policy objective of increasing access to health care. For Democrats, increased Medicaid enrollment provides tangible proof of the program's success in reaching its target population. In this view, expanding Medicaid enrollment supports work by improving individuals' access to preventative services and primary care. Healthier beneficiaries, in short, will be more productive and better able to support themselves. Democrats frequently attack work requirements as thinly veiled efforts to reduce the number of individuals eligible for Medicaid.

Republicans stress the importance of earned success—or dignity through hard work. Republicans contend that generous eligibility for Medicaid

Democratic Lawmakers Oppose "Unlawful" Medicaid Work Requirements

In February 2018, more than 170 Democratic members of Congress wrote to Secretary of Health and Human Services (HHS) Alex Azar, expressing their opposition to the Trump administration's support for work requirements for able-bodied adults eligible for Medicaid.

> Waivers with ideologically driven policies such as work requirements, mandatory drug testing, lock-out periods, coverage time limits, onerous premiums, and cost-sharing not only undermine, but exceed the statutory authority provided to the Secretary under Section 1115 and contravene longstanding Congressional intent. Far from promoting health, these types of policies will make it difficult for families struggling to make ends meet to access the care they need and are entitled to under Title XIX. Ultimately, this leads to poorer health for individuals and difficulty in maintaining successful employment, costing the system more in the long run and negatively impacting the overall health of our communities. That is why past Democratic and Republican Administrations have resoundingly rejected these types of waiver requests on the basis that such provisions would not further the program's statutory purposes of promoting health coverage and access. . . .
>
> Such actions to tie health coverage to work are motivated purely on the basis of ideology and mistaken assumptions about what Medicaid is and who it covers. Medicaid is a part of the lives of more than 70 million elderly, low-income, disabled adults and children that depend on the program to help provide them piece of mind and financial security to move their families out of poverty. The reality is that CMS's recent actions ignore a fundamental truth: most of those who can work, are working, but may fall through the cracks and lose their coverage due to harsh and inflexible implementation of this ideologically-driven policy.

Source

House Democrats. 2018. Letter to Alex Azar, Secretary, U.S Department of Health and Human Services. February 18. Accessed March 10, 2021. https://energycommerce.house.gov/sites/democrats.energycommerce.house.gov/files/documents/HHS.2018.02.14.%20Letter%20on%20Medicaid%20work%20requirements.pdf.

undermines individuals' work ethic and fosters dependency, not self-sufficiency. In this view, the success of social welfare programs is not measured by how many people enroll in public programs but rather by how few people actually need government assistance. Thus, Republicans regard rising Medicaid enrollment as evidence of steadily worsening policy problem, not a policy success. Republicans believe that work requirements will cut costs, encourage self-sufficiency, and foster a sense of dignity among beneficiaries. Finally, Republicans argue state Medicaid programs should reflect local preferences and circumstances.

According to Many Democrats . . .

- Requiring Medicaid beneficiaries to work is illegal and undermines Medicaid's primary goal of promoting access to health insurance for low-income Americans.
- Medicaid supports work by helping individuals to be healthier and thus more productive. Increased enrollment is evidence that the program is providing health security to more Americans.
- Work requirements for Medicaid are punitive and stigmatizing.
- Work requirements for Medicaid threaten the health and financial well-being of vulnerable individuals. Many deserving individuals with medical needs will lose coverage because of a lack of information or complicated reporting requirements.

According to Many Republicans . . .

- The success of social programs such as Medicaid is best measured by how few individuals need assistance.
- Public programs such as Medicaid foster dependency and discourage work.
- Work requirements for Medicaid build character and promote personal responsibility.
- Medicaid costs are a growing burden on state budgets. States should have the flexibility to insist that recipients contribute to society in exchange for publicly funded health insurance benefits.

Overview

Work requirements for public assistance programs have a long history in social policy. Some critics compare the Trump administration's new policy to Elizabethan "poor laws" in 16th-century England, which drew a distinction between the "industrious" and "idle" poor. "While the deserving poor were to be aided, the idle poor were to be punished" (Chokshi and Katz 2018). In the late 20th century, American social welfare policy often incorporated work expectations as a condition for receiving public benefits. Congress approved work requirements for food assistance programs in the 1980s and subsequently instituted work requirements for housing assistance in the 1990s (Baughman 2018). During the 1992 presidential campaign, Bill Clinton promised to "end welfare as we know it" (Carcasson 2006). Four years later, he brokered a historic bipartisan compromise with Republicans in Congress to enact a sweeping overhaul of the nation's welfare system. The Personal Responsibility and Work Opportunity Act (Pub. L. 104-193) transformed "the nation's welfare system into one that requires work in exchange for time-limited assistance. The law contains strong work requirements, a performance bonus to reward states for moving welfare recipients into jobs . . . and supports for families moving from welfare to work" (U.S. Department of Health and Human Services 1996).

The new law ratified changes already underway at the state level in many parts of the country. In fact, by 1995, 40 states had implemented work requirements through state waivers (Baughman 2018). In short, linking work and welfare enjoyed widespread, bipartisan support among policy makers and the public in the late 1990s. Some Democrats, however, raised concerns that work requirements would "cut off" deserving individuals from needed benefits (Kilborn and Verhovek 1996). This fear proved unfounded, according to a Council of Economic Advisors report that found that the Clinton administration's welfare reforms "reduced dependence and increased work for single mothers with children and they did so with little evidence of harm and some evidence of benefit to their children" (Haskins 2018).

Two decades later, Paul Ryan (R-WI), the chair of the House Budget Committee, developed a policy report entitled *Expanding Opportunity in America*. The report—which became a social policy manifesto for House Republicans in 2014—declared that "the welfare system creates a strong incentive to hover around or below the poverty line, unless you can hit a much higher rung on the income ladder in one short leap." As a result, "instead of helping people look for work, many federal programs end up discouraging people from finding work" (Ryan 2014). To address this alleged flaw, Ryan proposed a broad series of reforms to the federal safety net, including Medicaid, which had expanded considerably after Democrats passed the Affordable Care Act (ACA), also known as Obamacare, in 2010 (Ryan 2014). Republicans in Congress—and many Republican governors and Republican-controlled legislatures—had staunchly opposed the expansion of Medicaid under the ACA. By embracing work requirements, Republican legislators and governors sought to reassure constituents that the long-term costs of Medicaid expansion could be managed and that they were determined to implement reforms to make sure the program did not undermine personal responsibility and individual initiative.

During the Obama administration federal officials in the U.S. Department of Health and Human Services (HHS) soundly rejected requests by states to impose work requirements on Medicaid beneficiaries. The administration's Medicaid director, Vikki Wachino, declared in 2015, "Because Medicaid is a health coverage program, requiring employment may not be a condition of eligibility" (Wheaton 2015). Rep. Paul Westerman (R-AR) responded to the Obama administration's stance by introducing the State Flexibility and Workforce Requirement Act of 2015 (H.R. 886) "to permit States to impose workforce requirements for individuals made eligible for medical assistance under the amendments made by the Affordable Care Act." The bill was referred to committee, but no action was taken. Work requirements for Medicaid remained a political nonstarter through 2016. Administration officials remained fully committed to expanding, not limiting, access to Medicaid for all eligible individuals.

With the election of Donald Trump to the presidency in 2016, Medicaid work requirements gained traction at both the state and federal levels. Republicans controlled both houses of Congress and the presidency and soon introduced legislation to repeal and replace the ACA, the Obama administration's signature domestic policy achievement. The first bill—the American Health Care Act (AHCA; H.R. 1628)—faced significant opposition from both conservative and moderate Republicans in the House of Representatives in the Spring of 2017. House Speaker Paul Ryan introduced a "manager's amendment" in an effort to address a wide range of concerns raised by the Republican caucus. Notably, the amendment allowed states to impose a work requirement (modeled on the Transitional Aid to Needy Families (TANF) program) "on non-disabled, non-elderly, non-pregnant adults as a condition of Medicaid coverage" (Jost 2017). In addition to public- or private-sector employment, individuals could use education and job training programs, participation in community service programs, and providing childcare to individuals engaged in community service programs to fulfill the new requirements.

The AHCA passed the House by a slim margin (217–213) in May 2017, marking the first time Congress had endorsed work requirements for Medicaid. However, the legislation failed to pass the Senate. With no Democratic support for repealing the ACA, Republicans needed to maintain party unity, but unity proved elusive in both chambers. On the one hand, the conservative members of the House Freedom Caucus demanded dramatic cuts in Medicaid, which had been expanded under the ACA. For many Republican governors—such as Ohio's John Kasich—Medicaid expansion offered a way to increase access to health insurance. GOP senators also faced intense pressure to preserve Medicaid expansion in their own states. In addition, the Senate favored a more moderate "skinny repeal" than the bill the House passed (Bacon 2017).

Drawing upon the House blueprint, Republican senators drafted a substitute bill to repeal and replace the ACA in June 2017. This revised bill—the Better Care Reconciliation Act (BCRA)—also incorporated a provision allowing states to introduce Medicaid work requirements. The Senate rejected the BCRA by a margin of 57–43 in July 2017. The last gasp for integrating Medicaid work requirements into a comprehensive repeal-and-replace bill was the Graham-Cassidy proposal in September 2017. Section 122 of the act authorized states to impose work requirements as a condition of eligibility (Cassidy 2017). Three Republican senators—Rand Paul (R-KY), John McCain (R-AZ), and Susan Collins (R-ME)—refused to support the bill; by a thin margin, the ACA survived.

With no path forward for work requirements through a comprehensive reform bill, Republicans in Congress decided to press ahead with a more incremental approach. In May 2017, Sen. John Kennedy (R-LA) introduced S. 1150, the Medicaid Reform and Personal Responsibility Act, to require all states to establish work requirements for able-bodied Medicaid beneficiaries. Kennedy argued, "We need a program that is not optional for the states. My governor[, John Bel Edwards (D),] doesn't want to do it. I believe in more freedom, and he believes in more free stuff. I am not criticizing him; I am just describing him. This program should not be optional for governors" (Kennedy 2018).

Despite the failure of Republican efforts to repeal and replace the ACA, public opinion polls indicate that Medicaid work requirements are popular with the public. A June 2017 Kaiser Family Foundation poll found that 70 percent of the public supported "allowing states to impose work requirements for Medicaid." Work requirements enjoyed strong bipartisan support, as 56 percent of Democrats and 82 percent of Republicans endorsed changes that allowed states "to require adults without disabilities to work in order to get health insurance through Medicaid" (Kirzinger et al. 2017).

The legislative impasse did not stifle the Trump administration's interest in imposing work requirements. Instead, officials in the Centers for Medicare and Medicaid Services (CMS) embraced the administrative tools provided by Section 1115 of the Social Security Act to encourage state-level experimentation with work requirements for Medicaid. In January 2018, Brian Neale, the Trump administration's Medicaid director, announced "a new policy designed to assist states in their efforts to improve Medicaid enrollee health and well-being through incentivizing work and community engagement among non-elderly, non-pregnant adult Medicaid beneficiaries who are eligible for Medicaid on a basis other than disability" (Neale 2018). Under this policy, individuals would be required to submit documentation of their participation in employment, job search activities, job training, or schooling for a minimum number of hours per week. The administration justified the new policy by touting the benefits of social determinants of health on individuals' health and well-being. In his letter to state Medicaid directors, Neale noted that "targeting certain health determinants, including productive work and community engagement, may improve health outcomes. For example, higher earnings are positively correlated with longer lifespan. One comprehensive review of existing studies found strong evidence that unemployment is generally harmful to health" (Neale 2018).

The Trump administration acknowledged that the new policy was "a shift from prior agency policy regarding work and other community engagement as a condition of Medicaid eligibility or coverage, but it is anchored in historic CMS principles that emphasize work to promote health and well-being" (Neale 2018). In particular, the new policy encouraged states to apply for waivers that would align Medicaid requirements with existing Supplemental Nutritional Assistant Program (SNAP) or TANF work requirements; individuals who were already enrolled in or compliant with TANF or SNAP work requirements (as well as those exempt from such requirements) would be considered in compliance (Neale 2018).

Liberal think tanks such as the Center for Budget and Policy Priorities objected to the use of the Medicaid waiver process to impose work requirements: "Medicaid's core mission is to provide comprehensive health coverage to low-income people so they can get needed health services. Section 1115 of the Social Security Act allows states to deviate from certain federal Medicaid requirements, but only when necessary to implement demonstration projects that promote Medicaid's objectives" (Sarlin 2018). Since the new requirements placed limits on access to health care services for individuals who did not meet reporting requirements, critics argued that the Trump administration's actions were inconsistent with past practice in previous Democratic and Republican administrations and ran counter to the Medicaid program's statutory purpose of improving access to health care for low-income populations. In addition, critics of the new policy worried that many "able-bodied" adult Medicaid beneficiaries lived with one or more serious health conditions, including cognitive limitations and mobility issues that would make it difficult to obtain work (Schmidt and Hoffman 2018). Since a failure to comply with work requirements would result in the loss of health insurance, opponents argued that the new policy posed significant health risks for many Medicaid beneficiaries (Schmidt and Hoffman 2018).

Waivers had a strong appeal for governors and legislators in red states, though, because "work requirements are seen as a critical element in winning or maintaining support from conservative legislators for Medicaid expansion" (Wilson and Thompson 2018). Most states required enrollees to document 80 hours of work or community engagement each month to maintain eligibility, although New Hampshire required 100 hours per month for individuals up to age of 65. Some states (e.g., Arizona, Arkansas, and Wisconsin) exempted any individuals age 50 and over from the new requirements, but a majority of approved waivers extended participation to individuals up to age 60.

Arkansas was the first state to introduce new work and reporting requirements for Medicaid beneficiaries. More than two-thirds (67 percent) of Arkansas's Medicaid enrollees were exempt from the new reporting and work requirements. Able-bodied individuals subject to reporting requirements must report their work and community engagement activities to the state monthly; failure to properly file a report for three months triggers a loss of Medicaid benefits. After the new policy went into effect on June 1, 2018, more than 18,000 Medicaid beneficiaries lost coverage due to noncompliance. Only 13 percent of individuals subject to reporting requirements had successfully reported 80 hours of qualifying activities (Rudowitz, Musumeci, and Hall 2019). For critics of the new policy, such a low level of compliance suggested that most beneficiaries remained unaware of the new requirements or their implications. However, state officials defended the implementation of the work requirements, noting that all recipients had received notice of the policy by mail, email, and telephone (Sanger-Katz 2018).

The rollout of work requirements in Arkansas was plagued by technical glitches; many beneficiaries who lost coverage encountered difficulties using the online portal to report their hours (Musumeci, Rudowitz, and Lyons 2018). Interviews with beneficiaries revealed that the most vulnerable enrollees (e.g., homeless individuals and persons with mental and physical disabilities) experienced the greatest difficulty completing the new requirements; most beneficiaries—particularly individuals with less computer literacy and limited internet access—found the new reporting requirements to be confusing (Musumeci, Rudowitz, and Lyons 2018).

The high number of Medicaid beneficiaries in Arkansas who lost coverage because of the new reporting requirements raised concerns in Washington. The nonpartisan Medicaid and CHIP Payment and Access Commission (MACPAC) wrote that "the low level of reporting is a strong warning signal that the current process may not be structured in such a way that provides individuals an opportunity to succeed, with high stakes for beneficiaries who fail" (Howell 2018). MACPAC officials urged state officials to suspend Medicaid program disenrollments until compliance with the reporting requirements improved. An evaluation of the implementation of work requirements in Arkansas found that the new reporting requirements were "associated with significant losses in health insurance coverage in the initial 6 months of the policy but no significant change in employment. Lack of awareness and confusion about the reporting requirements were common" (Sommers et al. 2019). Notably, one out of three Arkansas Medicaid beneficiaries 30–49 years of age had not heard of the policy, and nearly half of adult beneficiaries were unsure about whether the new requirements applied to them (Sommers et al. 2019). Furthermore, the study's authors found that the implementation of work requirements in Arkansas reduced the proportion of residents with Medicaid coverage and increased the percentage of uninsured individuals in the state.

After Arkansas implemented its waiver, Medicaid enrollment declined, and the percentage of residents without health insurance increased. Opponents of work requirements in other states cited Arkansas as a cautionary tale, noting that many individuals may lose coverage despite their best efforts. Drawing upon Arkansas's experience, the Michigan League for Public Policy described the state's proposed work requirements as "a reprehensible, costly, and mean-spirited policy" (Spangler 2019). "A lot of folks are working, but they're in jobs that don't have consistent hours. In the service industry for example . . . people often have volatile schedules that are dependent on forces outside their control. Now they could lose access to health care when they're doing everything they can to work" (Spangler 2019).

Medicaid work requirements faced several legal challenges. The Trump administration approved Kentucky's request for a waiver to institute work requirements in 2017, but the state's new policy was challenged in court in *Stewart v. Azar*. In June 2018, a federal district court rejected the state's plan and instructed HHS to reconsider several provisions of the waiver (Rosenbaum 2018). In order to implement work requirements, the Court argued states must demonstrate that waivers are consistent with Medicaid's central purpose of providing coverage for low-income individuals and families. Changes to Medicaid, in other words, may not be made without first considering the impact it will have on coverage for beneficiaries (Rosenbaum 2018). Advocacy groups in New Hampshire also challenged the Trump administration's approval of work requirements, arguing the administration sought to "bypass the legislative process and act unilaterally to fundamentally transform Medicaid . . . threatening irreparable harm to the health and welfare of the poorest and most vulnerable in our country" (Meyer 2019).

In March 2019, District Court Judge James Boasberg set aside the Trump administration's approval of Medicaid work requirements in Arkansas and Kentucky as an "arbitrary and capricious" policy that led to thousands of residents losing health coverage. Officials in both states staunchly defended their new mandates and vowed to keep fighting in the courts. Gov. Asa Hutchinson of Arkansas declared, "If we give up on this, then we give up on the opportunity to lead nationally on this important program that gives Arkansans a better opportunity for training, for access to the marketplace and the jobs that they want and that they've proven they are capable of handling" (Davis 2019). That same month, however, New Hampshire's work requirement proposal, Granite Advantage, was also set aside by Judge Boasberg.

After the Trump administration appealed Boasberg's decision, the Arkansas and Kentucky work requirements were reconsidered by the U.S. Court of Appeals for the D.C. Circuit. In February 2020, the court unanimously rejected the Trump administration's approval of work requirements in Arkansas in *Gresham v. Azar*. As Judge David Sentelle—who was appointed to the court by President Reagan—noted, the Medicaid statute "includes one primary purpose, which is providing health care coverage without any restriction geared to healthy outcomes, financial independence or transition to commercial coverage" (Pradhan and Luthi 2020).

Upon taking office in January 2021, President Joe Biden issued an executive order to "protect and strengthen Medicaid" that signaled his desire to repeal Trump administration policies that "may reduce coverage under or otherwise undermine Medicaid" or "present unnecessary barriers" to individuals (Musumeci 2021). In February 2021, the Biden administration sent letters notifying Arkansas, New Hampshire, and other states with approved Medicaid work requirement waivers; it planned to rescind previous guidance that encouraged states to implement waivers, noting that policies aimed at disenrolling individuals from health care coverage were inconsistent with federal policies designed to combat COVID-19. In particular, the Families First Coronavirus Response Act banned states that received enhanced federal funding from implementing work requirements in the midst of a public health emergency (Musumeci 2021).

The COVID-19 pandemic posed new challenges for state work requirements, as stay-at-home orders and an economic shutdown made it difficult, if not impossible, for Medicaid beneficiaries to obtain employment or perform community service activities. In Utah, which had just implemented its work requirements in January 2020, the Department of Health suspended the community engagement program in April 2020 in response to the COVID-19 pandemic. Utah's community engagement policy required roughly 30 percent of the state's adult Medicaid beneficiaries "to complete an online job assessment, online training programs, and 48 job searches within the first three months of eligibility in order to continue to receive benefits" (Utah Department of Health 2020). Utah's Medicaid director noted, "During this time of increasing cases of COVID-19, a 'Stay Safe, Stay Home' directive, and rising unemployment, it is important that Medicaid members be able to continue their health coverage" (Utah Department of Health 2020). As of early 2021, the future of Medicaid work requirements remains uncertain.

Democrats on Medicaid Work Requirements

Democrats argue that imposing work requirements on Medicaid beneficiaries is illegal and inconsistent with long-standing Medicaid program objectives. Soon after the Trump administration announced its new work and community engagement guidelines, more than 170 Democratic members of Congress wrote to Health and Human Services (HHS) Secretary Alex Azar in February 2018 to express their "[deep concern] that linking health coverage to a work requirement not only will undermine access to health care but contradicts the plain text and purpose of Title XIX of the Social Security Act and Congress's longstanding intent for the Medicaid program" (House Democrats 2018). Since the goal of Medicaid is to promote access to health care, Democrats argued that work requirements are inconsistent with congressional intent.

Democrats argued that instead of promoting coverage—which previous Section 1115 waivers sought to do—Medicaid work requirements were designed to limit access to health insurance for noncompliant beneficiaries. In Mississippi, for example, "according to the state's own calculations, approximately 20,000 low income parents—many of whom are black mothers—will still lose Medicaid coverage over the next five years" (Cummings and Krishnamoorthi 2018). As a result of the disproportionate impact of the policy on Black mothers, Democrats warned that imposing work requirements could run afoul of Title VI of the Civil Rights Act, which prohibits discrimination on the basis of race for federally administered programs and services.

Democrats expressed growing frustration with the Trump administration's actions and raised concerns about the implementation of work requirements in Arkansas—the first state to implement the new work and community engagement requirements. Rep. Cedric L. Richmond (D-LA) argued, "Imposing work requirements on Medicaid recipients is counterproductive and most likely illegal. The last thing Americans who have fallen on hard times need is to lose their health care so Washington Republicans can take a political victory lap at their expense" (Timmons 2018).

In February 2019, Sen. Ron Wyden (D-OR) and Rep. Frank Pallone (D-NJ) wrote to HHS Secretary Alex Azar to express their "serious concerns with the [Trump] Administration's ongoing promotion and approval of harmful Medicaid waivers that undermine access to health care and violate the plain text and purpose of Title XIX of the Social Security Act and Congress's longstanding intent for the Medicaid program." Both legislators urged the Trump administration to "faithfully administer the Medicaid program and put a halt to any and all Section 1115 demonstration requests that jeopardize the health and financial security of millions of low-income Americans" (Pallone and Wyden 2019). The new elected Democratic majority in the House of Representatives also challenged the Trump administration's proposal to mandate Medicaid work requirements for all states in its 2020 budget. Pallone (D-NJ) described the Trump administration's proposed changes to Medicaid as "illegal efforts to kick vulnerable Americans off Medicaid through work requirements, lock outs and red tape" (Pallone 2019).

Democrats warned that the new policy, if implemented, could have dire consequences for vulnerable populations. As Reps. Elijah Cummings (D-MD) and Raja Krishnamoorthi (D-IL) warned in a letter to HHS Secretary Alex Azar and CMS Administrator Seema Verma in August 2018, "Work requirements—especially in these non-expansion states—could result in coverage losses for low income individuals who become ineligible for Medicaid, but are unable to afford private insurance" (Cummings and Krishnamoorthi 2018). In Mississippi, for example, they noted "a mother working 20 hours per week at minimum wage would earn $580 per month. This would make her ineligible for Medicaid because her monthly earnings would exceed the state's threshold for Medicaid eligibility by $113" (Cummings and Krishnamoorthi 2018). Pallone and Wyden further argued that "Medicaid 1115 waiver demonstrations that adopt restrictive conditions on eligibility like work requirements threaten to impede access to critical care for millions of Americans. We unfortunately are now seeing these concerns play out in real life in the state of Arkansas where thousands of individuals have been forced off and locked out of their Medicaid coverage" (Wyden and Pallone 2019).

In 2019, Maine's newly elected Democratic governor, Janet Mills, rejected the terms of the Section 1115 waiver sought by her Republican predecessor, Paul LePage, that would have imposed work requirements on the state's Medicaid beneficiaries. In a statement, Mills noted that "Maine's low unemployment rate, its widely dispersed population, and our lowest per capita income in New England make mandates—without appropriate supports like vocational training and specific exemptions for groups like people undergoing treatment—problematic" (Lawler 2019). Mills also challenged the underlying assumptions of the waiver, noting that "mounting evidence demonstrates that work requirements only impose burdensome mandates on people without increasing workforce participation" (Lawler 2019). In December 2019, Kentucky's newly elected Democratic governor, Andy Beshear, also rescinded Medicaid work requirements previously approved by the Trump administration. He argued that he made the move because the state's continued participation in the Medicaid work requirement scheme would "cost Kentucky money, lives and jobs" (Campo-Flores 2019).

Republicans on Medicaid Work Requirements

Policies to promote work are a key element of Republicans' larger anti-poverty strategy. Instead of fostering dependency, Republicans believe that Medicaid could—and *should*—encourage able-bodied individuals to become self-sufficient by obtaining full-time employment and private health insurance coverage. Speaking to the NAACP during the 2000 presidential campaign, George W. Bush declared, "America must close the gap of hope between communities of prosperity and communities of poverty" (Bush 2000). "We must put government squarely on the side of opportunity," Bush argued, so that "instead of helping people cope with their need, we will help them move beyond it" (Bush 2000). Fifteen years later, Arthur Brooks—the president of the American Enterprise Institute, a leading conservative think tank—sounded a similar theme. Brooks argued that "government technocrats have spent trillions of dollars standing up sprawling bureaucracies that have succeeded only in making poverty marginally less painful. They have failed to make it less permanent" (Brooks 2016).

Beginning in 2017, the Trump administration signaled that it intended to use these themes to support its ideas for Medicaid reform—most notably the imposition of work requirements for "able-bodied" recipients. Alex Azar, the secretary of Health and Human Services (HHS), testified before the House Energy and Commerce Committee: "We believe it's a fundamental aspect for able-bodied adults, if you are receiving free health care from the taxpayer, that it's not too much to ask [that] you would engage in some form of community activity" (Cunningham 2019).

Furthermore, Republicans contend that such expectations are consistent with Medicaid's original purpose. When the Medicaid program was created in 1965, President Lyndon Johnson declared that its goal was "not only to relieve the symptoms of poverty, but to cure it and, above all, prevent it" (Cunningham 2017). In the Trump administration's view, "If we are going to live up to the promise of Medicaid, we need to do more than simply pay for health-care services. . . . It's why we believe community engagement requirements are actually in the spirit of Johnson's idea" (Cunningham 2017).

Republicans believe that expanding public entitlement programs such as Medicaid encourages dependency and discourages work. In a 2018 report, the Buckeye Institute, a conservative public policy think tank, argued that "without a work requirement for Medicaid, studies have shown that the program tacitly encourages such recipients to stay home and not go to work" (Hederman and Kidd 2018). Instead of expanding entitlement programs, Republicans say that they seek to "make the safety net unnecessary for most people. Only a culture of opportunity, fueled with a policy agenda of education reform, private job creation, and entrepreneurship can truly set people up to flourish" (Brooks 2015). "Our true measure of success is the number of people who don't need government assistance," stated Ryan in 2014. "A minimum definition of success for our low-income programs—indeed, success for all of our programs—should be all able-bodied Americans earning enough money to place them above the poverty line and on a sustainable trajectory towards advancing their career" (Ryan 2014).

As a result, Republicans argue that providing benefits to able-bodied individuals with no obligations reinforces what George W. Bush described as the "soft bigotry of low expectations" (Bush 2000). Senator Mike Lee (R-UT) provided a representative summary of his party's stance when he said that "today's poverty programs place artificial restraints on those who are trying to get ahead, build careers and provide better lives for themselves and their families. Successful welfare programs are those that make poverty more temporary, not more tolerable, and we need to move current policy in that direction" (Lee 2018). Thus, requiring individuals to work or develop their job skills to receive Medicaid benefits establishes an expectation that otherwise healthy individuals should be able to support themselves. Sen. John Kennedy (R-LA), Lee's colleague in the Senate, contended in 2018 that "of the 70 million people on Medicaid, 28 million aren't elderly or disabled and they still aren't working. We spend about $150 billion a year to take care of these people that could have a job. Many of these folks would like to know the dignity of work, but they need a little help getting that job" (Kennedy 2018).

Republicans say that work requirements build character and develop marketable job skills. "For the able-bodied, work should be a condition of assistance," explained Ryan. "But more broadly, federal aid shouldn't just require people to find a job; it should put them on a path to build a career" (Ryan 2014). In particular, supporters of work requirements note that "time on the job makes employees more knowledgeable, more skilled, more qualified, more valuable to current employers and more marketable to future ones" (Hederman and Kidd 2018). Thus, "requiring Medicaid enrollees to work or work more will contribute to their financial well-being. Not only will work requirements yield higher lifetime earnings, but research also shows a strong correlation between income and health" (Hederman and Kidd 2018).

Medicaid Work Requirements Offer a Helping Hand, Not a Slap in the Face

In January 2018, Sen. John Kennedy (R-LA) defended Kentucky Governor Matt Bevin's efforts to implement a work requirement for Medicaid beneficiaries after the state's policy was challenged in court by the Southern Poverty Law Center, the National Health Law Program, and the Kentucky Equal Justice Center.

> Gov. Matt Bevin should be applauded for attempting to rein in the out-of-control costs of the Medicaid program. Instead, he's being sued.
>
> A work requirement for Medicaid doesn't ask mothers with children in their arms to work. It doesn't ask the elderly to work. It simply asks able-bodied adults to get a job, enroll in job training or do volunteer work in order to receive tax-payer funded Medicaid. I don't think that's asking too much. Medicaid is supposed to help able-bodied adults become healthy and sufficient and be an off-ramp from poverty, not a parking lot. A work requirement is a helping hand, not a slap in the face, and I support Gov. Bevin's efforts to make it a reality.

Source

Kennedy, John. 2018. "Press Release: Sen. John Kennedy (R-LA) Issues Statement In Support Of Kentucky Governor's Medicaid Work Requirement Efforts." January 25. Accessed March 11, 2021. https://www.kennedy.senate.gov/public/press-releases?ID=0FB009F7-AE39-491C-84D4-0F67DFBADE7C.

By emphasizing themes of personal responsibility, character development, and workforce readiness, Medicaid expansion proposals that incorporated mandatory work requirements redefined the political conversation in predominantly Republican states. Governor Hutchison said that Medicaid work requirements are "supposed to be an incentive and encouragement for people to work versus an incentive for people to just receive government benefits and not be part of a working culture of Arkansas" (Wheaton 2015). Governor Herbert of Utah echoed this assessment. Herbert declared, "I wanted to be able to say 'if you want taxpayers to fund your health care, then you need to go out and be involved in a work program, no ifs, ands or buts.' I've been accused by the Obama administration: 'Well, you're trying to turn this health care program into a work program.' And I've said, 'You're right'" (Wheaton 2015).

Republican governors pointed to the power of work to transform individual lives. Former New York Lt. Gov. Betsy McCaughey, who became a conservative commentator, described the push for Medicaid work requirements as "a national movement to dignify work, not dependence" (McCaughey 2018). In Ohio, Lt. Gov. Jon Husted argued that the state's new work requirements "give Ohioans the opportunity to live up to their God-given potential and pursue their own version of the American dream" (Porter 2019). This view regards work requirements as a win-win proposition that benefits both individuals and society. The goal of the new policy, argued Sen. John Kennedy (R-LA), is "not to throw people out in the cold, but to say let us help you get a job. It's better for our fellow Americans to know the dignity of work, and it's better for the American taxpayer. The Administration needs to loudly and aggressively say that the free market will lift you out of poverty" (Kennedy 2018).

New Hampshire's Gov. John Sununu defended his state's work requirements, arguing that "community engagement and work requirement will help bring more people into the workforce, empowering individuals with the dignity of work, self-reliability and access to high-quality healthcare" (Meyer 2018).

After the Trump administration approved Ohio's waiver request in March 2019, Gov. Mike DeWine declared the state's new requirements "are intended to put those able-bodied adults served by the Medicaid expansion on a pathway to full employment. Our next step is to focus on connecting Medicaid expansion recipients with opportunity. The opportunity to grow, to learn new skills, and to engage with their community" (Porter 2019). After Arkansas Works—the state's mandatory work requirement for Medicaid beneficiaries—was blocked by a federal judge in 2019, Governor Hutchinson continued to defend the new rules, even after thousands of residents lost health insurance coverage because they failed to comply with reporting requirements. "The goal of this requirement was not to reduce enrollment. It was to connect recipients to existing resources to help them improve their circumstances and move up the economic ladder" (Campo-Flores and Armour 2019).

Finally, Republicans strongly believe that states should be encouraged to experiment with work requirements, and other possible reforms, to adapt Medicaid programs to local circumstances. This philosophy of devolving responsibility for Medicaid policy to the states is designed to provide states with flexibility to develop different approaches to control Medicaid spending. McCaughey described the motivation for state experimentation in blunt terms: "Allowing states to impose conditions for Medicaid will curb the enrollment explosion." She urged Americans to "disregard the hysterical warnings that imposing conditions on Medicaid is heartless. It's a promising first step to avert a national crisis" (McCaughey 2018).

Several states that applied for waivers expected enrollment would decline, not increase, as a result of implementing work requirements for Medicaid benefits. In Kentucky, for example, state officials projected that Medicaid enrollment among able-bodied adults would decline by 15 percent over a five-year period (Sarlin 2018). By decreasing the number of individuals who are eligible to receive Medicaid benefits, work requirements limit overall Medicaid spending. Arkansas, the first state to implement work requirements in 2018, projected cost savings of $30 million as a result of reduced enrollment (Pear 2018).

Robert B. Hackey and Shannon McGonagle

Further Reading

Armour, Stephanie, and Brett Kendall. 2020. "Appeals Court Rejects Trump Administration's Approval of Work Requirements for Medicaid." *Wall Street Journal*, February 14. Accessed April 2, 2020. https://www.wsj.com/articles/appeals-court-rejects-trump-administration-approval-of-work-requirements-for-medicaid-11581694579.

Bacon, Perry. 2017. "Why the Senate's Obamacare Repeal Failed." FiveThirtyEight, July 28. Accessed October 23, 2020. https://fivethirtyeight.com/features/why-obamacare-repeal-failed/.

Ballotpedia. 2017. "American Health Care Act of 2017." Accessed February 28, 2019. https://ballotpedia.org/American_Health_Care_Act_of_2017.

Baughman, Allyson. 2018. "A History of Work Requirements." Accessed March 13, 2019. www.publichealthpost.org/viewpoints/history-of-work-requirements/.

Brooks, Arthur. 2016. *The Conservative Heart*. New York: Harper Collins/Broadside Books.

Bush, George W. 2000. "Text: George W. Bush's Speech to the NAACP." *Washington Post*, June 10. Accessed March 10, 2021. https://www.washingtonpost.com/wp-srv/onpolitics/elections/bushtext071000.htm.

Campo-Flores, Arian. 2019. "Kentucky's New Governor Ends Medicaid Work Requirement." *Wall Street Journal*, December 16. Accessed May 18, 2020. https://www.wsj.com/articles/kentuckys-new-governor-ends-medicaid-work-requirement-11576533315.

Campo-Flores, Arian, and Stephanie Armour. 2019. "The Medicaid Experiment in Arkansas: Thousands Lost Coverage, Few Gained Jobs." *Wall Street Journal*, October 13. Accessed May 18, 2020. https://www.wsj.com/articles/the-medicaid-experiment-in-arkansas-thousands-lost-coverage-few-gained-jobs-11570964402.

Carcasson, Martin. 2006. "Ending Welfare as We Know It: President Clinton and the Rhetorical Transformation of the Anti-Welfare Culture." *Rhetoric and Public Affairs* 9, no. 4: 655–692. Accessed March 10, 2021. https://www.jstor.org/stable/41940106.

Cassidy, Bill. 2017. "Graham-Cassidy Section by Section." Accessed February 28, 2019. https://www.cassidy.senate.gov/imo/media/doc/Section%20by%20Section%20Final.pdf.

Chokshi, Dave, and Mitchell Katz. 2018. "Medicaid Work Requirements—English Poor Law Revisited." *JAMA Internal Medicine* 178, no. 11: 1555–1557. Accessed March 18, 2019. doi:10.1001/jamainternmed.2018.4193.

Cummings, Elijah, and Raja Krishnamoorthi. 2018. Letter to Alex Azar, Secretary, U.S., Department of Health and Human Services. August 23. Accessed March 10, 2021. https://s3.amazonaws.com/assets.fiercemarkets.net/public/004-Healthcare/MedicaidworkreqsAzar.pdf.

Cunningham, Paige. 2017. "The Health 202: Work Requirements Are on Their Way for Medicaid." *Washington Post*, November 8. Accessed March 17, 2019. https://www.washingtonpost.com/news/powerpost/paloma/the-health-202/2017/11/08/the-health-202-work-requirements-are-on-their-way-for-medicaid/5a01ff5e30fb0468e76541ae/.

Cunningham, Paige. 2019. "The Health 202: Utah Is Testing the Trump Administration's Dreams of Limiting Medicaid Spending." *Washington Post*, March 13. Accessed March 16, 2019. https://www.washingtonpost.com/news/powerpost/paloma/the-health-202/2019/03/13/the-health-202-utah-is-testing-the-trump-administration-s-dreams-of-limiting-medicaid-spending/5c880bce1b326b2d177d6067.

Davis, Andy. 2019. "Arkansas Governor Urges Fight for Work Requirement." *Arkansas Democrat Gazette*, March 29. Accessed August 29, 2019. https://www.arkansasonline.com/news/2019/mar/29/governor-urges-fight-for-work-requireme/?latest.

DeLauro, Rosa, and Linda Sanchez. 2018. "Opinion: Work Requirements Don't Actually Work." Roll Call, June 18. Accessed March 18, 2019. http://www.rollcall.com/news/opinion/opinion-work-requirements-dont-actually-work.

Gitis, Ben, and Tara O'Neil Hayes. 2017. "The Value of Introducing Work Requirements to Medicaid." American Action Forum, May 2. Accessed February 28, 2019. https://www.americanactionforum.org/research/value-introducing-work-requirements-medicaid/.

Goldstein, Amy. 2018. "Trump Administration Again Permits Kentucky to Impose Work Requirement for Medicaid Recipients." *Washington Post*, November 20. Accessed March 23, 2019. https://www.washingtonpost.com/national/health-science/trump-administration-again-permits-kentucky-to-impose-work-requirement-for-medicaid/2018/11/20/04a097c0-ed2b-11e8-96d4-0d23f2aaad09_story.html.

Goldstein, Amy. 2020. "Appeals Court Unanimously Strikes Down Medicaid Work requirements." *Washington Post*, February 14. Accessed April 2, 2020. https://www.washingtonpost.com/health/appeals-court-unanimously-strikes-down-medicaid-work-requirements/2020/02/14/2fe1007a-4f43-11ea-b721-9f4cdc90bc1c_story.html.

Gresham et al. v. Azar. 2020. No. 19-5094. Accessed May 18, 2020. https://www.splcenter.org/sites/default/files/opinion.pdf.

Haskins, Ron. 2018. "Trump's Work Requirements Have Been Tested Before. They Succeeded." *Washington Post*, July 25. Accessed March 22, 2019. https://www.washingtonpost.com/opinions/trumps-work-requirements-have-been-successful-before--under-bill-clinton/2018/07/25/cbfbcdc0-9039-11e8-8322-b5482bf5e0f5_story.html.

Hederman, Rea, and Andrew Kidd. 2018. "Data Proves that Medicaid Needs Work Requirements." The Hill, December 3. Accessed March 10, 2021. https://thehill.com/opinion/healthcare/419488-data-proves-that-medicaid-needs-work-requirements.

House Democrats. 2018. Letter to Alex Azar, Secretary, U.S Department of Health and Human Services. February 18. Accessed March 10, 2021. https://energycommerce.house.gov/sites/democrats.energycommerce.house.gov/files/documents/HHS.2018.02.14.%20Letter%20on%20Medicaid%20work%20requirements.pdf.

Howell, Tom. 2018. "Advisory Board 'Highly Concerned' about Medicaid Lockouts." *Washington Times*, November 8. Accessed March 22, 2019. https://www.washingtontimes.com/news/2018/nov/8/advisory-board-highly-concerned-about-medicaid-loc/.

Jost, Timothy. 2017. "What's in the Manager's Amendment to the AHCA?" *Health Affairs* (blog), March 21. Accessed February 28, 2019. https://www.healthaffairs.org/do/10.1377/hblog20170321.059314/full/.

Kaiser Family Foundation. 2019. "Medicaid Waiver Tracker: Approved and Pending Section 1115 Waivers by State." Accessed August 29, 2019. https://www.kff.org/medicaid/issue-brief/medicaid-waiver-tracker-approved-and-pending-section-1115-waivers-by-state/.

Kennedy, John. 2018. "Sen. Kennedy (R-LA) Presses Sec. Azar on Medicaid Work Requirements." Accessed February 16, 2019. https://www.kennedy.senate.gov/public/2018/5/sen-kennedy-r-la-presses-health-and-human-services-sec-azar-on-medicaid-work-requirements.

Kilborn, Peter, and Sam Howe Verhovek. 1996. "Clinton's Welfare Shift Ends Tortuous Journey." *New York Times*, August 2. Accessed March 13, 2019. https://www.nytimes.com/1996/08/02/us/clinton-s-welfare-shift-ends-tortuous-journey.html.

Kirzinger, Ashley, Bianca DiJulio, Liz Hamel, Bryan Wu, and Mollyann Brodie. 2017. "Kaiser Health Tracking Poll—June 2017: ACA, Replacement Plan, and Medicaid." Accessed

March 18, 2019. https://www.kff.org/health-reform/poll-finding/kaiser-health-tracking-poll-june-2017-aca-replacement-plan-and-medicaid/.

Lawler, Emily. 2019. "Gov. Whitmer Eyes Changes to Medicaid Work Requirements." MLive, February 8. Accessed March 17, 2019. https://www.mlive.com/news/2019/02/gov-whitmer-eyes-changes-to-medicaid-work-requirements.html.

Lee, Mike. 2018. "Welfare Reform." Accessed February 19, 2019. https://www.lee.senate.gov/public/index.cfm/welfare-reform-and-upward-mobility.

McCaughey, Betsy. 2018. "Why Work Requirements Are Good for Medicaid." *New York Post*, January 16. Accessed February 16, 2019. https://nypost.com/2018/01/16/why-work-requirements-are-good-for-medicaid/.

Meyer, Harris. 2018. "N.H. Democrats Blast Medicaid for Changing Work Requirements." Modern Healthcare, December 5. Accessed March 17, 2019. https://www.modernhealthcare.com/article/20181205/TRANSFORMATION01/181209961/n-h-democrats-blast-medicaid-for-changing-work-requirements.

Meyer, Harris. 2019. "New Hampshire's Medicaid Work Requirement Challenged in Court." Modern Healthcare, March 20. Accessed March 23, 2019. https://www.modernhealthcare.com/government/new-hampshires-medicaid-work-requirement-challenged-court.

Mills, Janet. 2019. "In Lieu of Medicaid Restrictions, Governor Mills Directs DHHS & Labor to Promote Work Opportunities." Accessed March 17, 2019. https://www.maine.gov/governor/mills/news/lieu-medicaid-restrictions-governor-mills-directs-dhhs-labor-promote-work-opportunities-2019.

Musumeci, MaryBeth. 2021. "Medicaid Work Requirements at the U.S. Supreme Court." February 11. Accessed March 10, 2021. https://www.kff.org/policy-watch/medicaid-work-requirements-at-u-s-supreme-court/.

Musumeci, MaryBeth, Robin Rudowitz, and Barbara Lyons. 2018. "Medicaid Work Requirements in Arkansas: Experience and Perspectives of Enrollees." Kaiser Family Foundation. Accessed March 22, 2019. https://www.kff.org/medicaid/issue-brief/medicaid-work-requirements-in-arkansas-experience-and-perspectives-of-enrollees/.

Obasi, Olivia. 2018. "The New Work Requirement for Medicaid." American Bar Association, June 1. Accessed March 10, 2021. https://www.americanbar.org/groups/health_law/publications/aba_health_esource/2017-2018/june-2018/medicaid/.

Pallone, Frank. 2019. "Pallone Remarks at HHS Budget Hearing with Secretary Azar." U.S. House of Representatives, Committee on Energy and Commerce. Press Release, March 12. Accessed March 10, 2021. https://energycommerce.house.gov/newsroom/press-releases/pallone-remarks-at-hhs-budget-hearing-with-secretary-azar.

Pallone, Frank, and Ron Wyden. 2019. "Pallone, Wyden Call on Trump Administration to Stop Allowing Harmful Medicaid Waivers." U.S. House of Representatives, Committee on Energy and Commerce. Press Release, February 21. Accessed March 10, 2021. https://energycommerce.house.gov/newsroom/press-releases/pallone-wyden-call-on-trump-administration-to-stop-allowing-harmful-medicaid.

Pear, Robert. 2018. "Federal Panel Alarmed as Thousands Are Dropped from Medicaid in Arkansas." *New York Times*, September14. Accessed March 16, 2019. https://www.nytimes.com/2018/09/14/us/politics/arkansas-medicaid-work-requirements.html.

Pelham, Victoria. 2018. "Slow Down Medicaid-for-Work Approvals, Federal Advisors Urge." Bloomberg Law, October 25. Accessed March 10, 2021. https://news.bloomberglaw.com/health-law-and-business/slow-down-medicaid-for-work-approvals-federal-advisers-urge.

Porter, Stephen. 2019. "Ohio Medicaid Work Requirements OK'd as Legality of Similar Programs Questioned." Health Leaders, March 15. Accessed March 18, 2019. https://www.healthleadersmedia.com/strategy/ohio-medicaid-work-requirements-okd-legality-similar-programs-questioned.

Pradhan, Rachana, and Susannah Luthi. 2020. "Appeals Court Rejects Trump-Approved Medicaid Work Requirements." Politico, February 14. Accessed May 18, 2020. https://www.politico.com/news/2020/02/14/appeals-court-rejects-trump-approved-medicaid-work-requirements-115221.

Rosenbaum, Sara. 2018. "Medicaid Work Requirements: Inside the Decision Overturning Kentucky HEALTH's Approval." *Health Affairs* (blog), July 2. Accessed February 19, 2021. https://www.healthaffairs.org/do/10.1377/hblog20180702.144007/full/.

Rudowitz, Robin, MaryBeth Musumeci, and Cornelia Hall. 2019. "January State Data for Medicaid Work Requirements in Arkansas." Kaiser Family Foundation, February 25. Accessed March 22, 2019. https://www.kff.org/medicaid/issue-brief/state-data-for-medicaid-work-requirements-in-arkansas/.

Ryan, Paul. 2014. *Expanding Opportunity in America: A Discussion Draft from the House Budget Committee.* July 24. Accessed March 10, 2021. https://republicans-budget.house.gov/uploadedfiles/expanding_opportunity_in_america.pdf.

Sanger-Katz, Margot. 2018. "One Big Problem with Medicaid Work Requirement: People Are Unaware It Exists." *New York Times*, September 24. Accessed March 22, 2019. https://www.nytimes.com/2018/09/24/upshot/one-big-problem-with-medicaid-work-requirement-people-are-unaware-it-exists.html.

Sarlin, Benjy. 2018. "Critics Say Trump's Plan to Put Medicaid Recipients to Work Is a Bad Idea. Here's Why." NBC News, January 11. Accessed March 17, 2019. https://www.nbcnews.com/politics/white-house/critics-say-trump-s-plan-put-medicaid-recipients-work-bad-n836846.

Schmidt, Harald, and Allison K. Hoffman. 2018. "The Ethics of Medicaid's Work Requirements and Other Personal Responsibility Policies." *JAMA* 319, no. 22: 2265–2266. Accessed March 22, 2019. doi:10.1001/jama.2018.3384.

Sommers, Benjamin, Anna Goldman, Robert Blendon, E. John Orav, and Arnold M. Epstein. 2019. "Medicaid Work Requirements—Results from the First Year in Arkansas. *New England Journal of Medicine* 381, no. 11: 1073–1082. Accessed May 18, 2020. https://www.nejm.org/doi/full/10.1056/NEJMsr1901772.

Spangler, Todd. 2019. "Even Working Michiganders Could See Health Care Seized under New Rules." *Detroit Free Press*, January 10. Accessed March 17, 2019. https://www.freep.com/story/news/local/michigan/2019/01/10/michigan-medicaid-work-requirements/2537407002/.

Sununu, Chris. 2019. "Governor Chris Sununu Statement on Medicaid Ruling." Press Release, July 29. Accessed March 10, 2021. https://www.governor.nh.gov/news-and-media/governor-chris-sununu-statement-medicaid-ruling.

Timmons, Heather. 2018. "The Catch in Trump's New Medicaid Policy." Quartz, January 11. Accessed March 22, 2019. https://qz.com/1177705/the-medicaid-work-requirement-comes-with-catch-22/.

U.S. Department of Health and Human Services. 1996. "The Personal Responsibility and Work Opportunity Reconciliation Act of 1996." Accessed October 24, 2018. https://aspe.hhs.gov/report/personal-responsibility-and-work-opportunity-reconciliation-act-1996.

Utah Department of Health. 2020. "Medicaid Expansion Community Engagement Requirement Suspended." April 2. Accessed May 18, 2020. https://medicaid.utah.gov/Documents/pdfs/4.3.20_NR_CEsuspension.pdf.

Weiss, Debra. 2020. "DC Circuit Strikes Down Medicaid Work Requirements in Arkansas." ABA Journal, February 14. Accessed April 2, 2020. https://www.abajournal.com/news/article/dc-circuit-strikes-down-medicaid-work-requirements-in-arkansas.

Wheaton, Sarah. 2015. "GOP Warms to Obamacare—If Americans Work for It." Politico, April 30. Accessed February 19, 2019. https://www.politico.com/story/2015/04/obamacare-republicans-work-requirements-117486.

Wilson, J. Craig, and Joseph Thompson. 2018. 'Nation's First Medicaid Work Requirement Sheds Thousands from Rolls in Arkansas." *Health Affairs Blog*, October 2. Accessed March 10, 2021. https://www.healthaffairs.org/do/10.1377/hblog20181001.233969/full/.

Medicare Drug Pricing

At a Glance

Enacted in 1965, Medicare provides health insurance coverage to more than 60 million Americans. Although 85 percent of Americans qualify for Medicare benefits when they reach the age of 65, 15 percent of beneficiaries are disabled individuals under the age of 65 who receive Social Security cash payments; the remainder include more than 520,000 Americans living with end-stage renal disease (e.g., kidney failure). When Medicare was enacted in 1965, it did not include coverage for prescription drugs outside of the hospital setting. Over the next four decades, however, the growing burden of prescription drug costs for senior citizens spurred repeated calls to add a prescription drug benefit to Medicare.

The passage of the Medicare Modernization Act (MMA) in 2003 marked the largest expansion of the program since its creation in 1965. The MMA established a voluntary prescription drug benefit program known as Medicare Part D that relied on competition among private insurers to control drug spending; the law included a "noninterference clause" that expressly barred Medicare from negotiating drug prices with drug manufacturers. Medicare provided prescription drug coverage to more than 45 million beneficiaries in 2019 at a cost of $88 billion (Kaiser Family Foundation 2019a). Medicare beneficiaries could choose from wide array of stand-alone Medicare Part D prescription drug plans and Medicare Advantage plans that included prescription drug coverage (Kirzinger et al. 2019).

The cost of prescription medications remains one of the public's top health policy priorities. In a 2019 survey by the Kaiser Family Foundation, 81 percent of Democrats and 70 percent of Republicans viewed the cost of prescription drugs as "unreasonable." Furthermore, nearly one in four (23 percent) Americans over the age of 65 said it was "very difficult" to afford their medications (Kirzinger et al. 2019). Over the course of the 2010s, proposals to control the cost of prescription drugs demonstrated strong bipartisan appeal. In his 2020 State of the Union address, President Donald Trump also urged Congress to "get something on drug pricing done quickly and done properly" (Grogan 2020). Democrats and Republicans introduced several proposals to curb drug prices in the 116th Congress, but none commanded a bipartisan majority in both chambers. While both parties agree on the need to lower the high cost of drugs, Democrats and Republicans hold very different views on how to reach this goal.

Democrats blame the pharmaceutical industry for the high cost of prescription drugs. In their view, the patent system confers a monopoly on drug makers, leading to excess profits at the expense of patients and taxpayers. Democrats assert that if the federal government leveraged its purchasing power to negotiate lower prices with drug makers, Medicare could save billions of dollars each year and lower out-of-pocket costs for beneficiaries. As markets for brand-name drugs are not competitive, Democrats prescribe regulation rather than market competition to control the high cost of drugs—whether in the form of reference pricing, which would cap drug prices in the United States based on the average price of drugs in other nations—or proposals to require Medicare to negotiate prices with pharmaceutical manufacturers. Regardless of their intraparty policy differences, Democrats envision a larger role for the federal government to ensure that seniors can access lifesaving medications at an affordable cost.

In contrast, Republicans favor private initiatives rather than public solutions to lower pharmaceutical prices. Republicans celebrate the leadership role of the U.S. pharmaceutical industry, which leads the world in drug discovery, and they note that drug manufacturers must earn a profit to fund the search for promising new cures for various diseases and other maladies. Republicans also regard the current Medicare Part D system—which created a voluntary drug benefit administered by private insurers and pharmacy benefits managers (PBMs)—as a demonstrable success. Republicans argue that Medicare drug price negotiations such as the ones endorsed by Democrats would require the creation of a formulary (a list of approved drugs) that would inevitably limit available drugs for patients. Republicans also contend that government price setting would lead pharmaceutical companies to lower spending on research and development, which would slow the rate of progress in drug development. Republicans say that market-based solutions offer the best prospects for decreasing drug costs while supporting ongoing research and innovation.

According to Many Democrats . . .

- Drug manufacturers earn excessive profits at the expense of seniors and taxpayers.
- The federal government should leverage its purchasing power to bargain for lower drug prices.
- The dysfunctional market for prescription drugs demands a larger role for government in negotiating prices or setting limits on what drug companies can charge.

According to Many Republicans . . .

- Drug manufacturers need to earn a profit to fund the search for new cures.
- Medicare Part D's competitive model provides beneficiaries with a choice of plans at a reasonable cost; government price setting is coercive and limits consumer choice.
- Market competition, not government regulation, is the key to controlling Medicare prescription drug costs.

Overview

As enacted in 1965, Medicare did not include an outpatient prescription drug benefit. Despite overwhelming Democratic majorities in both the House and the Senate, fiscal concerns led legislators to drop their support for prescription coverage (Oliver, Lee, and Lipton 2004). Two years after Medicare became law, however, President Lyndon B. Johnson appointed a Task Force on Prescription Drugs to explore the challenges associated with adding a Medicare prescription drug benefit. The task force's final report, issued in February 1969, found that "a drug insurance program under Medicare is needed by the elderly and would be both economically and medically feasible" (Oliver, Lee, and Lipton 2004). However, the Nixon administration shelved the proposal. Medicare beneficiaries would have to wait until 2003 for a federally funded prescription drug benefit.

Expanding benefits took a back seat to cost containment in the 1970s and 1980s. To fight inflation, President Richard Nixon imposed nationwide wage and price controls in 1971; these continued in the health care industry even after they were lifted elsewhere in the economy. This experience led pharmaceutical manufacturers to be wary of future government regulation of drug prices (Oliver, Lee, and Lipton 2004). Numerous proposals to pass a national health insurance plan in the Nixon, Ford, and Carter administrations died in Congress.

The Reagan administration successfully lobbied Congress to enact the Medicare Catastrophic Coverage Act (Pub. L. 100-360), which included a new Medicare prescription drug benefit, in 1988 (Himmelfarb 1995). The new benefits relied on a progressive financing system in which more affluent beneficiaries contributed more than lower- and middle-income individuals. Led by the National Coalition to Preserve Social Security and Medicare, upper-income seniors clamored for the repeal of the new law (Himmelfarb 1995). A year after its passage, Congress obliged and overwhelmingly voted to repeal most of the new provisions, including the outpatient prescription drug benefit (Oliver, Lee, and Lipton 2004). As a result, millions of seniors continued to incur high out-of-pocket costs for prescription drugs.

Health care reform dominated the American political landscape in the early 1990s. In 1993, President Bill Clinton proposed an outpatient prescription drug benefit to Medicare as part of his administration's comprehensive health care reform bill. Clinton's Health Security Act faced withering opposition from congressional Republicans, health insurance companies, and physicians and never came up for a vote. Republicans portrayed the Clinton plan as an unaffordable "big government" boondoggle. As Senate Minority Leader Robert Dole argued, "We will have a crisis if we take the President's medicine—a massive overdose of government control" (Dole 1994). By 1994, the campaign for comprehensive health care reform was dead. Drug costs, however, continued to increase at a rapid pace, far exceeding the rate of inflation and the overall increase in medical costs (Oliver, Lee, and Lipton 2004). After the election of George W. Bush to the presidency in 2000, expanding Medicare coverage for prescription drugs attracted bipartisan interest. As Sen. Chuck Grassley (R-IA) noted, "Medical advances in delivering health care have moved us light years beyond 1965, but the Medicare program has not been changed to reflect those health care advances" (Grassley 2002).

In 2003, the passage of the Medicare Prescription Drug, Improvement, and Modernization Act—or Medicare Modernization Act (MMA)—created a new voluntary prescription drug plan for Medicare beneficiaries. In advance of the 2004 presidential election, passing a Medicare prescription drug benefit became the top domestic priority for the Bush administration and congressional Republicans. Senior citizens were a key demographic for Republican efforts to hold on to the presidency and Congress, resulting in a no-holds-barred battle over the bill. As Sen. Chuck Hagel (R-NE) noted, "I have never seen a bill with so much intensity, so much political pressure" (Tapper and Morris 2006).

Republicans and Democrats were split on what form the new benefit should take. Democrats favored a publicly operated drug plan in which Medicare would leverage its purchasing power by negotiating prices with drug manufacturers. In contrast, Republicans favored a market-driven approach in which competing private plans would offer consumers a range of options to purchase covered drugs. The cost of the new program was also a major sticking point. Republicans dismissed Democratic proposals as unaffordable. Even the Bush administration's plan had difficulty attracting support from fiscal conservatives in the Republican caucus. As Rep. Pat Toomey (R-PA) observed, "There is no mechanism to contain the cost of this bill. And you know in the history of every entitlement program in American history, they end up costing far more than the initial projections" (Tapper and Morris 2006).

The MMA passed by a razor-thin margin of 216–215 in the House after a controversial late-night vote that was held open by the Speaker for nearly three hours to allow senior Bush administration officials to lobby wavering members on the floor (Tapper and Morris 2006). At the bill signing ceremony, a jubilant President George W. Bush declared, "We passed reforms of Medicare to give patients prescription drugs and give seniors choices. . . . Our government is finally bringing prescription drug coverage to the seniors of America" (Tapper and Morris 2006).

Nevertheless, the MMA received a "muted reception" from seniors. An ABC News/*Washington Post* poll conducted in December 2003 revealed that only one in four (26 percent) seniors approved of the new law, while nearly half (47 percent) disapproved (ABC News 2003). The mixed reception to the new law can be traced to the unusual design of the prescription drug benefit itself. To control costs—and remain within the budgeted $400 billion cost over 10 years—the MMA included a "doughnut hole" in its benefits design. After meeting a $250 deductible, Medicare-approved drug plans would pay 75 percent of beneficiaries' drug costs up to a limit of $2,250, after which individuals would be responsible for the next $3,600 in out-of-pocket expenses (Doherty 2004). This design raised concerns for individuals with chronic illnesses who took multiple medications, as they would exhaust their covered benefits much sooner than others.

The new drug benefit, known as Medicare Part D, offered seniors the opportunity to purchase private prescription drug plans underwritten by the federal government. Public approval of the new program soared after its implementation in 2006 and has remained strong ever since. In 2019, one poll found that 9 out of 10 seniors were satisfied with their Medicare Part D plans, and 75 percent believed they were better off now than they were before they had prescription drug coverage through Part D (Morning Consult 2019). Medicare became one of the nation's leading purchasers of prescription drugs. The percentage of total U.S. prescription drug sales paid for by Medicare Part D increased from 18 percent in 2006 to 30 percent in 2017; prescription drugs accounted for 19 percent of total Medicare spending in 2016 (Kaiser Family Foundation 2019b). In 2020, the base premium for Medicare Part D beneficiaries was $32.74 (Kaiser Family Foundation 2019a).

Nevertheless, rising drug prices remain a significant cost driver for Medicare, as Part D spending has increased by more than 7 percent annually since 2006, driven by the high cost of specialty drugs, such as biologics (Frank and Nichols 2019). Many academic observers argued that Medicare should negotiate prices for such drugs with pharmaceutical manufacturers to control costs. As Richard Frank and Len Nichols (2019) wrote in the *New England Journal of Medicine*, "Using negotiation for a limited number of drugs is administratively feasible and not disruptive of the overall market. Common-sense policy calls for intervening when markets fail consumers and taxpayers."

However, price negotiation between the federal government and drug manufacturers was banned by the MMA's "noninterference" clause. Democrats had pressed for Medicare to play a larger role in setting drug prices, but under the law, the secretary of Health and Human Services (HHS) "may not interfere with the negotiations between drug manufacturers and pharmacies and PDP sponsors, and may not require a particular formulary or institute a price structure for the reimbursement of covered Part D drugs" (Cubanski et al. 2019). This provision reflected Republican beliefs in the power of competition to control drug costs.

Medicare Part D "Offers Consumers Better Choice, Better Coverage and Better Value"

Sen. Chuck Grassley, chair of the Senate Finance Committee, took to the floor to oppose Democratic proposals to repeal the Medicare noninterference clause in May 2019. Grassley celebrated the program's successes and cautioned against allowing the federal government to negotiate prices with drug manufacturers.

Let me explain why Congress kept the government out of the business of negotiating drug prices in the Medicare program. Some 16 years ago, I was a principal architect of the Medicare Part D program.

For the first time ever, Congress in 2003 added an outpatient prescription drug benefit to the Medicare program. Adding a prescription drug benefit for seniors was the right thing to do. But it needed to be done in the right way—right for seniors and right for the American taxpayer. By that, I mean allowing the forces of free enterprise and competition to drive costs down and drive value up. For the first time ever, Medicare recipients in every state had the voluntary decision to choose a prescription drug plan that fit their pocketbooks and their health care needs.

The Part D program has worked. Beneficiary enrollment and satisfaction are robust. The Part D marketplace offers consumers better choice, better coverage and better value. And yet, here we are again. It's been 13 years since Part D was implemented. And once again, I am hearing the same calls to put the government in the driver's seat. It's the same back seat drivers who think centralized government knows best. As the Senator who once again chairs the committee with jurisdiction over Medicare policy, I'm not going to let Congress unravel what's right about Medicare Part D.

Source

Grassley, Chuck. 2019. "Grassley On Medicare Part D Price Negotiation." News Release, May 22. Accessed March 8, 2021.https://www.grassley.senate.gov/news/news-releases/grassley-medicare-part-d-price-negotiation.

After Democrats regained control of Congress in the November 2006 midterm elections, they quickly submitted legislation to repeal the noninterference clause. H.R.4, the Medicare Prescription Drug Price Negotiation Act of 2007, required "the Secretary of Health and Human Services to negotiate lower covered Part D drug prices on behalf of Medicare beneficiaries." The Congressional Budget Office's score estimated that "H.R.4 would have a negligible effect on federal spending because we anticipate that the Secretary would be unable to negotiate prices across the broad range of covered Part D drugs that are more favorable than those obtained by PDPs under current law" (Congressional Budget Office 2007). Nevertheless, Democrats passed the bill in the House by a margin of 255–170 in January 2007, but the bill failed a procedural vote in the Senate and was not brought to the floor.

Although the passage of the Affordable Care Act (ACA), also known as Obamacare, in 2010 improved prescription drug coverage for Medicare Part D beneficiaries, it sidestepped the issue of drug pricing. As former Rep. Henry Waxman (D-CA) recalled, "The Obama administration decided to make a deal with the PhRMA to get them to support the legislation" (Owens 2016). The Pharmaceutical Research and Manufacturers Association (PhRMA) agreed to contribute $90 billion to underwrite the cost of expanding access to health insurance. However, PhRMA's support was contingent upon keeping Medicare drug price negotiation off the table. As PhRMA CEO Billy Tauzin quipped, "We had a choice to make sure it wasn't going to be a single-payer government system. If we were not at the table, it would be likely that we would become the meal" (Norman and Karlin-Smith 2016). Furthermore, Democrats had little leverage to press for drug pricing reform during the tumultuous debate over health care reform in 2009–2010. Ron Pollack, the executive director of Families USA, a health reform advocacy group, recalled that "we needed 60 votes in the Senate [to pass ACA]; we got 60. We needed 218 votes in the House; we got 219. Had structural changes to pharmaceutical pricing been in the bill, the Affordable Care Act would not have been enacted" (Norman and Karlin-Smith 2016).

The current structure of Medicare Part D relies on private negotiations between drug companies and pharmacy benefit managers for each participating insurer (Huetteman 2019). The Obama administration included a proposal to allow the secretary of HHS to negotiate the price of high-cost drugs and biologics covered by Part D with pharmaceutical manufacturers in its budget request to Congress (Kessler 2016). These proposals, however, fell victim to ongoing budget standoffs between the Republican-controlled Congress and the Obama administration. During the 2016 presidential campaign, Donald Trump, the Republican nominee, also bemoaned the lack of drug price negotiation by Medicare. On the campaign trail in 2016, Trump argued, "We're the largest drug buyer in the world. We don't negotiate. We don't negotiate" (Kessler 2016). For Trump, the inability of Medicare to negotiate prices was a missed opportunity, as the government passed up the opportunity to use its market power to bargain for lower prices with pharmaceutical manufacturers.

For their part, Democrats have pursued more progressive drug pricing reforms in recent years. The Lower Drug Prices Now Act (H.R.3)—later renamed for Rep. Elijah Cummings (D-MD)—passed the House by a margin of 230–192 in December 2019. H.R.3 proposed to cap prices for selected drugs at 120 percent of the average price paid for the same drug in a comparison group of countries (e.g., Canada, France, Germany). Drug companies that did not accept the maximum price would be assessed a fee equal to 65 percent of the gross sales for the drug in the first year (Dusetzina and Oberlander 2019). Pharmaceutical companies and their trade association decried the proposed bill, arguing that "Speaker Pelosi's radical plan would end the current market-based system that has made the United States the global leader in developing innovative, lifesaving treatments and cures" (Lovelace 2019). Despite winning strong support in the House, Senate Majority

"Negotiated Drug Pricing Should Be Enacted Now"

On September 26, 2019, Rep. Brian Higgins (D-NY) spoke on the House floor about the burden of rising prescription drug costs and argued that the federal government should be permitted to negotiate prescription drug prices.

> Mr. Speaker, this week, the Committee on Ways and Means released a report highlighting the disparities between the cost of prescription drugs in the United States and other developed nations.
>
> This report found that on average, drug prices in the United States were nearly four times higher than prices in similar countries.
>
> The sky-high cost of prescription drugs affects all of our communities, and too many Americans cannot afford the medications they need. The Medicare Program alone last year spent $135 billion for prescription drugs.
>
> It is a lot of money, but it is also a lot of leverage, a lot of leverage that should be used to negotiate lower drug prices for Medicare and for the American people. Negotiated drug pricing should be enacted now.

Source

Congressional Record, vol. 165, no. 156 (September 26, 2019): H7997. Accessed January 28, 2021. https://www.congress.gov/congressional-record/2019/9/26/house-section/article/h7997-9?q=%7B"search"%3A%5B"higgins+drug"%5D%7D&s=2&r=1.

Leader Mitch McConnell (R-KY) pronounced H.R.3 dead on arrival in the Senate. Sens. Chuck Grassley (R-IA) and Ron Wyden (D-OR) sought to forge a bipartisan compromise that would impose a cap on Medicare drug price increases that exceeded the rate of inflation. The Congressional Budget Office (CBO) estimated this bill, the Prescription Drug Pricing Reduction Act of 2019 (S.2543), would reduce federal spending on cost sharing for Medicare Part D beneficiaries by more than $70 billion over a 10-year period (Congressional Budget Office 2020). The bipartisan measure passed the Senate Finance Committee and won endorsements from Vice President Mike Pence and President Donald Trump, who pledged to sign it. However, more than nine months after it was first introduced, S.2543 still awaited a vote before the full Senate, and Democrats and Republicans expressed opposition to different elements of the bill. As Sen. Ron Wyden (D-OR) declared, "Democrats will not begin floor debate on this proposal until it is clear that amendments on two issues—preexisting conditions and negotiating power Medicare—will get votes on the Senate floor" (Wyden 2019). For Republicans such as Sen. Pat Toomey (R-PA), proposals to benchmark U.S. drug prices against a reference group of other nations were unacceptable. No further action on S.2543 was taken during the 116th Congress.

Public opinion polls during the 2010s have underscored the bipartisan appeal of proposals to increase government regulation of pharmaceutical prices, which most

Americans see as outrageously high due to high industry profits. An October 2019 poll by the Kaiser Family Foundation found 88 percent of the public—including 92 percent of Democrats and 85 percent of Republicans—favored "allowing the federal government to negotiate with drug companies to get a lower price on medications for people with Medicare" (Cubanski et al. 2019). A more pronounced partisan gap appeared on the question of reference pricing; only 52 percent of Republicans supported "lowering what Medicare pays for some drugs based on amounts in other countries where governments more closely control prices." In contrast, 73 percent of Democrats agreed with such an approach (Cubanski et al. 2019).

In part, the political appeal of regulating or taxing drug companies rests upon the unpopularity of the pharmaceutical industry's pricing strategy. A February 2019 poll found that 80 percent of Americans blamed "profits made by pharmaceutical companies" for rising prescription drug prices compared to 69 percent who cited the cost of research and development. Furthermore, while most Americans (71 percent) trust pharmaceutical companies to develop new, effective drugs, only 25 percent of the public believed that pharmaceutical companies priced their products fairly (Kirzinger et al. 2019). Upon closer inspection, however, public support for drug negotiation is more fluid. When drug negotiations are framed as a way to save money—either for beneficiaries or the federal government—8 out of 10 respondents support negotiations. When respondents were asked whether they would support negotiation if it could "lead to less R&D of new drugs" or "it could limit access to newer prescription drugs," more than 60 percent of the public opposed allowing the federal government to negotiate prices (Lopes et al. 2019).

Democrats on Medicare Drug Pricing

Democrats blame pharmaceutical manufacturers for the high cost of prescription drugs. The Roosevelt Institute, a progressive think tank, argued that "today's high-cost, high-profit pharmaceutical industry is structured to prioritize profits over the health care system, our economy, and our society" (Milani and Duffy 2019). Democrats contend that drug companies use the patent system, which confers monopoly powers on manufacturers of brand-name drugs, to reap enormous profits at the expense of seniors and taxpayers. On the presidential campaign trail in 2015, Hillary Clinton declared that "pharmaceutical companies can charge astronomical fees, far beyond anything it would take to recoup their investment" (Przybyla 2015).

Democrats also dismiss drug makers' claims that higher prices are necessary to fund medical innovation and research, noting that most basic research costs are underwritten by federal support of biomedical research and high costs for direct-to-consumer advertising of pharmaceuticals. As Rep. Matthew Cartwright (D-PA) explained, "We hear over and over again from big pharmaceutical companies . . . that these price hikes are necessary to pay for new research. . . . The simple truth is that the drug companies keep hiking their prices on us because they can get away with it" (Cartwright 2019). Democrats wave off pharmaceutical companies' objections that mandatory negotiations or price controls would stifle innovation as well. As Sen. Ron Wyden (D-OR) asked, "If lower prices would diminish R&D, why don't costly dividends? Why don't stock buybacks? Is the stock price more important than inventing the next miracle cure?" (Coombs 2019).

Democrats describe the cost of prescription drugs as unreasonable. As House Democratic leaders declared at the unveiling of H.R.3 in 2019, "The status quo on prescription drug prices is broken. Prescription drug companies are charging Americans prices that are three, four, or even ten times higher than what they charge for the same drug in other countries" (Lovelace 2019). Rep. Ro Khanna (D-CA) argued, "There is absolutely no reason for the big pharmaceutical companies to make Americans pay higher prescription drug prices than they charge our friends in Canada, Germany, and the UK" (Sanders 2019). Prescription drugs emerged as a major theme in the 2020 presidential campaign as well, with all the major Democratic candidates offering promises to make reducing drug prices a major priority in their administrations. As candidate Pete Buttigieg wrote, "Pharmaceutical companies are making tens of billions in profits while gouging Americans" (Buttigieg 2019).

Democrats also worry that the high cost of prescription drugs may force many seniors to skip doses or forego taking their prescription medications. Sen. Bernie Sanders (I-VT), who caucuses with the Democratic Party and ran for the party's presidential nomination in both 2016 and 2020, charged that "the United States pays by far the highest prices in the world for prescription drugs. This has created a health care crisis in which 1 in 5 American adults cannot afford to get the medicine they need" (Sanders 2019). The high cost of drugs, Democrats argued, forced seniors, particularly individuals taking multiple medications, to make painful choices. As Rep. Elijah Cummings (D-MD) declared, Americans "should not have to decide between paying their bills or paying for their prescriptions. We're a better country than that" (Sanders 2019). Rep. Dan Kildee (D-MI) expressed outrage that "Americans sometimes have to pay hundreds of dollars just to have that drug that was brought into this country, invented in the 1920s, and hasn't changed substantially. We have to make sure to pass H.R.3, which will make sure that Americans have access to prescription drugs at an affordable price" (Kildee 2019).

Over the past two decades, Democrats have also strongly supported proposals to repeal the Medicare noninterference clause. Congressional Democrats introduced legislation (H.R.4) in 2007 to grant the federal government the ability to negotiate drug prices with drug manufacturers for Medicare Part D enrollees. Rep. John Dingell (D-MI) observed that "common sense tells you that negotiating with the purchasing power of 43 million Medicare beneficiaries behind you would result in lower drug prices" (U.S. Senate, Committee on Finance 2007). On the presidential campaign trail in 2008, Barack Obama also pledged "to allow Medicare to negotiate for cheaper drug prices" (Jacobson 2010). More than a decade later,

Democratic candidates for the 2020 presidential nomination reaffirmed their commitment to Medicare drug price negotiation. As Pete Buttigieg wrote, "by empowering the federal government to negotiate drug prices on behalf of Medicare and our public plan, we will dramatically bring down the cost of drugs" (Buttigieg 2019). In short, Democrats believe that the federal government should leverage its purchasing power to bargain for lower prices with drug makers.

In 2019, leading House Democrats, including Rep. Bobby Scott (D-VA), Rep. Frank Pallone Jr. (D-NJ), and Rep. Richard Neal (D-MA), endorsed Medicare drug price negotiation for selected drugs. "For too long," they argued, "American families have been price gouged at the pharmacy counter, while consumers in other countries pay significantly less for the same drugs. This initial analysis proves that H.R.3 will effectively rein in the soaring cost of prescription drugs and level the playing field for American patients" (Energy and Commerce Committee 2019).

Democrats urge a larger role for government to fix what they see as a dysfunctional market for prescription drugs. Some Democrats, such as Sen. Elizabeth Warren (D-MA), called for public manufacturing of generic drugs to address market failure. In an op-ed, Warren described the high cost of medicines as a "public health crisis" that required aggressive enforcement of laws promoting competition and public manufacturing "to fix markets, not replace them" (Warren 2018). As Sen. Dick Durbin (D-IL) declared in 2019, "Giving Medicare the authority to negotiate on behalf of its beneficiaries is the right prescription for real savings on drug prices for America's seniors" (Durbin 2019). In this view, government provides a necessary counterbalance to the economic and political power of the pharmaceutical industry. In July 2019, Sens. Sherrod Brown (D-OH) and Debbie Stabenow (D-MI) urged their colleagues to pass "bold legislative measures that provides Medicare and Medicaid with the tools and authority necessary to address each component of the drug supply chain and meaningfully reduce the cost of prescription drugs for all Americans" (Brown 2019). Frustrated by the status quo, which ceded decisions over pharmaceutical pricing to drug manufacturers and private pharmacy benefits managers, Democrats argued that the federal government must flex its regulatory muscles to protect consumers from "unjustified price increases."

Republicans on Medicare Drug Pricing

Republicans say that they want to lower drug costs using the power of the free market, not regulation. They argue that the profit motive offers a powerful incentive for pharmaceutical companies to develop promising new cures and bring lifesaving drugs to consumers. They also argue that the federal government's purchasing power would lead to unfair negotiations, as pharmaceutical companies would have little recourse but to accept the government's offer because Medicare would become the nation's largest purchaser of drugs. As Sen. John Cornyn (R-TX) observed, "When you negotiate with somebody as the Federal Government, you are literally doing it with a gun to one's head or figuratively doing it with a gun to one's head. It is not a normal give-and-take negotiation" (Cornyn 2019).

Republicans point out that the process of drug development is inherently risky. The average cost of research and development to bring a new drug to market is $2.6 billion (Sullivan 2019b). Most drugs fail in clinical trials, and of those that do make it to market, few earn a profit. As a result, Republicans believe that drug manufacturers must earn a profit to fund continued drug discovery and innovation. "As a nation, we are incredibly blessed to live in a country where investment and innovation unlocks cures and treatments," said Sen. Chuck Grassley (R-IA). "The reason millions of Americans benefit from life-saving drugs in the first place is largely due to capitalism and the entrepreneurial spirit that drives innovation and opens new frontiers of modern medicine" (Grassley 2018).

Republicans warned that the reduced industry revenues that would follow if proposed Democratic reforms were implemented would stifle innovation and slow the search for promising new cures. As the *Wall Street Journal* (2019) editorialized, "Price controls are a prescription for less innovation, since they reduce the payoff on risky research and development. . . . Only about 12 percent of molecules that enter clinical testing ultimately obtain FDA approval, and those successes have to pay for the 88 percent that fail." Scott Gottlieb, the former commissioner of the Food and Drug Administration under the Trump administration, concurred, noting that the "high cost drugs lawmakers target are often the most innovative and potentially transformative new medications" (Gottlieb 2019).

Republicans thus portray federal negotiation of drug prices for Medicare and other programs as a slippery slope that will inevitably limit the availability of lifesaving medications for all Americans. The *Wall Street Journal* warned, "Government rationing and price controls on drugs are one major reason that countries with socialized medicine like the United Kingdom have lower cancer survival rates than the U.S." (*Wall Street Journal* 2020). Freedom Works, a conservative think tank, argued that "the United States leads the world in medical innovation, particularly in terms of breakthrough pharmaceuticals. Politicians and bureaucrats are lying to you if they claim that an inflation cap wouldn't harm innovation. . . . More than 60 percent of pharmaceuticals are developed in the United States, and an inflation cap would take a drastic toll on such critical innovation" (Brandon 2019). In this view price controls threaten access to lifesaving medicines.

Not surprisingly, Senate Majority Leader Mitch McConnell (R-KY) dismissed H.R.3, the 2019 prescription drug pricing bill passed by the Democrat-controlled House in 2019. "Socialist price controls will do a lot of left-wing damage to the healthcare system," he said. "And of course we're not going to be calling up a bill like that" (Everett 2019). McConnell's colleague Sen. John Thune (R-SD) shared a similar assessment of H.R.3, calling it "a huge intervention in the drug marketplace, with a lot of price-setting. And the government pretty much taking over a private industry. It's really bad policy and I think it's dead on arrival" (Everett

2019). Republicans cited a 2019 analysis of H.R.3 by the Congressional Budget Office (CBO), which projected that, if enacted, H.R.3 would result in fewer new drugs reaching the market over the next decade (Congressional Budget Office 2019). "CBO's report confirms House Democrats' 'dictate or destroy' price controls only serve to hurt the development of future cures and damage American innovation," insisted Rep. Kevin Brady (TX) (Sullivan 2019a). The Trump administration's Council of Economic Advisors also assailed H.R.3 as a threat to innovation: "Heavy-handed government intervention may reduce drug prices in the short term, but these savings are not worth the long-term cost of American patients losing access to new lifesaving treatments" (Council of Economic Advisors 2019).

Republicans view the current design of Medicare Part D as a policy success. As Sen. Mike Crapo (R-ID) noted in July 2019, "We worked really hard for years and years to set up the system in Part D so it will be a market-oriented system for pricing on drugs. And it has worked, and it has worked very effectively. Over 80 percent of Medicare beneficiaries are satisfied with their plan and the average premium remains about $30 a month" (U.S. Senate, Committee on Finance 2019). Private negotiation by pharmaceutical benefits managers provides beneficiaries with more choice at a lower cost. Republicans pointed out that premiums for Part D coverage were far below initial projections. As a coalition of conservative health policy think tanks noted in 2019, "The market-based structure of [Medicare] Part D is popular and successful. Since it was first created, federal spending has come in 45 percent below projections. . . . Monthly premiums are also just half the originally projected amount, while 9 in 10 seniors are satisfied with the Part D drug coverage" (Americans for Tax Reform 2019). As a result, while Republicans support private bargaining between prescription benefit managers (PBMs) and drug manufacturers over drug prices, most remained strongly opposed to the federal government using its leverage to negotiate or set prices for drugs. In 2019, Sen. Grassley, one of the original sponsors of the Medicare Modernization Act (MMA), insisted that "we must allow competition—not government mandates—to drive innovation, curb costs, expand coverage, and improve outcomes. It wouldn't work if the federal government interfered with the delivery of medicine and dictated which drugs would and would not be covered. That's why we wrote a non-interference clause in the law" (Grassley 2019).

In September 2019, McConnell denounced Democratic House Speaker Nancy Pelosi's proposal to require Medicare to negotiate drug prices with pharmaceutical manufacturers as "the same old one-size-fits-all, government-controlled philosophy we continue to see from Democrats: Forget about choice and competition. Forget about free enterprise and finding ways to unleash market forces to help consumers. Just give Washington bureaucrats more power to clumsily call the shots and manipulate markets from the top down" (House Republicans 2019). Although they were unable to block the passage of H.R.3, House Republicans offered a similar critique of the bill. House Minority Leader Kevin McCarthy (R-CA) characterized it as "a step toward nationalizing the drug industry and opening the door to a one-size-fits-all, government-controlled rationing of prescription drugs. This exacerbates the existing government policies that got us here in the first place while damaging the free market that has created these life changing medications and cures" (House Republicans 2019).

As a matter of principle, Republicans generally oppose government interference in the operation of free markets in health care. In this context, Medicare drug price negotiation, or proposals to benchmark the price of pharmaceuticals against other nations, represents an unwarranted interference in the marketplace. In contrast to this free market approach that relied on competing pharmaceutical benefits managers to negotiate prices with drug makers, Republicans argued that government-led negotiations amounted to what Rep. Devin Nunes (R-CA) described as "the seizure of medicines by an unhappy government" (Bluth 2019). The *Wall Street Journal* (2019) characterized H.R.3 as "a take it or leave it offer with a tax sword hanging over drug makers." The editors argued that "the concept of negotiated prices with government has always been a political ruse because the government has outsize leverage to coerce manufacturers" (*Wall Street Journal* 2019). Conservatives argue that competition, not regulation or price setting, is the only policy prescription that can control costs and preserve choice. Rep. Tom Reed (R-NY) declared, "The free market system is the tool that should be used to drive prices down. That is where the solution lies, rather than taking over this space with some kind of government fiat" (Bluth 2019). His colleague Rep. Tom Rice (R-SC) captured Republican thinking on pharmaceutical pricing: "The answer to high drug prices is to move towards more free market and less government control" (Bluth 2019).

Robert B. Hackey and Theresa Durkee

Further Reading

ABC News. 2003. "ABC News/Washington Post Poll: Medicare Reform." December 7. Accessed June 18, 2020. https://abcnews.go.com/images/pdf/883a37Medicare.pdf.

Americans for Tax Reform. 2019. "Coalition Opposes Inflationary Rebate Penalty in Medicare Part D." July 22. Accessed January 6, 2020. https://www.atr.org/sites/default/files/assets/ATR%20Coalition%20Letter%20Opposing%20Inflationary%20Rebate%20Penalty%20in%20Medicare%20Part%20D.pdf.

Bluth, Rachel. 2019. "Lawmakers United against High Drug Prices Bare Partisan Teeth." Kaiser Health News, March 7. Accessed December 30, 2019. https://khn.org/news/lawmakers-united-against-high-drug-prices-bare-partisan-teeth/.

Brandon, Adam. 2019. "Why Price Controls on Medicare Part D Are a Bad Prescription." FreedomWorks, August 27. Accessed January 6, 2020. https://www.freedomworks.org/content/why-price-controls-medicare-part-d-are-bad-prescription.

Brown, Sherrod. 2019. "Brown, Stabenow Lead Finance Dem Effort to Include Bold Drug Pricing Measures in Prescription Drug Bill." July 12. Accessed June 14, 2020. https://www.brown.senate.gov/newsroom/press/release/brown-stabenow-lead-finance-dem-effort-to-include-bold-drug-pricing-measures-in-prescription-drug-bill.

Buttigieg, Pete. 2019. "My Bold Plan for Affordable Prescription Drugs." *Boston Globe*, October 7. Accessed June 11, 2020. https://www.bostonglobe.com/opinion/2019/10/07/pete-buttigieg-bold-plan-for-affordable-prescription-drugs/LYqjKGuhzLrMGwX5QuIBmJ/story.html.

Cartwright, Matthew. 2019. "Prescription Drugs." *Congressional Record* (November 15): H8905. Accessed June 10, 2020. https://www.congress.gov/116/crec/2019/11/15/CREC-2019-11-15-pt1-PgH8905-3.pdf.

Congressional Budget Office. 2007. Letter to Rep. John Dingell. January 10. Accessed June 25, 2020. https://www.cbo.gov/sites/default/files/110th-congress-2007-2008/costestimate/hr410.pdf.

Congressional Budget Office. 2019. Letter to Rep. Frank Pallone. "Re: Effects of Drug Price Negotiation Stemming from Title 1 of H.R. 3, the Lower Drug Costs Now Act of 2019, on Spending and Revenues Related to Part D of Medicare." October 11. Accessed June 10, 2020. https://www.cbo.gov/system/files/2019-10/hr3ltr.pdf.

Congressional Budget Office. 2020. "Division A—Prescription Drug Pricing Reduction Act of 2019." March 13. Accessed June 24, 2020. https://www.cbo.gov/publication/56273.

Coombs, Bertha. 2019. "Americans Want Lower Prescription Prices, but Not if It Means Fewer Drugs, Survey Finds." CNBC, March 6. Accessed June 5, 2020. https://www.cnbc.com/2019/03/06/americans-want-lower-prescription-prices-but-not-fewer-drugs-survey.html.

Cornyn, John. 2019. "Prescription Drug Costs." *Congressional Record* (July 25): S5094–S5095. Accessed December 30, 2019. https://www.congress.gov/116/crec/2019/07/25/CREC-2019-07-25-pt1-PgS5094.pdf.

Council of Economic Advisors. 2019. "House Drug Pricing Bill Could Keep 100 Lifesaving Drugs from American Patients." December 11. Accessed March 2, 2021. https://trumpwhitehouse.archives.gov/articles/house-drug-pricing-bill-keep-100-lifesaving-drugs-american-patients/.

Cubanski, Juliette, Tricia Neuman, and Anthony Damico. 2019. "How Many Medicare Part D Enrollees Had High Out-of-Pocket Drug Costs in 2017?" Kaiser Family Foundation, June 21. Accessed November 5, 2019. https://www.kff.org/medicare/issue-brief/how-many-medicare-part-d-enrollees-had-high-out-of-pocket-drug-costs-in-2017/.

Cubanski, Juliette, Tricia Neuman, Sarah True, and Meredith Freed. 2019. "What's the Latest on Medicare Drug Price Negotiations?" Kaiser Family Foundation, October 17. Accessed June 11, 2020. https://www.kff.org/medicare/issue-brief/whats-the-latest-on-medicare-drug-price-negotiations/.

Doherty, Robert. 2004. "Assessing the New Medicare Prescription Drug Law." *Annals of Internal Medicine* 141, no. 5: 391–395. Accessed November 1, 2020. https://www.acpjournals.org/doi/10.7326/0003-4819-141-5-200409070-00100.

Dole, Robert. 1994. "Excerpts from the Republicans' Response to the President's Message." *New York Times*, January 26. Accessed November 1, 2020. https://www.nytimes.com/1994/01/26/us/state-union-republicans-excerpts-republicans-response-president-s-message.html.

Durbin, Dick. 2019. "Durbin, Schakowsky Introduces Legislation to Lower Drug Costs in Medicare through Price Negotiation & Competition." October 22. Accessed June 14, 2020. https://www.durbin.senate.gov/newsroom/press-releases/durbin-schakowsky-introduces-legislation-to-lower-drug-costs-in-medicare-through-price-negotiation-and-competition-.

Dusetzina, Stacie B., and Jonathan Oberlander. 2019. "Advancing Legislation on Drug Pricing—Is There a Path Forward?" *New England Journal of Medicine* 381 (November): 2081–2084. https://www.nejm.org/doi/full/10.1056/NEJMp1914044.

Energy and Commerce Committee. 2019. "Health Committee Chairs' Statement on CBO Analysis of H.R. 3." Press Release, October 11. Accessed June 10, 2020. https://energycommerce.house.gov/newsroom/press-releases/health-committee-chairs-statement-on-cbo-analysis-of-hr-3.

Everett, Burgess. 2019. "McConnell Warns Pelosi's Drug Pricing Plan Is DOA." Politico, September 19. Accessed June 5, 2020. https://www.politico.com/story/2019/09/19/mcconnell-pelosi-prescription-plan-1504496.

Frank, Richard G., and Len M. Nichols. 2019. "Medicare Drug-Price Negotiation—Why Now . . . and How." *New England Journal of Medicine* 381, no. 15 (October): 1404–1406. Accessed February 19, 2021. doi:10.1056/nejmp1909798.

Freed, Meredith, Juliette Cubanski, and Tricia Neuman. 2019. "A Look at Recent Proposals to Control Drug Spending by Medicare and Its Beneficiaries." Kaiser Family Foundation, November 26. Accessed June 24, 2020. https://www.kff.org/medicare/issue-brief/a-look-at-recent-proposals-to-control-drug-spending-by-medicare-and-its-beneficiaries/.

Gottlieb, Scott. 2019. "Price Controls Would Stifle Biotech Innovation." *Wall Street Journal*, December 11. Accessed June 11, 2020. https://www.wsj.com/articles/price-controls-would-stifle-biotech-innovation-11576107863.

Grassley, Chuck. 2002. "Grassley Fights for Prescription Drug Benefit." July 17. Accessed January 6, 2020. https://www.grassley.senate.gov/news/news-releases/grassley-fights-prescription-drug-benefit.

Grassley, Chuck. 2018. "Grassley Remarks on Transparency in Prescription Drug Pricing." November 29. Accessed January 4, 2020. https://www.grassley.senate.gov/news/news-releases/grassley-remarks-transparency-prescription-drug-pricing.

Grassley, Chuck. 2019. "Grassley on Medicare Part D Price Negotiation." May 22. Accessed January 4, 2020. https://www.grassley.senate.gov/news/news-releases/grassley-medicare-part-d-price-negotiation.

Grassley, Chuck. 2020. "Vice President Pence Endorses Grassley-Wyden Prescription Drug Bill." February 5. Accessed June 24, 2020. https://www.grassley.senate.gov/news/news-releases/vice-president-pence-endorses-grassley-wyden-prescription-drug-bill.

Grogan, Joe. 2020. "White House Principles for Reducing Drug Costs." *Wall Street Journal*, March 11. Accessed June 8, 2020. https://www.wsj.com/articles/white-house-principles-for-reducing-drug-costs-11583850048.

Himmelfarb, Richard. 1995. *Catastrophic Politics: The Rise and Fall of the Medicare Catastrophic Coverage Act of 1988*. University Park: Pennsylvania State University Press. Accessed February 19, 2021. http://www.psupress.org/books/titles/0-271-01465-2.html.

House Republicans. 2019. "Burying the Socialist Agenda: Speaker Pelosi's Prescription to Kill Drug Innovation and Access." September 23. Accessed June 6, 2020. https://www.gop.gov/burying-the-socialist-agenda-speaker-pelosis-prescription-to-kill-drug-innovation-and-access/.

Huetteman, Emmarie. 2019. "Pelosi Aims for Feds to Negotiate Drug Prices, Even for Private Insurers." Kaiser Health News, June 28. Accessed November 7, 2019. https://khn.org/news/pelosi-aims-for-feds-to-negotiate-drug-prices-even-for-private-insurers/.

Jacobson, Louis. 2010. "Health Care Law Takes Different Tack on Medicare Drug Negotiating." Politifact, April 9. Accessed June 10, 2020. https://www.politifact.com/truth-o-meter/promises/obameter/promise/73/allow-medicare-to-negotiate-for-cheaper-drug-price/.

Kaiser Family Foundation. 2019a. "An Overview of the Medicare Part D Prescription Drug Benefit." Accessed November 15, 2019. https://www.kff.org/medicare/fact-sheet/an-overview-of-the-medicare-part-d-prescription-drug-benefit/.

Kaiser Family Foundation. 2019b. "10 Essential Facts about Medicare and Prescription Drug Spending." Accessed November 5, 2019. https://www.kff.org/infographic/10-essential-facts-about-medicare-and-prescription-drug-spending/.

Kessler, Glenn. 2016. "Trump's Truly Absurd Claim He Would Save $300 Billion a Year on Prescription Drugs." *Washington Post*, February 18. Accessed June 25, 2020. https://www.washingtonpost.com/news/fact-checker/wp/2016/02/18/trumps-truly-absurd-claim-he-would-save-300-billion-a-year-on-prescription-drugs/.

Kildee, Dan. 2019. "Affordable Prescription Drugs for Americans." *Congressional Record* (November 15): H8884. Accessed June 10, 2020. https://www.congress.gov/116/crec/2019/11/15/CREC-2019-11-15-pt1-PgH8884-3.pdf.

Kirzinger, Ashley, Lunna Lopes, Bryan Wu, and Mollyann Brodie. 2019. "KFF Health Tracking Poll – February 2019: Prescription Drugs." Kaiser Family Foundation, March 1. Accessed March 2, 2021. https://www.kff.org/health-costs/poll-finding/kff-health-tracking-poll-february-2019-prescription-drugs/.

Kirzinger, Ashley, Tricia Neuman, Juliette Cubanski, and Mollyann Brodie. 2019. "Data Note: Prescription Drugs and Older Adults." Kaiser Family Foundation, August 9. Accessed June 8, 2020. https://www.kff.org/health-reform/issue-brief/data-note-prescription-drugs-and-older-adults/.

Lopes, Lunna, Liz Hamel, Audrey Kearney, and Mollyann Brodie. 2019. "KFF Health Tracking Poll—October 2019: Health Care in the Democratic Debates, Congress, and the Courts." Accessed June 25, 2020. https://www.kff.org/health-reform/poll-finding/kff-health-tracking-poll-october-2019/.

Lovelace, Berkeley, Jr. 2019. "House Speaker Pelosi Unveils Democrats' Broad Plan to Lower Prices on the Most Expensive Drugs." CNBC, September 19. Accessed December 30, 2019. https://www.cnbc.com/2019/09/19/nancy-pelosi-unveils-sweeping-plan-to-lower-prescription-drug-prices.html.

Milani, Katy, and Devin Duffy. 2019. "Profit over Patients." Accessed December 30, 2019. https://rooseveltinstitute.org/wp-content/uploads/2019/02/RI_Profit-Over-Patients_brief_021319-1.pdf.

Morning Consult. 2019. "Medicare Today: Nearly 9 in 10 Seniors Are Satisfied with Medicare Part D." Accessed December 30, 2019. http://medicaretoday.org/wp-content/uploads/2019/08/8.5.2019-Senior-Satisfaction-Survey-Fact-Sheet.pdf.

Norman, Brett, and Sarah Karlin-Smith. 2016. "The One That Got Away: Obamacare and the Drug Industry." Politico, July 13. Accessed June 5, 2020. https://www.politico.com/story/2016/07/obamacare-prescription-drugs-pharma-225444.

Oliver, Thomas, Philip Lee, and Helene Lipton. 2004. "A Political History of Medicare and Prescription Drug Coverage." *Milbank Quarterly* 82, no. 2: 283–354. Accessed December 30, 2019. https://www.ncbi.nlm.nih.gov/pmc/articles/PMC2690175/#b92.

Owens, Caitlin. 2016. "Why Prescription Drugs Aren't Part of Obamacare." Morning Consult, March 24. Accessed June 12, 2020. https://morningconsult.com/2016/03/24/why-prescription-drugs-arent-part-of-obamacare/.

Pharmaceutical Research and Manufacturers Association (PhRMA). 2019. "Medicare Monday: How Successful Negotiation Takes Place in Medicare." Accessed December 30, 2019. http://phrma-docs.phrma.org/sites/default/files/pdf/medicare-monday-negotiation.pdf.

Przybyla, Heidi. 2015. "Hillary Clinton Unveils Plan to Lower Prescription Drug Costs." *USA Today*, September 22. Accessed June 11, 2020. https://www.usatoday.com/story/news/politics/elections/2015/09/22/hillary-clinton-prescription-drug-plan/72598898/.

Sanders, Bernie. 2019. "Sweeping Plan to Lower Drug Prices Introduced in Senate and House." January 10. Accessed March 2, 2021. https://www.sanders.senate.gov/newsroom/recent-business/sweeping-plan-to-lower-drug-prices-introduced-in-senate-and-house.https://www.sanders.senate.gov/press-releases/sweeping-plan-to-lower-drug-prices-introduced-in-senate-and-house-2/.

Sullivan, Peter. 2019a. "CBO: Pelosi Bill to Lower Drug Prices Saves Medicare $345 Billion." The Hill, October 11. Accessed June 10, 2020. https://thehill.com/policy/healthcare/465491-cbo-pelosi-bill-to-lower-drug-prices-saves-medicare-345-billion.

Sullivan, Thomas. 2019b. "A Tough Road: Cost to Develop One New Drug Is $2.6 Billion; Approval Rate for Drugs Entering Clinical Development Is Less Than 12%." Policy & Medicine, March 21. Accessed June 11, 2020. https://www.policymed.com/2014/12/a-tough-road-cost-to-develop-one-new-drug-is-26-billion-approval-rate-for-drugs-entering-clinical-de.html.

Tapper, Jake, and Dan Morris. 2006. "Just How Did Medicare Bill Get Passed?" ABC News, January 6. Accessed June 18, 2020. https://abcnews.go.com/Nightline/story?id=128998&page=1.

U.S. Senate, Committee on Finance. 2007. "Prescription Drug Pricing and Negotiation: Overview and Economic Perspectives for the Medicare Prescription Drug Benefit." Hearing before the Committee on Finance, U.S. Senate, 110th Congress, January 11. Accessed January 6, 2020. https://www.finance.senate.gov/imo/media/doc/39938.pdf.

U.S. Senate, Committee on Finance. 2019. "Open Executive Session to Consider an Original Bill Entitled 'The Prescription Drug Pricing Reduction Act of 2019.'" July 25. Accessed January 6, 2020. https://www.finance.senate.gov/imo/media/doc/7-25-19%20--%20RX%20Drug%20Pricing%20Reduction%20Act%20of%202019.pdf.

Wall Street Journal. 2019. "Pelosi's Expensive Drug Bill." October 4. Accessed December 31, 2019. https://www.wsj.com/articles/pelosis-expensive-drug-bill-11570228189.

Wall Street Journal. 2020. "Where You Want to Get Cancer." January 9. Accessed June 6, 2020. https://www.wsj.com/articles/where-you-want-to-get-cancer-11578615274.

Warren, Elizabeth. 2018. "It's Time to Let the Government Manufacture Generic Drugs." *Washington Post*, December 17. Accessed June 14, 2020. https://www.washingtonpost.com/opinions/elizabeth-warren-its-time-to-let-the-government-manufacture-generic-drugs/2018/12/17/66bc0fb0-023f-11e9-b5df-5d3874f1ac36_story.html.

Wyden, Ron. 2019. "Wyden Statement at Finance Committee Hearing to Markup Prescription Drug Pricing Proposal." U.S. Senate, Committee on Finance, July 25. Accessed November 1, 2020. https://www.finance.senate.gov/imo/media/doc/Wyden%20Statement%20at%20Finance%20Committee%20Hearing%20to%20Markup%20Prescription%20Drug%20Pricing%20Proposal.pdf.

Physician-Assisted Death

At a Glance

Medical aid in dying, or physician-assisted death, has been the focus of highly contested ethical and moral debates among Republicans and Democrats for decades. In 1994, Oregon became the first state to allow terminally ill patients to end their own lives. In 1997, the U.S. Supreme Court ruled that the U.S. Constitution did not enshrine a right to die, but Oregonians voted to keep the act in place. As of 2020, medical aid in dying was legal in nine states as well as the District of Columbia. Although specific provisions differ from state to state, the laws legalizing the procurement of medical assistance in ending one's own life require a prognosis of six months or less to live, passage of mental health evaluations, and verbal and written requests by the patient who is seeking aid in dying.

Republicans tend to view medical aid in dying as a violation of the Hippocratic oath taken by physicians to do no harm. Arguing that aid-in-dying laws target vulnerable citizens, Republicans maintain that terminally ill patients may be experiencing financial or emotional pressure and that legalizing physician-assisted suicide exploits potentially compromised mental states. Additionally, Republicans argue that federal funds should not be used to subsidize medical aid in dying.

Democrats, on the other hand, view the ability of terminally ill patients to end their lives not as a violation of the Hippocratic oath but rather as a way for those patients to avoid unnecessary pain and suffering. Democrats assert that medical aid-in-dying laws do not put vulnerable patients at risk because safeguards ensure that terminally ill individuals are mentally capable of making appropriate end-of-life decisions. Additionally, Democrats consider medical aid in dying as critical to personal autonomy and bodily integrity, and they believe that terminally ill individuals should have the liberty to end what they perceive as intolerable suffering.

According to Many Democrats . . .

- Medical aid in dying does not violate the Hippocratic oath because it eliminates unnecessary suffering for terminally ill individuals.

- Legal and medical safeguards are in place to ensure that terminally ill individuals are mentally stable and autonomous when electing medical aid in dying.
- Medical aid in dying is central to personal autonomy and bodily integrity, and terminally ill individuals deserve to determine for themselves whether they want to end their own life under physician supervision.

According to Many Republicans . . .

- Medical aid in dying violates the Hippocratic oath taken by physicians to "do no harm."
- Medical aid in dying puts vulnerable individuals at risk and undermines the integrity of the health care system.
- Federal funds should not be used to pay for services related to medical aid in dying.

Overview

Physician-assisted death sits at the root of deeper divisions among Democrats and Republicans regarding governmental authority over decision-making at the end of life. The issue has sparked intense disagreement among Democrats and Republicans regarding the morality and legality of medical aid in dying. Although the positions espoused by both parties have shifted somewhat over time, Democrats have historically supported medical aid in dying, and Republicans have traditionally opposed the practice.

Legalization of medical aid in dying dovetailed with preexisting legal debates about constitutional rights to demand or refuse medical treatment at the end of life. A series of policy and court decisions during the George H. W. Bush (R) and Bill Clinton (D) presidential administrations set the stage in which states would evaluate medical aid in dying from the 1990s onward. In 1990, the U.S. Supreme Court issued an important ruling in *Cruzan v. Director, Missouri Department of Health*, which centered on an individual's constitutional right to refuse medical treatment and the state's right to require clear evidence before the termination of life support services for incompetent patients. In a 5–4 majority opinion issued by Chief Justice William Rehnquist, the court indicated that competent Americans had a constitutional right to refuse treatment. However, as Rehnquist also noted, "There is no automatic assurance that the view of close family members will necessarily be the same as the patient's would have been had she been confronted with the prospect of her situation while competent" (*Cruzan, by Cruzan v. Director, Missouri Department of Health* 1990).

In 1997, the U.S. Congress passed the Assisted Suicide Funding Restriction Act, sponsored by Rep. Ralph Hall (D-TX) and originally cosponsored by 87

Republican and 16 Democratic representatives. As Hall explained, "The bill has the modest goal of keeping the Federal Government out of the business of assisted suicide" (Hall 1997). The act, which prohibited the use of federal funds for any health service or coverage for medical aid in dying, passed by votes of 99–0 in the Senate and 398–16 in the House. When President Bill Clinton signed the act in April 1997, he emphasized his personal opposition to medical aid in dying: "I continue to believe that assisted suicide is wrong. While I have deep sympathy for those who suffer greatly from incurable illness, I believe that to endorse assisted suicide would set us on a disturbing and perhaps dangerous path" (Clinton 1997).

Meanwhile, the U.S. Supreme Court issued rulings in 1997 on two cases pertaining to physician-assisted death: *Washington v. Glucksberg* and *Vacco v. Quill*. In *Washington v. Glucksberg*, several physicians and a nonprofit organization that offered counseling services to individuals considering physician-assisted death challenged Washington State's ban on physician-assisted death. The Supreme Court held in a unanimous ruling that the state's ban was not unconstitutional and that assisted death was not protected as a fundamental liberty by the Fourteenth Amendment. The court concluded that while the U.S. Constitution may guarantee the right to refuse medical treatment, it did not guarantee a right to assisted death. Importantly, however, *Washington v. Glucksberg* left it to the states to decide how to regulate the practice.

The second case, *Vacco v. Quill*, came to the U.S. Supreme Court after physicians in New York challenged the constitutionality of the state's ban on physician-assisted death. The state allowed competent terminally ill adults to withdraw their own lifesaving treatment but prohibited physicians from doing so on their patients' behalf. In another unanimous ruling, the U.S. Supreme Court concluded that New York's ban was constitutional and within the state's regulatory interest. While *Washington v. Glucksberg* held that Washington State's ban did not violate the due process clause of the Fourteenth Amendment, in this case, the court held that New York's ban did not violate that amendment's equal protection clause (*Vacco, Attorney General of New York v. Quill* 1997). Because states had the constitutional authority to institute such bans, the matter of regulating medical aid in dying fell to the states.

Oregon

In 1994, Oregon became the first state to legalize medical aid in dying. The path to enactment of the Oregon Death with Dignity Act began in 1989 when state senator Frank Roberts (D) introduced several unsuccessful bills in support of medical aid in dying. Roberts retired from office in 1993 due to terminal cancer. The following year, the debate shifted from the legislative process to the ballot box. Oregon voters subsequently passed the Oregon Death with Dignity Act by a margin of 51–49 percent (*Oregon Blue Book* 2020). The first state law of its kind, Oregon's Death with Dignity Act spurred national attention. A legal injunction delayed implementation until the Ninth Circuit Court of Appeals lifted it in 1997. That year, Oregon voters also defeated Measure 51, a repeal initiative, by a margin of 60 percent to 40 percent (*Oregon Blue Book* 2020).

When Measure 51 failed, national lawmakers opposed to physician-assisted death sprang into action. Sen. Don Nickles (R-OK) introduced legislation to bar physicians from prescribing controlled substances approved by the Drug Enforcement Administration (DEA) for the purpose of medical aid in dying. Meanwhile, House Judiciary Committee Chairman Henry Hyde (R-IL) remarked, "I'm interested in medical doctors being healers . . . not social engineers serving as executioners" ("House Passes Bill" 1999). Senate Judiciary Committee Chairman Orrin Hatch (R-UT) weighed in as well: "To me, physician-assisted suicide is morally and ethically reprehensible, an abhorrent practice which our society can ill-afford to see as a viable alternative to compassionate care and treatment" (Burrell 1998).

Democrats in Congress responded to these developments by accusing Republicans of superseding states' rights—frequently a guiding principle of GOP politics. "You are imposing the government over the right of people to make decisions in their lives," said Rep. Barney Frank (D-MA). "Some of us believe an individual has the right to make a decision that life has become unbearable" ("House Passes Bill" 1999). Sen. Ron Wyden (D-OR) added, "Does this Congress meeting here in Washington, D.C., believe it is better equipped than the citizens of my state to make moral decisions about acceptable medical practice in Oregon?" (Burrell 1998). The U.S. Senate, under President Pro Tempore Strom Thurmond (R-SC) and Majority Leader Trent Lott (R-MS), took no action on Nickles's proposed legislation.

The matter ultimately reached the U.S. Supreme Court, which in 2005 heard arguments in the case of *Gonzales v. Oregon*. U.S. Attorney General Janet Reno, who served under Bill Clinton, had previously argued that the federal government could not prosecute physicians acting in accordance with the provisions of Oregon's law. But John Ashcroft, who served as U.S. attorney general under George W. Bush from 2001 to 2005, threatened to prosecute physicians who prescribed lethal doses to terminally ill patients in accordance with Oregon's law. Oregon Attorney General Hardy Myers (D) challenged Ashcroft's stance, and the state's Democratic members of Congress indicated public support of the state's position (Daly 2005).

The U.S. Supreme Court decided in favor of Oregon, 6–3, holding that the federal government did not have authority under the Controlled Substances Act to overrule state laws. Barbara Roberts (D), who was Oregon's governor at the same time her husband served in the state senate, later reflected that "end-of-life care has become better in Oregon. People know they have choices. As of 2014, 1,300 prescriptions have been written [for physician-assisted death], and 850 were used. Getting the prescription doesn't mean you have to use it. . . . There is a special place in my heart for the law and the benefits of death with dignity" (Sherman 2016).

Following the *Gonzales v. Oregon* ruling, other states, including Arizona, Rhode Island, and Washington, began considering legislation based on the Oregon model. States that legalized physician-assisted death did so in one of three ways—legislation, court mandate, or ballot initiative—with some variation with respect to prescribing methods and reporting processes. At the same time, however, public opinion on medical aid in dying remained politically divided. One 2007 Gallup poll, conducted the week of Dr. Jack Kevorkian's release from prison, reported that while 54 percent of Republicans considered assisted death to be morally unacceptable, 59 percent of Democrats responded that it was morally acceptable (Carroll 2007). Kevorkian, a physician colloquially known as "Doctor Death," had aided an estimated 130 terminally ill patients with ending their own lives (Childress 2012).

Washington

Fourteen years after Oregon voters legalized aid in dying, Washington voters did the same, making Washington the second state to legalize the practice by ballot initiative. In 2008, former Washington State Gov. Booth Gardner (D) filed an aid in dying initiative to be placed on the November ballot that year. Gardner cited Oregon when defending Ballot Initiative I-1000: "The Oregon Death with Dignity Act has passed the test of time. . . . None of the frightening outcomes predicted by opponents came true" (Gardner 2008). Moreover, as Gardner argued, "Based on their religious beliefs, many people think that a person should not under any circumstances choose to end their life. I respect this moral belief, but it should not be the basis for state law" (Gardner 2008). Another former Washington governor, John Spellman (R), voiced his disapproval: "Do you really think that, once implemented, assisted suicide will remain merely a 'personal choice,' isolated from not-so-subtle coercions of everyday life and magically protected from health care rationing?" (Spellman 2008).

Spellman's concern echoed broader concerns raised by other Republican critics, who feared that legalizing medical aid in dying would threaten vulnerable, terminally ill patients. The same day that Democratic presidential nominee Barack Obama won Washington by a 17-point margin over Republican nominee John McCain, Washington voters approved ballot initiative I-1000 by a 51–49 percent margin.

Like Oregon, Washington had a decades-long history debating the issue of medical aid in dying. The state's Natural Death Act of 1979 banned physician-assisted death, and Washington legislators and voters alike had rejected earlier legalization efforts. Most notably, in 1991, Bradley Robinson of Seattle introduced the Washington Aid in Dying Initiative, which called for legalizing assisted death in cases of medically terminal conditions. After the Washington State Legislature failed to take action on proposed legislation, Washington voters defeated a ballot initiative by a margin of 54 percent to 46 percent ("Washington Aid-in-Dying" 1991).

Traditionally blue states like Washington began to introduce medical aid-in-dying legislation following the *Gonzales* ruling—even as public opinion remained politically divided. While the percentage of U.S. adults considering physician-assisted death to be morally acceptable remained relatively stable between 2001 and 2011, a 2011 Gallup national poll indicated a clear partisan difference, with 51 percent of Democrats considering assisted death to be morally acceptable compared to only 32 percent of Republicans (Saad 2011).

These results indicated gradually warming acceptance to the concept of physician-assisted death among politically progressive Americans. But passage and implementation of medical aid-in-dying legislation remained difficult in blue states as well. For example, in 2012, Massachusetts voters defeated a ballot initiative that would have legalized assisted suicide by a margin of 51 percent to 49 percent (Span 2012). The result marked a significant departure from public polling as late as August that had indicated that 58 percent of voters supported the measure, including 61 percent of Democrats and 44 percent of Republicans, with only 24 percent of respondents opposed (Public Policy Polling 2012).

Montana

Montana represents an unusual case. It is a traditionally red state in which legalization of physician-assisted death was not the product of legislation or ballot initiative but court mandated. Montana state code already permitted terminally ill individuals to withdraw or withhold life-sustaining care at end of life via the Montana Rights of the Terminally Ill Act, which was enacted in 1985. The Montana Supreme Court's ruling in *Baxter v. Montana* in 2009 authorized assisted death in the state. Although the medical aid-in-dying cases heard by the U.S. Supreme Court—*Glucksberg v. Washington*, *Vacco v. Quill*, and *Gonzales v. Oregon*—all centered on constitutional rights, *Baxter v. Montana* did not. The case reached the Montana Supreme Court after a district court had ruled that Robert Baxter, a trucker from Billings, had a right to die by physician-assisted suicide. Ultimately, the Montana Supreme Court issued a narrower ruling based on statutory law. In its majority opinion, the court indicated that "we find nothing in Montana Supreme Court precedent or Montana statutes indicating that physician aid in dying is against public policy" (*Baxter v. State of Montana* 2009).

Not all Democratic legislators agreed with efforts to expand health rights to include medical aid in dying. As state representative Julie French (D) argued, "Before we deal with assisted suicide, we should make sure first and foremost that everybody has equal access [to health care services]" (Johnson 2009). The ruling protected physicians from prosecution if they helped terminally ill patients die but did not affirm that the state constitution guaranteed a right to medical aid in dying. Because the Montana Supreme Court ruled on statutory grounds, future legislative efforts to criminalize medical aid with dying remain possible in the state.

California

California legalized medical aid in dying in 2016 following public debate that shed light on inter- and intraparty differences. In 2015, California state senators Lois Wolk (D) and Bill Monning (D) introduced Senate Bill 128 in response to the well-publicized case of Brittany Maynard, a terminally ill 29-year-old California resident who relocated to Oregon to end her own life. The act outlined specific regulatory safeguards, including a written request for aid-in-dying drugs signed in the presence of a witness (Senate Bill No. 128 2015). Public opinion indicated widespread support for medical aid-in-dying legislation across the political spectrum: one 2015 University of California–Berkeley poll found that 82 percent of Democrats and 67 percent of Republicans supported the idea (Maclay 2015).

The bill only faced Republican opposition in the state senate and among some liberal members of the Assembly. One news report characterized liberal opposition to the bill as a rift among affluent white policy makers and Latino policy makers who represented agricultural and working-class communities (Greenhut 2015). Democratic assemblywoman Lorena Gonzalez highlighted what she considered the illusion of choice for financially vulnerable patients: "We have a health care system that is set up to cut costs" (Morain 2015). Republican policy makers such as state senator Bob Huff echoed similar concerns about socioeconomic pressure associated with medical aid in dying: "Let's call this for what it really is: It's not death with dignity. This is state-assisted death, physician-assisted death and relative-assisted death" (McGreevy 2015).

Gov. Jerry Brown (D) signed the California End of Life Option Act into law on October 5, 2015. "I do not know what I would do if I were dying in prolonged and excruciating pain," said Brown. "I am certain, however, that it would be a comfort to be able to consider the options afforded by this bill. And I wouldn't deny that right to others" (Pérez-Peña and Lovett 2015). The existence of regulatory safeguards as outlined in the law, and the right of a terminally ill individuals to have the choice of how to end their life, are two of the main principles taken by the Democratic party regarding medical aid in dying. The bill was enacted in June 2016, making California the fifth state to have right-to-die legislation. In May 2018, a state court judge invalidated the law, ruling that it had been improperly passed during a special legislative session (Anapol 2018). A state appeals court reinstated the law, a decision that was later affirmed by the California State Supreme Court when it declined to review the case.

Colorado

In November 2016, Colorado voters approved Proposition 106, the End of Life Option Act, by an overwhelming 2-to-1 margin (Brown 2016), and Gov. John Hickenlooper (D) signed the measure into law in December 2016. The measure limited eligibility to terminally ill individuals with less than six months to live, and like other state laws modeled after Oregon's legislation, required requestors to submit multiple requests to an attending physician, obtain a second opinion, and undergo a mental health consultation. Public reports indicated that the number of terminally ill Coloradans obtaining prescriptions through the measure increased steadily two years after passage, from 72 in 2017 to 125 in 2018 (Navarro 2019).

Maryland

During his Maryland gubernatorial campaign in 2014, Larry Hogan (R) expressed opposition to medical aid in dying (Wiering 2014). Following his reelection in 2018, the Democratic-majority Maryland General Assembly introduced a bill to legalize medical aid in dying. As the legislature prepared to debate the bill, Hogan acknowledged that the issue is "one that I really wrestle with from a personal basis" (Wood 2019b). Hogan's wrestling coincided with a greater sense of support among Maryland voters, as public opinion polling in early 2019 indicated that 62 percent of Marylanders favored the concept of providing medical aid in dying (Bonessi 2019). After the state's House of Delegates approved the bill in February 2019, state senators incorporated several amendments into the Senate version of the End-of-Life Option Act, which strengthened eligibility requirements by requiring requestors to have an irreversible condition that would "within a reasonable degree of medical certainty" lead to death within six months (*Washington Post* 2019).

The bill would have represented one of the strictest laws on medical aid in dying, but it failed with a tie vote in the Democratic-led Senate. After the vote, state senator Cheryl Kagan (D) tweeted her disappointment but emphasized that "votes crossed party and racial lines. The debate honored the significance of the issue." Indeed, one Republican supported the measure while nine Democrats voted against it. As the bill's sponsor, state senator Will Smith (D), acknowledged, "At the end of the day, this was about giving folks a modicum of autonomy when they're facing their end of life" (Rey 2019). During the same legislative session, Hogan allowed HB77, a bill that decriminalized attempted suicide, to become law without his signature, leaving the door open for future debate on assisted death in Maryland (Waldman 2019).

Democrats on Physician-Assisted Death

By 2020, physician-assisted death was legal in Washington, DC; seven traditionally blue states (California, Hawaii, Maine, New Jersey, Oregon, Vermont, and Washington); one traditionally red state (Montana); and one state (Colorado) that has shifted from Republican to Democratic dominance over the last two decades (CNN 2019). A number of Democratic-majority city councils, including those in Albuquerque, Santa Fe, and Las Cruces, New Mexico, have also affirmed their support for medical aid in dying (AP News 2018).

Democrats argue that assisted suicide does not violate the Hippocratic oath because it actually eliminates unnecessary suffering for terminally ill individuals. Following intense debate, Hawaii was the seventh jurisdiction to pass aid-in-dying legislation in 2018. Hawaii state senator Russell Ruderman (D) argued, "There is no reason to deny others the freedom to live and die as we choose" (Nanea 2018). When fellow Democratic senator Josh Green, a physician, voiced his support for the legislation, he also expressed concern regarding how he could balance upholding the Hippocratic oath while feeling obligated to alleviate his patients' suffering (Nanea 2018). Democratic majorities in both the state house of representatives and the state senate cleared the path toward passage, and the Our Care, Our Choice Act went into effect on January 1, 2019 (Gorman 2018).

In 2019, on the other side of the country, Gov. Andrew Cuomo (D) of New York explained, "It's a controversial issue, it's a difficult issue, but the older we get and the better medicine gets the more we've seen people suffer for too, too long" (Bump 2019). Cuomo's comments were in direct response to Gov. Phil Murphy (D) having signed a medical aid-in-dying law in New Jersey. According to one January 2019 Quinnipiac poll, 63 percent of New Yorkers supported assisted suicide, including a striking 69 percent of Democrats (Lovett 2019).

Democrats also maintain that medical aid in dying does not put vulnerable individuals at risk because legal and medical safeguards are in place to ensure that terminally ill individuals are mentally stable and autonomous. State laws may vary with respect to specifics, but states that have implemented medical aid-in-dying legislation have included procedural safeguards intended to ensure that requestors are mentally competent. For example, Hawaii's Our Care, Our Choice Act requires that terminally ill individuals make three medication requests, wait at least 20 days between such requests, and undergo a mental health consultation with two medical professionals before a patient could obtain a prescription (Span 2019). When Gov. David Ige (D) signed Hawaii's medical aid-in-dying legislation, he remarked, "I believe that we have clear safeguards in place. It is time for terminally ill, mentally competent Hawai'i residents who are suffering to make their own end-of-life choices with dignity, grace and peace" (Office of the Governor of the State of Hawai'i 2018).

In New Mexico, medical aid in dying returned to the legislative docket following the election of a Democratic governor and the expansion of the Democratic majority in the state house in the 2018 midterm elections (Lee 2019). Gov. Michelle Lujan Grisham voiced support for medical aid in dying while on the campaign trail. The proposal introduced by Rep. Deborah Armstrong (D) and state senator Liz Stefanics (D) in December 2018 incorporated safeguards that included a 48-hour postprescription waiting period and also required authorization from two medical professionals. The bill progressed through committee but failed to receive a vote during the 2019 legislative session.

Democrats contend that medical aid in dying is central to personal autonomy and bodily integrity. In this respect, terminally ill individuals deserve to have the choice of whether or not they want to end their own life under physician supervision. When Gov. Peter Shumlin (D) signed Vermont's aid-in-dying law in May 2013, he said, "Vermonters who face terminal illness and are in excruciating pain at the end of their lives now have control over their destinies. This is the right thing to do" (Muller 2013). Upon signing a bill passed in New Jersey's Democratic-led state assembly and state senate in 2019, Gov. Phil Murphy expressed similar sentiments, declaring that "signing this legislation is the decision that best respects the freedom and humanity of all New Jersey residents" (Murphy 2019).

Although states under Democratic control have taken a leading role in introducing and implementing medical aid-in-dying legislation, some Democrats have resisted the idea. For example, in 2013, Vermont policy makers legalized physician-assisted death by enacting Act 39, or the Vermont Patient Choice and Control at the End of Life Act, as a less restrictive adaptation of Oregon's law. Democrats and Republicans in the state senate were deadlocked between those who wanted a bill like Oregon's and those who wanted less government intervention. Arguments within the state Democratic party focused on the appropriate degree of government regulation: while state senator Claire Ayer (D) called the hybrid law a "compromise," another Democratic lawmaker, Peter Galbraith, argued that the law allowed for too much government involvement in the process (Hallenbeck 2013). In 2014, Gov. Dannel Malloy (D) of Connecticut also voiced his personal apprehension with medical aid in dying when it looked as if a Democratic-sponsored bill might reach his desk: "I don't think in society we should be viewed as encouraging suicide" (Pazniokas 2014). For almost a decade, the Connecticut General Assembly had considered medical aid-in-dying legislation, but none of these legislative efforts advanced out of committee (Altimari 2019). And although Gov. Phil Murphy signed medical aid-in-dying legislation in New Jersey in April 2019, he expressed similar personal misgivings: "While my faith may lead me to a particular decision for myself, as a public official I cannot deny this alternative to those who may reach a different conclusion" (Linge 2019).

In 2016, the New Mexico Supreme Court, composed of four elected Democratic judges and one Republican, issued a unanimous ruling that medical aid in dying was not a constitutional right. Justice Edward Chavez (D) wrote that the court recognized the "magnitude and importance of the very personal desire of a terminally ill patient to decide how to safely and peacefully exit a painful and debilitating life." He also conceded that the state "does not have an interest in preserving a painful and debilitating life that will end imminently" (Haywood 2016). Nonetheless, the court's decisive ruling was a disappointment to supporters of physician-assisted death options. Following that ruling, the New Mexico Legislature revisited the matter. In March 2017, however, the state senate defeated Senate Bill 252—which would have legalized medical aid in dying—by a 22–20 vote, with 15 Republicans voting nay (Terrell 2017).

Democratic control of the Maryland House of Delegates and Senate throughout the 2010s also did not lead to smooth passage of medical aid-in-dying legislation in the state. Several prospective bills failed to advance beyond committee during the decade. In March 2019, Maryland state senator Bobby Zirkin (D) argued that the initial version of the most recent bill was "flawed to its core." Zirkin supported the measure after stricter definitions and additional safeguards were incorporated, much to the chagrin of state senator Will Smith (D), the bill's sponsor, who concluded, "The bill does shift toward many more steps to go through . . . and maybe that's a

DC's Death with Dignity Act Exploits the Suffering and Vulnerable

On February 6, 2017, Rep. Keith Rothfus (R-PA) addressed the Speaker of the U.S. House of Representatives to express his strong opposition to Washington, DC's Death with Dignity Act.

The D.C. City Council recently passed a so-called Death with Dignity Act, which would allow adults who have been diagnosed with a terminal disease and who have been told they have 6 months or less to live to receive a prescription from their doctor to end their life. D.C.'s assisted suicide law, Mr. Speaker, threatens the inalienable rights of vulnerable citizens. Not only does the new D.C. statute tear at the tapestry of our Nation's founding, it directly contradicts the Hippocratic oath every physician takes, to do no harm.

I shudder to think of the lives that will be lost because our society tells the weak, the despairing, the suffering, or the hopeless that suicide is the best option for them. Laws similar to the D.C. Death with Dignity Act in the U.S. and Europe have resulted in individuals being pressured to end their lives, and insurance companies covering the reimbursements for suicide treatment but not for other care.

Allowing physicians to prescribe lethal medications to patients would mean we are abandoning our Nation's most vulnerable citizens and, instead, succumbing to a culture that is worse than the disease.

Source

Congressional Record, vol. 163, no. 20 (February 6, 2017): H998. Washington, DC: Government Printing Office. Accessed August 23, 2019. https://www.congress.gov/congressional-record/2017/2/6/house-section/article/h998-1.

good thing, and maybe that's not" (Wood 2019a). The state senate ultimately deadlocked on the revised bill, leading to its defeat during the 2019 legislative session. The tie vote marked the furthest that medical aid-in-dying legislation had advanced within the Maryland General Assembly. State delegate Shane Pendergrass (D) and state senator Jeff Waldsteicher (D) reintroduced the End-of-Life Option Act in both chambers in January 2020, but the legislature adjourned for the 2020 session due to the COVID-19 pandemic before taking action on the bill.

Republicans on Physician-Assisted Death

Republicans have raised ethical concerns with medical aid in dying, arguing that the practice threatens the integrity of the health care system by compelling medical professionals to harm terminally ill patients and potentially enabling family members to exploit their relatives' vulnerabilities for their own gain. Among the 44 states where assisted suicide is illegal, 30 awarded their electoral votes to Republican presidential nominee Donald Trump during the 2016 presidential election.

Republicans argue that physician-assisted death violates the Hippocratic oath to "do no harm." Gov. Paul LePage (R) of Maine, who held office from 2011 to 2019, vowed to veto any medical aid-in-dying legislation that came across his desk. In public statements, LePage described assisted death as an immoral act. As he explained, "Here we are talking about death with dignity and we're sitting there, human beings, passing judgment on who can live and who can die. No, I don't believe in it" ("LePage Says" 2017). LePage's sentiment mirrored that of Republicans on the other side of the country. When Hawaii's House Committee on Health and Human Services held hearings regarding HB-2739 in February 2018, the Honolulu County Republican Party testified against the proposed medical aid-in-dying legislation. As they argued, "No one, especially a doctor, should be permitted to kill intentionally or assist in killing intentionally. Physicians are sworn to eliminate illness and disease but never eliminate their patients" (Honolulu County Republican Party 2018).

Similarly, when the Maryland General Assembly moved forward with legislation in 2019, state senator Justin Ready (R) argued, "This crosses a very bright red line of where we should be going as a society, as a state" (Wood 2019a). Patricia Fenati, a Republican who sought but lost election to the Maryland House of Delegates in 2018, weighed in even more forcefully. In a February 2019 letter to the Montgomery County Republican Party, Fenati declared, "I believe Assisted Suicide is another term for Assisted Murder and it sets us high on a slippery slope leading to other uses of sympathetic murder and mercy killing" (Montgomery County Republican Party 2019).

Republicans argue that medical aid-in-dying legislation places vulnerable individuals at risk, undermining the integrity of the health care system. When the Maine Legislature deliberated over medical aid-in-dying legislation in 2017, state representative Deborah Sanderson (R) asked, "Do we know there is choice at the end when they self-administer? I think we would be naive to imagine that every family is perfect and there may not be an occasion for an alternative motive, an inheritance or financial gain" (Miller 2017). Similarly, when the Connecticut General Assembly revisited the matter in 2018, state senator Joe Markley (R) admitted, "My greatest fear is that people who are disabled or terminally ill will be pressured by family or insurance companies to take their own lives. Life is precious, and the laws in the state of Connecticut should continue to acknowledge that" (Connecticut Senate Republicans 2018). In 2019, New Mexico representative Gregg Schmedes (R) emphasized that despite procedural safeguards, the ability to self-administer lethal doses without a medical professional present could allow family members to carry out "the perfect crime" (Lee 2019).

In January 2019, Montana state representative Carl Glimm (R) introduced House Bill 284, which would criminalize medical aid in dying in Montana. He intended the bill "to send a message about suicide from young to old, from healthy to sick—that it's not a good option" (Ragar 2019). The bill passed in the house almost entirely along party lines in February 2019, with 41 of 46 Democrats voting nay and 52 of 53 Republicans voting yea. The bill died in the state senate in April 2019, leaving the court mandate intact.

Under a 2019 bill sponsored by Maine state representative Patty Hymanson (D) and state senator Marianne Moore (R), a terminally ill patient with a six-month prognosis would be allowed to receive a lethal dose from a physician for self-administration. The bill marked a second effort to pass physician-assisted death legislation in the state. State senator Roger Katz (R) sponsored a 2017 bill that passed on a bipartisan vote in the one-seat Republican-majority Senate, but ran aground on a bipartisan vote in the slim Democratic-majority House (Miller 2017).

The 2019 bill required requestors to submit one written and two oral requests to an attending physician, obtain a second opinion from another physician, and undergo a mental health consultation. State representative Abigail Griffin (R) offered her opposition, proclaiming, "This bill is an attack against the value of life.

Aid in Dying Respects Personal Liberty

On June 12, 2019, Gov. Janet Mills (D-ME) offered the following remarks when signing the Death with Dignity Act, which legalized physician-assisted death in the state of Maine:

> What is the balancing of rights then, when an individual, in the throes of suffering and facing certain death, but while still competent, wishes to end life, denying death its ultimate pain?
>
> Some argue that enactment of L.D. 1313 equates to the government authorizing taking life, or "playing god" with the lives of our citizens.
>
> It is not up to the government to decide who may die and who may live, when they shall die or how long they shall live. It is our duty to provide the most comprehensive end of life care possible, a task we have only recently begun to recognize. But what is the responsibility of society when compassionate end of life care may not be adequate or accessible?
>
> We also have a duty to prevent people from being victimized, to prevent discrimination against persons with disabilities, to make sure others do not take advantage of vulnerable citizens.
>
> Despite the narrowest of votes in the House of Representatives, L.D. 1313 appears to be favored by a majority of Maine people surveyed, and it includes some, though not all, safeguards to protect the decision-making of competent terminally ill patients and to protect misuse and abuse of lethal medications and the diversion of dangerous drugs.

Source

Mills, Janet. 2019. "Governor Mills Signs Death with Dignity Act." June 12. Accessed March 12, 2021. https://www.maine.gov/governor/mills/news/governor-mills-signs-death-dignity-act-2019-06-12.

Physician assisted suicide tells the elderly, disabled and dependent family members their lives are not valuable. It takes away their hope. It is not compassionate" (Griffin 2019). Following the 2018 midterm elections, Democrat Janet Mills succeeded Paul LaPage as governor and signed into law what LaPage had long vowed to veto (Span 2019).

Republicans also insist that federal funds should not be used to pay for services related to assisted death. One of the most prominent cases in this respect occurred after Washington, DC, became the sixth jurisdiction to enact medical aid-in-dying legislation. Mayor Muriel E. Bowser, a Democrat, signed the district's Death with Dignity Act on January 6, 2017, which was then transferred to Congress for review. A spokesman for the mayor stated that "we are committed to ensuring this legislation becomes law and will keep all options on the table to implement it should Congress attempt to meddle in our local affairs" (Portnoy and Davis 2017). Within the week, however, Sen. James Lankford (R) of Oklahoma and Rep. Brad Wenstrup (R) of Ohio condemned the law and introduced companion resolutions disapproving of the act (H.J. Res. 27 2016). Seventy-two cosponsors, all Republican, joined the joint resolution, but it never reached the floor of the U.S. House or Senate for a full vote.

Republican opponents did not give up. Next, House Republicans tried to repeal the law and bar funding to the city for implementation. In May 2017, language in President Trump's proposed 2018 federal budget barred Washington, DC, from using any funding of any kind for implementation. In July 2017, the House Appropriations Committee voted 28–24 to repeal the law and impose a spending ban via an amendment introduced by Rep. Andy Harris (R-MD). Harris argued that "encouraging patients to commit suicide deprives them of the opportunity to potentially be cured by new treatments that could ameliorate their condition and even add years to their lives, if not cure them completely" (Kinery 2017). In response, DC Council Member Mary M. Cheh (D) decried that the spending ban "would directly result in the prolonged suffering and pain of District residents" (Portnoy and Davis 2017). The 2018 federal budget resolutions passed by the U.S. House of Representatives and Senate in October 2017 did not include Harris's rider to repeal the District's Death with Dignity Act.

In September 2017, Representative Wenstrup introduced another concurrent resolution, cosponsored by five Republicans and five Democrats, which questioned assisted death more broadly. As the resolution concluded, "It is the sense of the Congress . . . that the Federal Government should not adopt or endorse policies or practices that support, encourage, or facilitate suicide or assisted suicide, whether by physicians or others" (H. Con. Res. 80 2017). During the first two years of implementation, only two DC residents ended their lives under the district's "death with dignity" legislation (Nirappil 2019).

While blue states have moved forward with medical aid-in-dying legislation, legislatures in several traditionally red states have either imposed more stringent bans on physician-assisted death or reaffirmed their opposition to medical aid in dying.

In April 2017, Alabama state representative Mack Butler (R) sponsored HB96, entitled the Assisted Suicide Ban Act. The act would "prohibit a person or a health care provider from providing aid in dying to another person and would provide civil and criminal penalties for violations" (Assisted Suicide Ban Act 2017). The bill passed the state house and senate by margins of 80–2 and 25–3, respectively, and garnered yea votes from the majority of Democrats and Republicans in both chambers. Gov. Kay Ivey (R) signed the bill into law in May 2017, making assisted death a felony in Alabama (Hill 2017). That same year, the South Dakota state senate adopted and the house of representatives concurred with Resolution 11, which affirmed that "the Legislature strongly opposes and condemns physician-assisted suicide" (State of South Dakota 2017).

Todd M. Olszewski and Morgan Bjarno

Further Reading

An Act to Enact the Maine Death with Dignity Act. LP 1313 HP 948. 129th Maine Legis. (2019). Accessed August 23, 2019. http://legislature.maine.gov/legis/bills/bills_129th/billtexts/HP094801.asp.

Altimari, Daniela. 2015. "Malloy Still Struggling with the Concept of 'Aid-in-Dying.'" *Hartford Courant*, March 17. Accessed August 23, 2019. https://www.courant.com/politics/capitol-watch/hc-gov-dannel-p-malloy-still-struggling-with-aidindying-20150317-story.html.

Altimari, Daniela. 2019. "Connecticut Lawmakers Won't Advance Bill Allowing Terminally Ill Patients to Obtain a Doctor's Help to End Their Lives." *Hartford Courant*, April 1. Accessed August 23, 2019. https://www.courant.com/politics/hc-pol-aid-in-dying-no-vote-20190401-hrpz3cnsrvgrtdthawuzi5udde-story.html.

Anapol, Avery. 2018. "California Judge Assisted Suicide." The Hill, May 16. Accessed August 23, 2019. https://thehill.com/policy/healthcare/387931-california-judge-overturns-assisted-suicide-law.

AP News. 2018. "New Mexico City Backs Assisted Suicide Legislation." Accessed August 23, 2019. https://www.apnews.com/7859df08299b40afa3945e32ffeee980.

Assisted Suicide Ban Act. AL HB96, 114th Cong. (2017). Accessed August 23, 2019. https://legiscan.com/AL/bill/HB96/2017.

Baxter v. State of Montana. 2009. 224 P.3d 1211. Accessed August 21, 2019. https://law.justia.com/cases/montana/supreme-court/2009/94adc027-086a-4b36-a80e-0aaf09a60127.html.

Bonessi, Dominique Maria. 2019. "Right-to-Die Bill Advances in Maryland House." WAMU 88.5, March 7. Accessed August 23, 2019. https://wamu.org/story/19/03/07/right-to-die-bill-advances-in-maryland-house/.

Brown, Jennifer. 2016. "Colorado Passes Medical Aid in Dying, Joining Five Other States." *Denver Post*, November 9. Accessed August 23, 2019. https://www.denverpost.com/2016/11/08/colorado-aid-in-dying-proposition-106-election-results/.

Bump, Bethany. 2019. "Cuomo Says He Would Support Aid in Dying Legislation." *Times Union*, April 10. Accessed August 23, 2019. https://www.timesunion.com/news/article/NY-Gov-Cuomo-says-he-would-support-aid-in-dying-13756237.php.

Burrell, Cassandra. 1998. "Physician-Assisted Suicide: Life-and-Death Fight." *Kitsap Sun*, August 3. Accessed August 21, 2019. https://products.kitsapsun.com/archive/1998/08-03/0032_physician-assisted_suicide__life-.html.

Camden, Jim. 1991. "Aid-in-Dying Initiative Trailing by 95,000." *Spokane Chronicle*, November 6. Accessed December 14, 2018. https://news.google.com/newspapers?id=BFpYAAAAIBAJ&sjid=EPoDAAAAIBAJ&dq=initiative119g:locwashington&pg=7131,746316.

Carroll, Joseph. 2007. "Public Divided over Moral Acceptability of Doctor-Assisted Suicide." Gallup, May 31. Accessed August 21, 2019. https://news.gallup.com/poll/27727/public-divided-over-moral-acceptability-doctorassisted-suicide.aspx.

Childress, Sarah. 2012. "The Evolution of America's Right-to-Die Movement." PBS, November 13. Accessed December 14, 2018. https://www.pbs.org/wgbh/frontline/article/the-evolution-of-americas-right-to-die-movement/.

Chokshi, Niraj. 2014. "Christie May Face a Decision on Assisted Suicide in New Jersey." *Washington Post*, November 19. Accessed August 23, 2019. https://www.washingtonpost.com/blogs/govbeat/wp/2014/11/19/christie-may-face-a-decision-on-assisted-suicide-in-new-jersey/.

Clinton, William J. 1997. "Statement on Signing the Assisted Suicide Funding Restriction Act of 1997." Accessed August 21, 2019. https://www.govinfo.gov/content/pkg/WCPD-1997-05-05/pdf/WCPD-1997-05-05-Pg617-4.pdf.

CNN. 2019. "Physician-Assisted Suicide Fast Facts." Accessed August 23, 2019. https://www.cnn.com/2014/11/26/us/physician-assisted-suicide-fast-facts/index.html.

Connecticut Senate Republicans. 2018. "Senator Joe Markley Stands against Assisted Suicide in CT." Accessed August 23, 2019. https://ctsenaterepublicans.com/2018/03/senator-joe-markley-stands-against-assisted-suicide-in-ct/#.XWPg0JNKgWr.

Cruzan, by Cruzan v. Director, Missouri Department of Health. 1990. 497 U.S. 261. Accessed August 21, 2019. https://www.law.cornell.edu/supremecourt/text/497/261.

Cunningham, Maurice T. 2014. "Defeating 'Death with Dignity': Morality and Message in a Massachusetts Referendum." *American Catholic Studies* 125, no. 2: 23–43. Accessed December 14, 2018. doi:10.1353/acs.2014.0042.

Daley, John. 2016. "After Contentious Fight, Colorado Voters Approve Aid-in-Dying Measure." NPR, November 10. Accessed December 14, 2018. https://www.npr.org/sections/health-shots/2016/11/10/501484312/colorado-voters-overwhelmingly-approves-aid-in-dying-measure.

Daly, Matthew. 2005. "Assisted Suicide Defended." *The Columbian* (Vancouver, WA), July 21: c2. Accessed February 19, 2021. https://infoweb.newsbank.com/apps/news/document-view?p=AMNEWS&docref=news/10B80E28D006C0B0.

Disapproving the Action of the District of Columbia Council in Approving the Death with Dignity Act of 2016. H.J. Res. 27, 115th Cong. (2016). Accessed August 23, 2019. https://www.congress.gov/bill/115th-congress/house-joint-resolution/27/text.

Gabriel, Trip. 1991. "A Fight to the Death." *New York Times*, December 8. Accessed December 14, 2018. https://www.nytimes.com/1991/12/08/magazine/a-fight-to-the-death.html.

Gardner, Booth. 2008. "'Death with Dignity' Initiative Deserves Dignified Consideration." *Seattle Times*, July 3. Accessed December 14, 2018. https://www.seattletimes.com/opinion/death-with-dignity-initiative-deserves-dignified-consideration/.

Gorman, Anna. 2016. "Aid-in-Dying Laws Only Accentuate Need for Palliative Care, Providers Say." Kaiser Health News, July 15. Accessed December 14, 2018. https://khn.org/news/aid-in-dying-laws-only-accentuate-need-for-palliative-care-providers-say/.

Gorman, Steve. 2018. "Hawaii Lawmakers Approve Medical Aid in Dying for Terminally Ill." Reuters, March 29. Accessed August 23, 2019. https://www.reuters.com/article/us-hawaii-dying/hawaii-lawmakers-approve-medical-aid-in-dying-for-terminally-ill-idUSKBN1H606J.

Greenhouse, Linda. 2005. "Justices Hear Arguments on Oregon's Assisted-Suicide Law." *New York Times*, October 5. Accessed December 14, 2018. https://www.nytimes.com/2005/10/05/politics/justices-hear-arguments-on-oregons-assistedsuicide-law.html.

Greenhut, Steven. 2015. "'Aid in Dying' Causes a Democratic Split." *San Diego Union-Tribune*, July 6. Accessed August 21, 2015, https://www.sandiegouniontribune.com/news/politics/sdut-assisted-suicide-democratic-split-whites-latinos-2015jul06-story.html.

Griffin, Abigail. 2019. "LD 1313 'An Act to Enact the Maine Death with Dignity Act.'" Accessed August 23, 2019. http://legislature.maine.gov/legis/bills/getTestimonyDoc.asp?id=117209.

H. Con. Res. 80, 115th Cong. (2017). Accessed August 23, 2019. https://www.congress.gov/115/bills/hconres80/BILLS-115hconres80ih.pdf.

HB 1536, 92nd Ark. Legis. (2019). Accessed August 23, 2019. http://www.arkleg.state.ar.us/assembly/2019/2019R/Bills/HB1536.pdf.

Hall, Ralph M. 1997. "Assisted Suicide Restriction Act." *Congressional Record*. Accessed August 23, 2019. https://www.congress.gov/crec/1997/03/11/CREC-1997-03-11-pt1-PgE431-2.pdf.

Hallenbeck, Terri. 2013. "Vermont Senate OKs End-of-life Legislation." *USA Today*, May 9. Accessed December 14, 2018. https://www.usatoday.com/story/news/politics/2013/05/09/vermont-physician-assisted-death-bill/2146617/.

Haywood, Phaedra. 2016. "New Mexico Supreme Court Rules against Physician-Assisted Suicide." *Santa Fe New Mexican*, June 30. Accessed August 23, 2019. https://www.santafenewmexican.com/news/health_and_science/new-mexico-supreme-court-rules-against-physician-assisted-suicide/article_6fee621d-e689-520d-a51f-974d08ec5ec2.html.

Hill, Samantha. 2017. "Assisted Suicide Ban Act Passed with Mixed Reactions." *Anniston Star*, June 27. Accessed August 23, 2019. https://www.annistonstar.com/news/state/assisted-suicide-ban-act-passed-with-mixed-reactions/article_7afca17c-5af9-11e7-8972-6b2876419a1d.html.

Honolulu County Republican Party. 2018. "Opposition to HB-2739." Accessed August 23, 2019. https://www.capitol.hawaii.gov/Session2018/Testimony/HB2739_TESTIMONY_HHS-JUD_02-27-18_.PDF.

"House Passes Bill to Bar Doctor-Assisted Suicide; No Senate Action Taken." In *CQ Almanac 1999*, 55th ed., 18-35-18-38. Washington, DC: Congressional Quarterly, 1999. Accessed February 19, 2021. http://library.cqpress.com/cqalmanac/cqal99-0000201193.

Johnson, Kirk. 2009. "Montana Court to Rule on Assisted Suicide Case." *New York Times*, August 31. Accessed August 21, 2019. https://www.nytimes.com/2009/09/01/us/01montana.html.

Kinery, Emma. 2017. "Republicans in Congress Attempt to Repeal D.C. Assisted Suicide Law." *USA Today*, July 17. Accessed August 23, 2019. https://www.usatoday.com/story/news/2017/07/17/d-c-assisted-suicide-law-targeted-gop/485209001/.

Lee, Morgan. 2019. "New Mexico Considers End-of-Life Legislation, Legalizing Medically Assisted Suicide." *Las Cruces Sun News*, January 21. Accessed August 23, 2019. https://www.lcsun-news.com/story/news/local/new-mexico/legislature/2019/01/21/medically-assisted-suicide-being-considered-new-mexico-legislature/2640221002/.

"LePage Says He Will Veto Assisted Suicide Bill." 2017. *Portland Press Herald*, April 18. Accessed August 23, 2019. https://www.pressherald.com/2017/04/18/lepage-says-he-will-veto-aid-in-dying-bill/?rel=related.

Linge, Mary Kay. 2019. "Phil Murphy Takes Step toward Making Assisted Suicide Legal in New Jersey." *New York Post*, April 13. Accessed August 23, 2019. https://nypost.com/2019/04/13/phil-murphy-takes-step-toward-making-assisted-suicide-legal-in-new-jersey/.

Lovett, Kenneth. 2019. "Advocates for Physician Assisted Suicide Dismiss Opposition from Catholic Church." *Daily News*, January 27. Accessed August 23, 2019. https://www.nydailynews.com/news/politics/ny-pol-physician-assisted-suicide-church-compassionate-care-20190127-story.html.

Maclay, Kathleen. 2015. "IGS Poll: Californians Support Medical Aid in Dying for Terminally Ill." Institute of Governmental Studies, September 3. Accessed August 21, 2019. https://igs.berkeley.edu/news/igs-poll-californians-support-medical-aid-in-dying-for-terminally-ill.

McGreevy, Patrick. 2015. "After Struggling, Jerry Brown Makes Assisted Suicide Legal in California." *Los Angeles Times*, October 5. Accessed August 23, 2019. https://www.latimes.com/local/political/la-me-pc-gov-brown-end-of-life-bill-20151005-story.html.

Miller, Kevin. 2017. "Maine House Rejects 'Death with Dignity' Bill." *Portland Press Herald*, May 23. Accessed August 23, 2019. https://www.pressherald.com/2017/05/23/house-rejects-death-with-dignity-bill/?rel=related.

Montgomery County Republican Party. 2019. "SB 311 Physician Assisted Suicide." Accessed August 23, 2019. https://www.mcgop.com/sb_311_physician_assisted_suicide.

Morain, Dan. 2015. "Struggling with a Life and Death Issue." *Sacramento Bee*, July 8. Accessed August 23, 2019. https://www.sacbee.com/opinion/opn-columns-blogs/dan-morain/article26831875.html.

Muller, Sarah. 2013. "Assisted Suicide: Vermont Governor Signs 'Death with Dignity' Measure." MSNBC, October 2. Accessed December 14, 2018. http://www.msnbc.com/the-last-word/assisted-suicide-vermont-governor-signs-dea.

Murphy, Philip D. 2019. "Statement upon Signing Assembly Bill No. 1504." Accessed August 23, 2019. http://d31hzlhk6di2h5.cloudfront.net/20190412/4b/cd/8b/1f/02854e1f1393a35250679633/A1504.pdf.

Nanea, Kalani. 2018. "Hawaii Senate Passes Medical Aid in Dying, Sending Legislation to Governor." *Honolulu Star-Advertiser*, March 29. Accessed December 14, 2018. http://www.staradvertiser.com/2018/03/29/breaking-news/hawaii-senate-passes-medical-aid-in-dying-sending-legislation-to-governor/.

Navarro, Natalia V. 2019. "More Terminally Ill People in Colorado Are Getting Prescriptions to End Their Lives." CPR News, February 4. Accessed August 23, 2019. https://www.cpr.org/2019/02/04/more-terminally-ill-people-in-colorado-are-getting-prescriptions-to-end-their-lives/.

Nirappil, Fenit. 2017. "DC Assisted Suicide Law Could Be Blocked under Trump's Budget." *Washington Post*, May 23. Accessed August 23, 2019. https://www.washingtonpost.com/local/dc-politics/dc-assisted-suicide-law-could-be-blocked-under-trumps-budget/2017/05/23/2e002ad0-3fd6-11e7-adba-394ee67a7582_story.html.

Nirappil, Fenit. 2019. "Two Terminally Ill D.C Residents Legally Ended Their Lives in 2018, Report Says." *Washington Post*, August 2. Accessed August 23, 2019. https://www.washingtonpost.com/local/dc-politics/two-terminally-ill-dc-residents-legally-ended-their-lives-in-2018-report-says/2019/08/02/8e244006-b534-11e9-8f6c-7828e68cb15f_story.html.

Office of the Governor of the State of Hawai'i. 2018. "Governor Signs Our Care, Our Choice Act, Allowing End of Life Choices for Terminally Ill." April 5. Accessed August 23, 2019. https://governor.hawaii.gov/newsroom/latest-news/office-of-the-governor-news-release-governor-signs-our-care-our-choice-act-allowing-end-of-life-choices-for-terminally-ill/.

Oregon Blue Book. 2020. "Initiative, Referendum and Recall." Accessed February 7, 2021. https://sos.oregon.gov/blue-book/Documents/elections/initiative.pdf.

Pazniokas, Mark. 2014. "Malloy Skeptical on Assisted-Suicide Bill." CT Mirror, March 14. Accessed November 1, 2020. https://ctmirror.org/2014/03/14/malloy-skeptical-on-assisted-suicide-bill/.

Pérez-Peña, Richard, and Ian Lovett. 2015. "California Governor Signs Assisted Suicide Bill into Law." *New York Times*, December 21. Accessed February 18, 2019. https://www.nytimes.com/2015/10/06/us/california-governor-signs-assisted-suicide-bill-into-law.html.

Portnoy, Jenna, and Aaron C. Davis. 2017. "House Republicans Promise New Line of Attack on D.C.'s Assisted Suicide Law." *Washington Post*, February 15. Accessed August 23, 2019. https://www.washingtonpost.com/local/dc-politics/house-republicans-promise-new-line-of-attack-on-dcs-assisted-suicide-law/2017/02/15/6ce97dde-f399-11e6-8d72-263470bf0401_story.html?utm_term=.5c9b04f553bb&tid=a_mcntx.

Public Policy Polling. 2012. "Obama Holds Modest Lead in Massachusetts." Accessed August 21, 2019. https://www.publicpolicypolling.com/wp-content/uploads/2017/09/PPP_Release_MA_082212.pdf#page=2.

Ragar, Shaylee. 2019. "Bill Would Criminalize Doctor-Assisted Death." Montana Public Radio, January 29. Accessed August 23, 2019. https://www.mtpr.org/post/bill-would-criminalize-doctor-assisted-death.

Rey, Diane. 2019. "End-of-Life Act Fails in Senate by Tie Vote." *Maryland Reporter*, March 28. Accessed August 23, 2019. https://marylandreporter.com/2019/03/28/end-of-life-option-act-fails-in-senate-by-tie-vote/.

Saad, Lydia. 2011. "Doctor-Assisted Suicide Is Moral Issue Dividing Americans Most." Gallup, May 31. Accessed August 21, 2019. https://news.gallup.com/poll/147842/doctor-assisted-suicide-moral-issue-dividing-americans.aspx.

Senate Bill No. 128. 2015. "End of Life." Accessed December 14, 2018. https://leginfo.legislature.ca.gov/faces/billNavClient.xhtml?bill_id=201520160SB128.

Sherman, Barbara. 2016. "Gov. Roberts Speaks Frankly about Oregon's Death with Dignity Law." Pamplinmedia.com, December 15. Accessed December 14, 2018. https://pamplinmedia.com/rc/64-features/336666-215574-gov-roberts-speaks-frankly-about-oregons-death-with-dignity-law-.

Span, Paula. 2012. "How the 'Death with Dignity' Initiative Failed in Massachusetts." *New York Times*, December 6. Accessed August 21, 2019. https://newoldage.blogs.nytimes.com/2012/12/06/how-the-death-with-dignity-law-died-in-massachusetts/.

Span, Paula. 2019. "Aid in Dying Soon Will Be Available to More Americans. Few Will Choose It." *New York Times*, July 8. Accessed August 23, 2019. https://www.nytimes.com/2019/07/08/health/aid-in-dying-states.html?searchResultPosition=5.

Spellman, John. 2008. "I-1000 Could Remove Personal Choice." SeattlePI, October 21. Accessed August 21, 2019. https://www.seattlepi.com/local/opinion/article/I-1000-could-remove-personal-choice-1288960.php.

State of South Dakota. 2017. "Journal of the Senate." February 7. Accessed November 1, 2020. https://mylrc.sdlegislature.gov/api/Documents/44041.html#page=5.

Terrell, Steve. 2017. "Handful of Senate Dems Help Republicans Defeat Aid-in-Dying Bill." *Santa Fe New Mexican*, March 15. Accessed August 23, 2019. https://www.santafenewmexican.com/news/legislature/handful-of-senate-dems-help-republicans-defeat-aid-in-dying/article_a0976f58-7d70-558a-8234-0a7eed8afcdf.html.

Vacco, Attorney General of New York v. Quill. 1997. 521 U.S. 793. Accessed August 21, 2019. https://caselaw.findlaw.com/us-supreme-court/521/793.html.

Waldman, Tyler. 2019. "Gov. Hogan Vetoes Eight Bills, Allows Dozens of Others to Become Law." WBAL News Radio, May 24. Accessed August 23, 2019. https://www.wbal.com/article/390983/3/gov-hogan-vetoes-eight-bills-allows-dozens-of-others-to-become-law.

"Washington Aid-in-Dying, Initiative 119 (1991)." 1991. Ballotpedia. Accessed December 14, 2018. https://ballotpedia.org/Washington_Aid-in-Dying,_Initiative_119_(1991).

Washington Post. 2019. "Maryland Comes Agonizingly Close to Passing Death-with-Dignity Legislation." March 28. Accessed August 23, 2019. https://www.washingtonpost.com/opinions/maryland-comes-agonizingly-close-to-passing-death-with-dignity-legislation/2019/03/28/f7a5cef2-50bf-11e9-a3f7-78b7525a8d5f_story.html.

Wiering, Maria. 2014. "Larry Hogan Passionate about Job Creation, Welcomes Church Input." Archdiocese of Baltimore, October 8. Accessed August 23, 2019. https://www.archbalt.org/larry-hogan-passionate-about-job-creation-welcomes-church-input/.

Wood, Pamela. 2019a. "Medically Assisted Suicide Bill Advances in Maryland, but with Changes That Frustrate Advocates." *Baltimore Sun*, March 22. Accessed August 23, 2019. https://www.baltimoresun.com/politics/bs-md-medical-suicide-advances-20190322-story.html.

Wood, Pamela. 2019b. "Medically Assisted Suicide Bill Moves Forward in Maryland General Assembly." *Baltimore Sun*, March 1. Accessed August 23, 2019. https://www.baltimoresun.com/politics/bs-md-death-bill-vote-20190301-story.html.

Preexisting Conditions

At a Glance

Prior to the implementation of the Affordable Care Act (ACA) in 2014, most insurers required individuals with preexisting health conditions to fill out detailed questionnaires about past conditions or known risk factors (e.g., cancer, chronic diseases, pregnancy). This process of risk assessment—known as *underwriting*—was commonplace in the individual and small group health insurance markets. Insurers used this information to predict subscribers' use of medical services and to set premiums. Many private insurers declined to offer coverage to individuals with multiple risk factors, excluded coverage for treatment related to preexisting conditions, or charged higher premiums or deductibles to subscribers with known risks (Claxton et al. 2016). Some individuals in high-risk occupations or with unusually expensive conditions (e.g., hepatitis C, HIV/AIDS, lupus) were effectively "uninsurable" because the expected cost of their medical care exceeded what insurers could reasonably charge in premiums. In 2019, an estimated 53.8 million Americans under the age of 65 lived with one or more preexisting conditions that could limit their ability to purchase health insurance in the individual health insurance marketplace. In addition, nearly half (45 percent) of families had at least one nonelderly adult with a "declinable medical condition" (Claxton et al. 2019).

The ACA, commonly known as Obamacare, prohibited the use of underwriting to assess the risk of potential subscribers and required insurers to sell policies to all individuals, regardless of their claims history, gender, or health status. In addition, insurers could no longer impose annual limits or a lifetime cap on covered benefits (Kaiser Family Foundation 2012). These policy changes transformed the market for individual health insurance. By establishing a comprehensive set of "essential health benefits" for all insurers, the ACA effectively ended the practice of excluding preexisting medical conditions or treatments from coverage (Kaiser Family Foundation 2012).

Although the public remains sharply divided about the ACA, a 2019 Kaiser Family Foundation poll indicated that protections for persons with preexisting conditions enjoyed broad bipartisan support. A majority of Democrats (88 percent) and Republicans (62 percent) agreed that it was "very important" to "prohibit private health insurance companies from denying coverage because of a pre-existing medical condition" (Kirzinger, Muñana, and Brodie 2019). A decade after the ACA became law, the question dividing the parties was no longer *whether* to protect patients with preexisting conditions but rather *how* to do so.

Democrats regard the passage of the ACA as a historic milestone in the quest to protect patients with preexisting conditions. They note that before 2010 millions of Americans lived in fear that they would be denied insurance coverage in the individual insurance marketplace. During the first presidential debate in September 2020, former Vice President Joe Biden warned that without the ACA, health insurance coverage for 100 million people would be in jeopardy (Page 2020). As a result, Democrats view the insurance market reforms introduced by the ACA as a matter of basic fairness. Without these protections, millions of vulnerable Americans would suffer from health-based discrimination. Since illness can strike at any time, Democrats believe all Americans benefit from the ACA's insurance market reforms. They see Republican efforts to repeal the ACA—and the Trump administration's support for overturning it in court—as actions that would disproportionately harm the chronically ill, pregnant women, and other patients with underlying risk factors. As Biden pointed out, without the ACA's protections, insurers would be "able to charge women more for the same exact procedure a man gets" (Page 2020). Democrats regard proposals to repeal or weaken the ACA as a step backward that would permit insurers to raise premiums or deny coverage to millions of Americans.

Republicans steadfastly opposed the ACA, which failed to win a single Republican vote in 2010. This hostility toward Obamacare, the passage of which was one of the major triumphs of the Democratic president's two terms in office, has not diminished over time. Republicans condemn the ACA as both an unwarranted intrusion on individual liberty and an unprecedented increase in the size and power of the federal government. Republicans also contend the ACA unnecessarily limits consumer choice by mandating a one-size-fits-all approach to insurance benefit design. In addition, Republicans argue that the ACA's insurance market reforms increased insurance premiums for *all* subscribers. They see the rising cost of health insurance, not discrimination by insurers, as the principal threat to affordable health insurance. Republicans say that they seek to increase competition in the insurance marketplace by encouraging the development of more affordable—and less comprehensive—insurance products. President Donald Trump promised that his America First Healthcare Plan would offer Americans "a better and less expensive plan that will always protect individuals with preexisting conditions" (Trump 2020). Although Republicans defend the need to protect patients with preexisting conditions, they argue that states, not the federal government, should take the lead in crafting solutions.

According to Many Democrats . . .

- The Affordable Care Act (ACA) ensured equitable access to health insurance for all Americans by banning discrimination against patients with preexisting conditions.
- The ACA made health insurance more affordable for patients with chronic diseases and other high-cost medical conditions.
- Insurers must be strictly regulated to protect access to care for vulnerable patients.

According to Many Republicans . . .

- The Affordable Care Act (ACA) should be repealed and replaced; insurance market reforms have increased premiums and limit consumer choice.
- The rising cost of health insurance, not discrimination by insurers, is the principal threat to health care access.
- States need more flexibility to create high-risk pools for vulnerable patients to ensure access to care for patients with preexisting conditions without increasing premiums for all subscribers.

Overview

Government efforts to assist individuals with preexisting health conditions first appeared in the 1970s. Millions of Americans purchased coverage in the individual insurance market, where premiums were based on individuals' likelihood of using medical care, which depended on such factors as age, family medical history, past personal medical history, and health risk behaviors such as smoking. In 1976, Connecticut and Minnesota became the first states to create high-risk pools for individuals who had been denied coverage by insurers in the individual health insurance market. Over the next two decades, two dozen states established similar plans; total plan enrollment in state high-risk pools exceeded 91,000 in 1996 (Pollitz 2017).

That same year, Congress passed the Health Insurance Portability and Accountability Act (HIPAA). The new law included protections for individuals with preexisting protections who were enrolled in employer-based health insurance plans. Under HIPAA, employer-sponsored plans were not allowed to exclude medical conditions from coverage. HIPAA also guaranteed individuals who lost group-based insurance the right to purchase individual health insurance without any exclusions for preexisting conditions. HIPAA also prohibited employers and health insurers from discriminating against employees and their dependents based on their health status or genetic information (American Cancer Society 2020). While HIPAA made it easier for individuals with preexisting conditions to switch health plans or change jobs without losing coverage, it did nothing to address the affordability of insurance coverage. Furthermore, HIPAA's requirements did not apply to subscribers purchasing coverage in the individual market who were not previously covered by a group health insurance plan (American Cancer Society 2020).

After HIPAA passed in 1996, 10 additional states established high-risk pools. Enrollment varied widely. Four states enrolled more than 20,000 subscribers, but relatively few individuals with preexisting conditions were covered through state high-risk pools before 2010. Furthermore, most plans charged significantly higher premiums to subscribers and often excluded coverage of preexisting conditions for up to a year. Nearly all state plans also included a lifetime cap on covered benefits, which significantly impacted subscribers with ongoing, expensive health conditions (Pollitz 2017). State high-risk pools improved access to coverage for some individuals who were previously shut out of the individual health insurance market, but the high cost of premiums and limits on coverage attracted few enrollees. Nationally, total enrollment in state high-risk pools totaled only 226,615 individuals in 2011 (Pollitz 2017).

The passage of the Affordable Care Act (ACA) in 2010 transformed the individual health insurance marketplace. Beginning in 2014, provisions in Obamacare "required insurers to cover high-risk individuals via the 'guaranteed-issue' and 'community-rating' provisions." The guaranteed-issue provision requires insurers to "accept every employer and individual in the State that applies for . . . coverage. . . . The community-rating provision prohibits insurers from charging higher rates to individuals based on age, sex, health status, or other factors" (O'Connor 2018). The ACA also established a new national high-risk pool: the Federal Pre-Existing Condition Insurance Program (PCIP). This program was a stopgap measure until the new health insurance marketplaces, which would offer community-rated plans to individuals without exclusions, were fully operational. PCIP plans were available in all states; 27 states elected to create their own plans, while the federal government operated PCIP plans for the remaining states and the District of Columbia in 2011 (Pollitz 2017). Once the health insurance marketplaces became fully operational in 2014, PCIP enrollment declined rapidly, as most subscribers elected to purchase coverage—typically with advanced premium tax credits—through the annual open enrollment process.

The ACA survived several legal and legislative challenges after President Obama signed it into law in March 2010. Two legal challenges, *National Federation of Independent Business (NFIB) v. Sebelius* (2012) and *King v. Burwell* (2015), made their way to the U.S. Supreme Court. In each case, the justices upheld the ACA in a 5–4 decision, maintaining the law's protections for individuals with preexisting conditions. Over a five-year period (2011–2015), House Republicans passed more than 60 bills to repeal and replace the ACA (Acosta and Holmes 2016). Democrats, however, blocked further action on repeal-and-replace legislation until 2014.

When Republicans regained control of the Senate in the 2014 midterm elections, they held majorities in both houses of Congress for the first time in Obama's presidency. Congress thus quickly passed the Restoring Americans' Health Care Freedom Act (H.R.3762) by a margin of 240–189 in the House and 52–48 in the Senate (House Republicans 2020). The Republican bill—sponsored by Rep. Tom Price (R-GA), who later served as the secretary of Health and Human Services in the Trump administration—sought to repeal the financial underpinnings of the ACA. As a budget reconciliation bill, H.R. 3762 was not subject to a Senate filibuster. President Obama vetoed the bill on January 8, 2016, saving the ACA (and protections for individuals with preexisting conditions) once again.

The election of Donald Trump in 2016 emboldened Republicans to mount a direct assault on the ACA. With control over both the House and the Senate, congressional Republicans expressed confidence that after several years of concerted opposition, they finally had the votes to repeal Obamacare. Their first proposal, the American Health Care Act (AHCA), was introduced by House leadership in March 2017. The AHCA maintained the ACA's consumer protections but allowed insurers to raise premiums by 30 percent for individuals who did not maintain continuous coverage. The nonpartisan Congressional Budget Office (CBO) estimated that up to 26 million Americans would lose insurance coverage under the law (mostly because the AHCA would end Medicaid expansion that had taken place under Obamacare) and that premiums would rise 15–20 percent in the individual health insurance market (Congressional Budget Office 2017a). The AHCA was the most unpopular piece of legislation in decades, with fewer than a third of all voters supporting the bill (Alter and Edwards 2017). After this initial effort failed to win a majority within the House Republican caucus, a revised version that afforded states more flexibility passed the Republican-controlled House by a vote of 217–213 on May 4, 2017 (Mattina 2017).

Advocates for patients living with preexisting conditions dominated the debate over the future of the ACA in the U.S. Senate during the summer of 2017. Self-described "Trach Mommas" from Louisiana and "little lobbyists" representing pediatric patients rallied against proposals "that would allow insurers to impose lifetime caps on benefits, which could make seriously ill patients essentially uninsurable in the private market" (Alter and Edwards 2017). A grassroots movement emerged as tens of thousands of patients living with cancer, diabetes, and various hereditary conditions mobilized to defend the ACA from Republican legislation. Patient advocates staged sit-ins in Senate offices during the summer recess. Activists targeted prominent Republican senators, and nearly protesters in wheelchairs were arrested in a mass demonstration outside of Senate Majority Leader Mitch McConnell's office in June (Alter and Edwards 2017).

Some of the most poignant and powerful lobbying efforts came from "pint-sized petitioners" known as the "little lobbyists." Parents drove their children hundreds of miles to testify before congressional committees. As House Minority Leader

Nancy Pelosi (D-CA) noted, the little lobbyists "have made all the difference in the world. . . . You do not want to stand in between one of these moms and the good health care of her child." As the parent of one child testified, "Without the Affordable Care Act, Charlie would have exceeded her lifetime cap before ever coming home from the hospital and would have been uninsurable" (Pear 2017). Late-night host Jimmy Kimmel also weighed into the debate over the AHCA. In an emotional monologue after the birth of his son Billy, who was diagnosed with a heart murmur. Kimmel declared, "No parent should ever have to decide if they can afford to save their child's life. It just shouldn't happen. Not here" (Adamczyk 2017).

The Republican-led Senate declined to take up the House bill and instead drafted its own version of the legislation: the Better Care Reconciliation Act (BCRA). The Senate bill prohibited waivers of the ACA's protections for patients with preexisting conditions, but the CBO estimated that it would increase the number of people who are uninsured by 22 million in 2026 relative to the number under current law (Congressional Budget Office 2017b). The BCRA struggled from the start, failing to even garner support from a majority of Republican senators. After repeal efforts foundered in the Senate, Sens. Lindsey Graham (R-SC) and Bill Cassidy (R-LA) mounted a last-ditch effort to rally support for a compromise bill. The Graham-Cassidy proposal also fell short, as three Republican senators—Rand Paul (R-KY), John McCain (R-AZ), and Susan Collins (R-ME)—refused to support the bill, thus denying the Republicans a necessary majority for passage (all Democrats voted against the bill). With no path forward, Senate Majority Leader Mitch McConnell pulled the bill on September 26, effectively ending Republican efforts to repeal the ACA in its entirety. In the wake of their defeat, Republicans refocused their efforts on repealing the individual health insurance mandate penalty during the fall of 2017. In the end, McConnell described the failed effort to end Obamacare as "the one disappointment of this Congress from a Republican point of view" (Sullivan 2018).

Democrats used the 2018 midterms as a referendum on health care reform. By 2018, more Americans held a favorable (50 percent) than unfavorable (41 percent) view of the ACA (Kirzinger, Muñana and Brodie 2018). During the summer of 2018, surveys by the Kaiser Family Foundation found that three-quarters of Democrats (74 percent) and nearly half (49 percent) of Republican voters said that a candidate's position on preexisting conditions was either the "most important factor" or a "very important" factor in shaping their voting decision (Kirzinger, Muñana and Brodie 2018). Ironically, then, Republican efforts to repeal and replace Obamacare backfired, as Democrats "focused attention on the law's protections for people with preexisting medical conditions and urged voters to envision the consequences of losing those safeguards" (Sullivan 2018).

This political strategy helped Democrats retake control of the House in the 2018 midterm elections. "Health care was on the ballot, and health care won," said Rep. Nancy Pelosi (D-CA), who reclaimed her position as Speaker after the midterms

(Sullivan 2018). In the wake of the 2018 midterm elections, conservative commentators noted that "Republicans who didn't pay attention to the implications of gutting Obamacare walked into the buzz-saw of pre-existing conditions, which was a very effective issue for Democrats" (Sullivan 2018).

The June 2018 retirement of Justice Anthony Kennedy from the Supreme Court rekindled speculation about the future of the ACA. During the confirmation hearing for now Supreme Court Justice Brett Kavanaugh in 2018, advocates warned that his appointment would jeopardize protections for preexisting conditions. Justin Wise, a 13-year-old boy with an inherited genetic disorder, testified before the Senate Judiciary Committee on behalf of "every American whose life could change tomorrow with a new diagnosis." For these 130 million Americans, Wise warned that "if you destroy protections for pre-existing conditions, you leave me and all kids and adults like me without care and without the ability to afford our care. All because of who we are. We deserve better than that" (Wise 2018). Wise urged the senators to remember that "we must have justices on the Supreme Court who will save the Affordable Care Act, safeguard pre-existing conditions, and protect our care" (Wise 2018).

The passage of the Tax Cuts and Jobs Act (TCJA) in December 2017 set the stage for yet another legal challenge to the ACA. In the Supreme Court's 2012 ruling in *NFIB v. Sebelius*, Chief Justice John Roberts upheld the ACA's individual mandate as an exercise of Congress' taxing power. Failure to comply with the individual mandate, Roberts noted, "triggered a tax" on the uninsured. Once the TCJA reset the penalty to $0 for not purchasing insurance, plaintiffs argued that this rationale ceased to exist, for the ACA no longer raised any revenue for the government—an essential feature of any tax.

In his decision in *Texas v. United States*, Judge Reed O'Connor, a conservative federal district court judge in Texas, wrote that "the individual mandate is no longer fairly readable as an exercise of Congress' Tax Power and continues to be unsustainable under Congress' Interstate Commerce Power. The Court therefore finds the Individual Mandate, unmoored from a tax, is unconstitutional" (O'Connor 2018). For its part, the Trump administration announced that it would no longer defend the ACA's insurance market reforms, such as guaranteed issue or community rating, in court.

The ongoing uncertainty over the future of the ACA led many states to enact stand-alone legislation to protect individuals with preexisting conditions in the event that GOP efforts to torpedo Obamacare ever succeeded. In 2019, 11 states either required insurers to offer coverage to individuals with preexisting conditions or mandated minimum benefits comparable to ACA-compliant health plans. In other states, legislators sought to establish high-risk pools to cover individuals with expensive medical conditions (Armour 2019). In May 2019, the Democratic-controlled House of Representatives also passed the Protecting Americans with Pre-Existing Conditions Act (H.R.986) to "revoke guidance issued by the Trump Administration in October 2018 that encourages states to approve health plans that do not cover preexisting conditions" (Beyer 2019). This bill never received a hearing in the Republican-controlled Senate.

By the summer of 2019, a clear majority of Democrats and Republicans expressed strong support for key provisions of the ACA—including legal protections for people with preexisting medical conditions. A Kaiser Family Foundation health tracking poll in July 2019 found that 88 percent of Democrats and 62 percent of Republicans favored regulations to prohibit "private insurance companies from denying coverage because of a pre-existing medical condition" (Kirzinger, Muñana and Brodie 2019). In addition, a majority of Democrats (76 percent) and Republicans (55 percent) supported rules that prohibited private insurers from "charging sick people higher premiums than healthy people." Prohibitions on insurers' ability to deny coverage to pregnant women or to set dollar limits on coverage for subscribers won strong support from Democrats, but fewer than half of Republicans agreed with these regulations (Kirzinger, Muñana and Brodie 2019). By October 2020, Kaiser tracking polls revealed a sharp partisan divide over whether President Trump had a plan to maintain protections for people with preexisting conditions. Nine out of ten Democrats did "not think President Trump has a plan to maintain protections for people with pre-existing health conditions." In contrast, 85 percent of Republicans believed President Trump "has a plan" to preserve these protections (Kirzinger et al. 2020).

A year after Judge O'Connor's original ruling in *Texas v. United States*, the Fifth Circuit Court of Appeals upheld the district court's finding that the ACA was no longer a constitutional exercise of Congress' tax power (Jost 2019). The future of the ACA's individual insurance market reforms remains uncertain; in March 2020, the U.S. Supreme Court announced that it would hear the latest challenge to the ACA during its 2020–2021 term. The death of Supreme Court Justice Ruth Bader Ginsburg in September 2020 brought the ACA's protections for preexisting conditions to the forefront of the 2020 presidential campaign. Justice Ginsburg had voted to uphold the ACA during each legal challenge over the past decade. The Senate confirmation hearings over the Trump administration's nominee to succeed Ginsburg on the Court, Judge Amy Coney Barrett, focused heavily on the impact of her appointment on the future of the ACA. As Sen. Dianne Feinstein (D-CA), the ranking Democrat on the Senate Judiciary Committee, noted, "The stakes are extraordinarily high for the American people both in the short term and for decades to come. . . . Most importantly, health care coverage for millions of Americans is at stake" (Hughes and Kendall 2020). In October 2020, a Kaiser Family Foundation health tracking poll found strong bipartisan support for maintaining the ACA's preexisting condition protections. A majority of Democrats (91 percent) and Republicans (66 percent) opposed a Supreme Court decision that would "overturn the ACA's protections for people with pre-existing conditions" (Kirzinger et al. 2020). Support for these protections had increased significantly since 2019.

Democrats on Preexisting Conditions

For Democrats, the passage of the Affordable Care Act (ACA) was a watershed moment in health care reform. As Rep. Donna Shalala (D-FL) wrote, "The ACA was a leap, not just a step, toward a better healthcare system for all Americans" (Shalala 2019). Democrats' support for patients living with preexisting conditions reflected the party's long-standing commitment to improving access to health care for all Americans. In this view, the ACA's insurance market reforms ended decades of discrimination against vulnerable patients.

Not surprisingly, then, Democrats characterize Republican efforts to limit or repeal Obamacare as misguided, callous, and driven by partisan hostility toward President Obama and his eight years in the White House. Rep. Ann Kuster (D-NH) declared that "the Trump Administration continues to try to undermine the Affordable Care Act and take us back to a time when Americans could be charged more or denied coverage because of their medical history" (Kuster 2019). At a hearing in October 2019, Kuster noted that "before the Affordable Care Act, Americans could be denied their health insurance coverage if they had any kind of a preexisting condition. I think about it in my family, I'll just start at the beginning of the alphabet—asthma, allergies, Alzheimer's, cancer, diabetes, the list goes on and on. And in fact, over 50% of Americans have a deniable condition" (Kuster 2019).

Democrats view Republican efforts to repeal and replace the ACA as a threat to health equity. As House Ways and Means chair Rep. Richard Neal (D-MA) observed, "The ACA's impact is undeniable—an end to discrimination against people with pre-existing conditions, the removal of barriers to preventative services, and 20 million more Americans with insurance" (Ways and Means Committee 2019). During the vice presidential debate in October 2020, Sen. Kamala Harris argued that President Donald Trump "is in court right now . . . trying to get rid of the Affordable Care Act, which means that you will lose protections, if you have pre-existing conditions" (*USA Today* 2020). Harris left viewers with no doubt about the health consequences of the 2020 presidential election. She warned, "If you have a pre-existing condition, heart disease, diabetes, breast cancer, they're coming for you. If you love someone who has a pre-existing condition—they're coming for you" (*USA Today* 2020).

Democrats have also characterized Republican efforts to challenge the ACA in court as a matter of life or death for patients with preexisting conditions. Without the ACA's protections, patients' ability to purchase affordable insurance coverage would vary from state to state. As the nation grappled with the coronavirus pandemic in March 2020, for example, House Speaker Nancy Pelosi (D-CA) declared, "The Affordable Care Act is an essential pillar of health and financial security for American families, and its protections are even more critical during a dangerous epidemic. But even in the middle of the coronavirus crisis, the Trump Administration continues to ask the court to destroy protections for people with pre-existing

Maintaining Critical Health Care Protections

In October 2019, Sen. Kyrsten Sinema (D-AZ) took to the Senate floor to highlight the experiences of Arizonans with preexisting conditions. Sinema urged her colleagues to defend the "critical health care protections" included in the Affordable Care Act.

> Not long ago, insurance companies were allowed to deny care, or overcharge Americans based on the fact that those Americans had been sick before or had been born with a chronic condition. Arizonans who had previously been treated for skin cancer or diabetes were told that no insurance company would cover them, or that the insurance plans they'd purchased would not cover their pre-existing condition, despite promises of comprehensive coverage. Beyond major illnesses, even Arizonans with common conditions like high blood pressure, high cholesterol, asthma, and even acne, were denied the coverage they needed.
>
> Until recently, insurance companies had also been allowed to charge consumers high prices for insurance plans, only to leave out coverage for essential health benefits that virtually all Americans eventually need, like prescription drug costs, ambulance costs, and hospital stays—critical needs that consumers rightly expect will be covered. Insurance is supposed to be there when people need it. Hardworking Americans who play by the rules and pay their monthly premiums shouldn't have the rug pulled out from under them at the very moment they need health care. That's why such discrimination against people with pre-existing health conditions is now banned, and why health insurance plans are now required to cover essential health benefits. And that's why it is so disturbing that the administration and some members of Congress have begun moving backwards, allowing insurance companies to again sell plans to Americans that lack the very health protections consumers need.

Source

Sinema, Kyrsten. 2019. "Sinema Speaks on Senate Floor Defending Arizonans' Critical Health Care Protections." October 19, 2019. Accessed March 8, 2021. https://www.sinema.senate.gov/sinema-speaks-senate-floor-defending-arizonans-critical-health-care-protections.

conditions and tear away health coverage from tens of millions of Americans" (Pelosi 2020b). In September 2020, Sen. Chuck Schumer (D-NY) announced his opposition to the nomination of Judge Amy Coney Barrett to the U.S. Supreme Court, warning colleagues that "a vote by any Senator for Judge Amy Coney Barrett is a vote to strike down the Affordable Care Act and eliminate protections for millions of Americans with pre-existing conditions. By nominating Judge Amy Coney Barrett to the Supreme Court, President Trump has once again put Americans' healthcare in the crosshairs" (Schumer 2020).

Democrats argue that without the ACA, millions of Americans living with pre-existing conditions would no longer have access to affordable health insurance and, by extension, to health care. During the debate over repealing the ACA in 2017, Pelosi (D-CA) charged that the "Republican plan to gut essential health benefits and protections for pre-existing conditions make it impossible for millions of Americans to afford the health coverage they desperately need. This is deadly" (Pelosi 2017). Democrats continued to reinforce their support for protecting individuals with preexisting conditions before the midterm elections in 2018 and on the presidential campaign trail in 2020. Rep. Nancy Pelosi declared, "House Republicans' assault on protections for Americans with pre-existing conditions was one of the . . . cruelest parts of their Trumpcare legislation. In every district across America, families spoke out with the stories of their loved ones, frightened and angry that the GOP would try to make health coverage completely unaffordable for those in the most need of it" (Pelosi 2018). One year later, during his unsuccessful quest for the Democratic presidential nomination, Sen. Bernie Sanders (D-VT) declared, "Trump has an idea on health care . . . if you have cancer, you have heart disease, you have diabetes. If Trump gets his way the cost of health insurance for you will be so high that many people literally will not be able to afford it. Thousands of people will literally die. That's Trump's health insurance plan" (Sanders 2019). When the Trump administration announced that it would not defend the ACA in court against legal challenges brought primarily by conservative lawmakers, officials, and organizations, Rep. Jim McGovern (D-MA) charged that, in doing so, "the Trump Administration doubled down on their efforts to take insurance coverage away from millions of Americans and roll back protections for those with pre-existing conditions like cancer, asthma, and diabetes" (McGovern 2019).

Democrats argue that without strict regulation, insurers would quickly revert to the same discriminatory practices they employed before the passage of the ACA in 2010. As 2020 presidential nominee Joe Biden declared, "Because of Obamacare, over 100 million people no longer have to worry that an insurance company will deny coverage or charge higher premiums just because they have a pre-existing condition—whether cancer or diabetes or heart disease or a mental health challenge. Insurance companies can no longer set annual or lifetime limits on coverage" (Biden for President 2020).

As a result, Democrats believe that regulations such as guaranteed issue and prohibitions on coverage limits by insurers must be defended to protect access to care for vulnerable patients. As Rep. Donna Shalala (D-FL) recalled, "Before Jan. 1, 2014, when the bulk of the ACA went into effect, Americans were completely at the mercy of an inequitable and unfair healthcare system: Insurers could place lifetime limits on covering essential benefits; drop your coverage if you got sick; or simply deny you coverage for 'pre-existing' conditions. The ACA not only removed these outrageous barriers to getting health insurance, it gave all Americans, irrespective of provider, access to better quality and more affordable health insurance" (Shalala 2019).

Because patients with preexisting conditions represent a financial burden for insurers, Democrats warn that repealing the ACA will place patients at risk.

Speaking on the 10th anniversary of President Barack Obama signing the ACA into law, Rep. Nancy Pelosi (D-CA) warned that "if President Trump succeeds in striking down the ACA in court, gone is the ban on insurers putting limits on your health care, gone are guaranteed essential health benefits and free preventive services . . . and gone are the lifesaving protections for more than 130 million Americans with pre-existing conditions" (Pelosi 2020a).

Republicans on Preexisting Conditions

Republicans in Congress have professed strong support for patients living with preexisting conditions throughout the debate over repealing and replacing the Affordable Care Act (ACA). As Sen. John Kennedy (R-LA) declared, "I don't know a single person, Republican or Democrat, who thinks we shouldn't cover pre-existing conditions" (Tillis 2019). Sen. John Barrasso (R-WY) concurred, noting that "as a doctor and the husband of a breast cancer survivor, I know firsthand how important it is to make sure that patients with pre-existing conditions have the ability to get the care they need" (Tillis 2019). Republicans, however, regarded the ACA's insurance market reforms as a heavy-handed approach in protecting vulnerable patients. Furthermore, the ACA, in this view, was not necessary to protect vulnerable patients. Senate Majority Leader Mitch McConnell (R-KY) insisted that "there is nobody in the Senate not in favor of covering pre-existing conditions. And if [the ACA] were . . . to go away, we would act quickly on a bipartisan basis to restore it" (Hohmann 2019). Rep. Don Bacon (R-NE) agreed, arguing that "you've got to have a framework for pre-existing conditions. You can't just wipe everything away and have nothing there" (Armour and Peterson 2019).

Instead of the ACA's sweeping regulation of the individual insurance market, Republicans have favored freestanding legislation to guarantee protections for patients with preexisting conditions. In 2019, Republican senators introduced the Protect Act (S.1125), a bill to amend HIPAA to guarantee the availability of health insurance coverage regardless of preexisting conditions. In his 2020 State of the Union address, President Donald Trump reaffirmed his support for individuals living with preexisting conditions and declared that "I've also made an ironclad pledge to American families: We will always protect patients with pre-existing conditions" (Palmer 2020).

Republicans viewed the ACA as an unjustified and unaffordable example of governmental overreach. "Instead of imposing arrogant and paternalistic mandates," House Speaker Paul Ryan (R-WI) argued that Republicans wanted to replace the ACA with legislation that "would increase choice and competition, creating a vibrant market where every American will have access to quality, affordable coverage" (Ryan 2017). Even though Republicans failed to repeal the ACA in 2017, they remained staunchly opposed to its insurance mandates. Speaking in 2019, Sen. Thom Tillis (R-NC) declared, "The one-size-fits-all approach being pushed by Democrats is a government takeover of our health care system" (Tillis 2019). After the passage of the Tax Cuts and Jobs Act (TCJA) in 2017, 20 states mounted a new legal challenge to the ACA in the case of *Texas v. United States*. While the Trump administration refused to defend the ACA in court, President Trump argued that essential protections for patients would remain intact because Texas and other states "want to put [in] something that's much better. . . . And they've all pledged that pre-existing conditions, [will be] 100 percent taken care of" (Zeballos-Roig 2020). Facing criticism that his administration's support for a lawsuit challenging

Repealing the ACA Offers Hope for the American Health Care System

On May 10, 2017, Rep. Phil Roe (R-TN) hailed the passage of H.R. 1628, the American Health Care Act (AHCA), which sought to repeal and replace the Affordable Care Act. Roe reassured his constituents that Americans with preexisting conditions would be protected from health-based discrimination.

I've been opposed to Obamacare from the start, in large part because as a doctor, I've seen first-hand what happens when you take power out of the hands of patients and their doctors and centralize it in the hands of government bureaucrats. . . . One thing I've heard consistently since this debate started is how much people are concerned about losing their health insurance due to a pre-existing condition. There's no doubt about it: the last thing you want to be doing when your loved one is sick or dying is worrying about whether you are covered. As a doctor, I can't tell you how frustrating it is to have to jump through all the bureaucratic hurdles to get life-saving care approved. I want to protect people with pre-existing conditions—but we believe there is a better way to achieve these protections without driving up the cost of health insurance and making coverage unaffordable for millions of Americans.

That's why I'm proud to say, despite a great deal of misinformation being circulated, the AHCA continues strong protections for people with pre-existing conditions. The AHCA requires insurers to cover individuals regardless of their health status, while also prohibiting insurers from charging higher premiums because of one's illness. Individuals who maintain health insurance will be protected by a "community rating" that prohibits charging higher premiums, and individuals who don't maintain continuous coverage will have to pay a 30 percent surcharge—instead of taxing you on the front end if you fail to purchase government-approved coverage. We also added an amendment to give states the flexibility to experiment with better plan designs that can lower premiums, stabilize the insurance market or improve conditions for people with pre-existing conditions.

Source

Roe, Phil. 2017. "Hope for the American Health Care System." Press Release, May 10, 2017. Accessed March 8, 2021. https://www.legistorm.com/stormfeed/view_rss/1090599/member/981.html.https://roe.house.gov/news/documentsingle.aspx?DocumentID=398163.

the constitutionality of the ACA would place millions of Americans at risk, in September 2020, President Trump issued an executive order "to affirm it is the official policy of the United States government to protect patients with preexisting conditions. So we're making that official. . . . Democrats like to constantly talk about it, and yet preexisting conditions are much safer with us than they are with them. And now we have it affirmed. This is affirmed, signed, and done so we can put that to rest" (Trump 2020). Congress, however, has yet to pass legislation guaranteeing protections for individuals with preexisting conditions in the event that the Supreme Court finds the ACA to be unconstitutional.

Republicans contend that the rising cost of health insurance, not discrimination by insurers, is the principal shortcoming in the individual health insurance marketplace. As Sen. Bill Cassidy (R-LA) declared in 2017, "We are going to protect those with pre-existing conditions, but we will do it by lowering premiums and not by giving crumby coverage, but rather by having adequate coverage" (Cassidy 2017a). In short, Republicans believe that increased competition will lower prices and increase the availability of affordable insurance options for consumers. Former Rep. Tom Price, who served as the secretary of Health and Human Services in the Trump administration, argued that "under ObamaCare, insurers are either running for the exit doors or proposing huge premium increases. Americans instead deserve a market where companies clamor to offer competitive plans to as many customers as possible" (Price 2017). Sen. Bill Cassidy (R-LA) added, "The greatest barrier to coverage for pre-existing conditions under Obamacare is unaffordable health insurance and too high deductibles" (Tillis 2019).

Republicans noted that rising costs affected all Americans, not just individuals with preexisting conditions, and portrayed the ACA's insurance market reforms as a cure worse than the disease itself. "The insurance packages being offered to most Americans are so expensive that they can't afford them," asserted Sen. Sonny Perdue (R-GA). "Premiums and deductibles have skyrocketed and priced people out of the market. . . . If you can't actually afford insurance, you're not protected from anything" (Tillis 2019).

Furthermore, Republicans disputed Democratic claims that tens of millions of Americans faced health-based discrimination. While millions of Americans lived with preexisting conditions, Republicans pointed out that most were covered by employer-sponsored plans. As a result, Republicans dismissed Democratic claims that millions of Americans would lose coverage if the ACA was repealed as a shameless scare tactic. As the *Wall Street Journal* (2017) editorialized, "Liberals are inflating the pre-existing conditions panic with images of patients pushed out to sea on ice floes, but the GOP plan will ensure everyone can get the care they need." During the first presidential debate in 2020, President Donald Trump dismissed former Vice President Joe Biden's warning that 100 million Americans with preexisting conditions would be at risk without the protections conferred by the ACA. "There aren't 100 million people with pre-existing conditions," Trump declared.

"Joe, the hundred million people is totally wrong. I don't know where you got that number" (Page 2020).

Republicans emphasized the need for state flexibility in crafting policy solutions. Republicans touted a familiar policy tool—state high-risk insurance pools—as the best way to provide "uninsurable" individuals access to coverage. As House Speaker Paul Ryan (R-WI) recalled, "For decades, many states successfully served high-risk populations by segmenting them from the market into 'risk pools' and directly subsidizing their coverage. This gave the most vulnerable Americans access to affordable coverage and stabilized markets, but without requiring higher premiums on healthier individuals to offset the costs" (Ryan 2017). Critics of the ACA noted that "forcing insurance companies to accept all applicants and offer the same premiums regardless of health status would be a good deal for people with costly conditions and a bad deal for everyone else" (Manning 2018). By removing individuals with preexisting conditions from the insurance risk pool, Republicans argued that premiums would fall for most subscribers and that more insurers would enter the individual insurance marketplace. As Sen. Ron Johnson (R-WI) noted, "Returning more health care decisions to the states and ensuring equal treatment for states like Wisconsin that spend taxpayer dollars wisely will allow local leaders to tailor their health care system to the needs of its citizens while maintaining protections for those with high-cost and pre-existing conditions" (Cassidy 2017b). The result, Republicans argued, would be lower premiums for most families as insurers were unshackled from the ACA's minimum essential coverage standards and insurance market reforms such as guaranteed issue requirements.

Robert B. Hackey and Shannon Rowe

Further Reading

Acosta, Jim, and Karen Holmes. 2016. "Obama Vetoes Obamacare Repeal Bill." CNN, January 8. Accessed April 15, 2020. https://www.cnn.com/2016/01/08/politics/obama-vetoes-obamacare-repeal-bill/index.html.

Adamczyk, Alicia. 2017. "Jimmy Kimmel Tearfully Explains Why It's Wrong to Deny Health Coverage for Pre-Existing Conditions." Money, May 2. Accessed February 7, 2021. https://money.com/jimmy-kimmel-baby-obamacare/.

Alter, Charlotte, and Haley Sweetland Edwards. 2017. "The United Patients of America." *Time*, July 13. Accessed April 20, 2020. https://time.com/4856231/the-united-patients-of-america/.

American Cancer Society. 2020. "HIPAA (The Health Insurance Portability and Accountability Act of 1996)." Accessed March 23, 2020. https://www.cancer.org/treatment/finding-and-paying-for-treatment/understanding-health-insurance/health-insurance-laws/what-is-hipaa.html.

Armour, Stephanie. 2019. "As Court Case Imperils Affordable Care Act, Some States Prepare Contingency Plans." *Wall Street Journal*, October 21. Accessed March 11, 2020. https://www.wsj.com/articles/as-court-case-imperils-affordable-care-act-some-states-prepare-contingency-plans-11571650207.

Armour, Stephanie, and Kristina Peterson. 2019. "Trump Administration Renews Attempt to Topple Affordable Care Act." *Wall Street Journal*, March 26. Accessed March 8, 2021. https://www.wsj.com/articles/trump-administration-renews-attempt-to-topple-affordable-care-act-11553634899.

Beyer, Don. 2019. "House Passes Bill to Protect Individuals with Preexisting Conditions, Pushback against President Trump's Sabotage of the ACA." May 10. Accessed April 13, 2020. https://beyer.house.gov/news/documentsingle.aspx?DocumentID=4327.

Biden for President. 2020. "Health Care." Accessed March 8, 2020. https://joebiden.com/healthcare.

Cassidy, Bill. 2017a. "ICYMI: Cassidy Explains #KimmelTest." Accessed March 11, 2020. https://www.cassidy.senate.gov/newsroom/press-releases/icymi-cassidy-explains-kimmeltest.

Cassidy, Bill. 2017b. "Senators Introduce Graham-Cassidy-Heller-Johnson." September 13. Accessed March 11, 2020. https://www.cassidy.senate.gov/newsroom/press-releases/senators-introduce-graham-cassidy-heller-johnson.

Claxton, Gary, Cynthia Cox, Anthony Damico, Larry Levitt, and Karen Pollitz. 2016. "Pre-Existing Conditions and Medical Underwriting in the Individual Insurance Market Prior to the ACA." Kaiser Family Foundation, December 12. Accessed March 22, 2020. www.kff.org/health-reform/issue-brief/pre-existing-conditions-and-medical-underwriting-in-the-individual-insurance-market-prior-to-the-aca/.

Claxton, Gary, Cynthia Cox, Anthony Damico, Larry Levitt, and Karen Pollitz. 2019. "Pre-Existing Condition Prevalence for Individuals and Families." Kaiser Family Foundation, October 4. Accessed March 26, 2020. https://www.kff.org/health-reform/issue-brief/pre-existing-condition-prevalence-for-individuals-and-families/.

Congressional Budget Office. 2017a. "American Health Care Act." March 13. Accessed April 15, 2020. https://www.cbo.gov/publication/52486.

Congressional Budget Office. 2017b. "Better Care Reconciliation Act." July 20. Accessed October 14, 2020. https://www.cbo.gov/publication/52941.

Demko, Paul, and Adam Cancryn. 2018. "Trump's Losing Fight against Obamacare." Politico, August 1. Accessed March 8, 2020. https://www.politico.com/story/2018/08/01/trump-obamacare-health-insurance-719300.

Hamel, Liz, Ashley Kirzinger, Cailey Muñana, and Mollyann Brodie. 2020. "5 Charts about Public Opinion on the Affordable Care Act and the Supreme Court." Kaiser Family Foundation, September 22. Accessed October 14, 2020. https://www.kff.org/health-reform/poll-finding/5-charts-about-public-opinion-on-the-affordable-care-act-and-the-supreme-court/.

Hohmann, James. 2019. "Trump Might Win a Pyrrhic Victory against Obamacare, as the Balance of Judicial Power Shifts His Way." *Washington Post*, July 10. Accessed March 8, 2020. https://www.washingtonpost.com/news/powerpost/paloma/daily-202/2019/07/10/daily-202-trump-might-win-a-pyrrhic-victory-against-obamacare-as-the-balance-of-judicial-power-shifts-his-way/5d24bf7e1ad2e552a21d5326/.

House Republicans. 2020. "H.R. 3762, Restoring Americans' Healthcare Freedom Reconciliation Act (Veto Override)." Accessed April 15, 2020. https://www.gop.gov/bill/h-r-3762-restoring-americans-healthcare-freedom-reconciliation-act-veto-override/.

Hughes, Siobhan, and Brett Kendall. 2020. "Republicans, Democrats Clash at Confirmation Hearing for Amy Coney Barrett." *Wall Street Journal*, October 12. Accessed October 14, 2020. https://www.wsj.com/articles/politics-dominates-as-amy-coney-barretts-confirmation-hearings-begin-in-senate-11602495000.

Jost, Timothy. 2019. "Fifth Circuit Sends Affordable Care Act Case Back to the District Court, Prolonging Uncertainty." Commonwealth Fund, December 19. Accessed April 15, 2020. https://www.commonwealthfund.org/blog/2019/fifth-circuit-sends-affordable-care-act-case-back-to-district-court.

Kaiser Family Foundation. 2012. "Summary of Coverage Provisions in the Patient Protection and Affordable Care Act." Accessed March 10, 2020. https://www.kff.org/health-costs/issue-brief/summary-of-coverage-provisions-in-the-patient/.

Kendall, Brent. 2020. "Amy Coney Barrett Faces Lawmakers' Questions." *Wall Street Journal*, October 13. Accessed October 14, 2020. https://www.wsj.com/articles/amy-coney-barrett-to-face-lawmakers-questions-11602581406.

Kirzinger, Ashley, Lunna Lopes, Audrey Kearney, and Mollyann Brodie. 2020. "KFF Health Tracking Poll—October 2020: The Future of the ACA and Biden's Advantage on Health Care." Kaiser Family Foundation, October 16. Accessed October 16, 2020. https://www.kff.org/health-reform/report/kff-health-tracking-poll-october-2020/.

Kirzinger, Ashley, Cailey Muñana, and Mollyann Brodie. 2018. "Kaiser Health Tracking Poll—July 2018." Kaiser Family Foundation, July 25. Accessed March 22, 2020. https://www.kff.org/health-reform/poll-finding/kaiser-health-tracking-poll-july-2018-changes-to-the-affordable-care-act-health-care-in-the-2018-midterms-and-the-supreme-court/.

Kirzinger, Ashley, Cailey Muñana, and Mollyann Brodie. 2019. "KFF Health Tracking Poll—July 2019: The Future of the ACA and Possible Changes to the Current System, Preview of Priorities Heading into 2nd Democratic Debate." Kaiser Family Foundation, July 30. Accessed October 16, 2020. https://www.kff.org/health-reform/poll-finding/kff-health-tracking-poll-july-2019/.

Kuster, Ann. 2019. "In Hearing, Kuster Holds Trump Administration Official Accountable for Efforts to Sabotage Access to Health Care." October 23. Accessed April 13, 2020. https://kuster.house.gov/media-center/press-releases/in-hearing-kuster-holds-trump-administration-official-accountable-for.

Manning, Hadley. 2018. "Republicans Shouldn't Embrace ACA Rules about Pre-Existing Conditions." The Hill, November 27. Accessed March 8, 2021. https://thehill.com/opinion/healthcare/418449-republicans-shouldnt-embrace-aca-rules-about-pre-existing-conditions.

Mattina, Christina. 2017. "Infographic: Update—A Brief History of ACA Repeal and Replace Efforts." *American Journal of Managed Care*, September 27. Accessed March 22, 2020. https://www.ajmc.com/newsroom/infographic-update-a-brief-history-of-aca-repeal-and-replace-efforts.

McGovern, Jim. 2019. "Statement on the Trump Administration's Latest Attempt to Undermine the Affordable Care Act." March 26. Accessed April 3, 2020. https://mcgovern.house.gov/news/documentsingle.aspx?DocumentID=398326.

O'Connor, Reed. 2018. "Memorandum Opinion and Order—*Texas, et al. v. United States of America, et al.*" Civil Action No. 4:18-cv-00167-O. December 18. Accessed March 31, 2020. https://assets.documentcloud.org/documents/5629711/Texas-v-US-Partial-Summary-Judgment.pdf.

Page, Susan. 2020. "Read the Full Transcript of Vice Presidential Debate between Mike Pence and Kamala Harris." *USA Today*, October 8. Accessed October 13, 2020. https://www.usatoday.com/story/news/politics/elections/2020/10/08/vice-presidential-debate-full-transcript-mike-pence-and-kamala-harris/5920773002/.

Palmer, Ewan. 2020. "Trump Accused by People with Pre-Existing Conditions of Lying about Protecting Them during State of the Union Address." *Newsweek*, February 5.

Accessed April 13, 2020. https://www.newsweek.com/trump-state-union-obamacare-exisitng-conditions-1485804.

Pear, Robert. 2017. "'Little Lobbyists' Help Save the Health Care Law, for Now." *New York Times*, September 30. Accessed April 3, 2020. https://www.nytimes.com/2017/09/30/us/politics/little-lobbyists-obamacare.html.

Pelosi, Nancy. 2017. "Pelosi Remarks at Press Conference on GOP Attacks on Pre-Existing Condition Protections in Trumpcare." May 3. Accessed March 21, 2020. https://pelosi.house.gov/news/press-releases/pelosi-remarks-at-press-conference-on-gop-attacks-on-pre-existing-condition.

Pelosi, Nancy. 2018. "Pelosi Remarks at Press Conference Announcing Letters to Trump Administration Demanding Documents on New Attack on Pre-Existing Conditions Protections." June 13. Accessed March 22, 2020. https://pelosi.house.gov/news/press-releases/pelosi-remarks-at-press-conference-announcing-letters-to-trump-administration.

Pelosi, Nancy. 2020a. "Pelosi Remarks on 10th Anniversary of Affordable Care Act & Unveiling of Take Responsibility for Workers and Families Act." March 23. Accessed April 13, 2020. https://pelosi.house.gov/news/press-releases/pelosi-remarks-on-10th-anniversary-of-affordable-care-act-unveiling-of-take.

Pelosi, Nancy. 2020b. "Pelosi Statement on Supreme Court Decision to Hear ACA Lawsuit." March 2. Accessed April 13, 2020. https://www.speaker.gov/newsroom/3220.

Pollitz, Karen. 2017. "High Risk Pools for Uninsurable Individuals." Kaiser Family Foundation, February 22. Accessed April 20, 2020. https://www.kff.org/health-reform/issue-brief/high-risk-pools-for-uninsurable-individuals/.

Price, Thomas. 2017. "ObamaCare's Victims Need Relief Now." *Wall Street Journal*, June 28: A17.

Ryan, Paul. 2017. "Keeping Our Promise to Repeal ObamaCare." *Wall Street Journal*, March 22. Accessed March 8, 2020. https://www.wsj.com/articles/keeping-our-promise-to-repeal-obamacare-1490222397.

Sanders, Bernie. 2019. "Transcript: Sen. Bernie Sanders on 'Face the Nation.'" CBS News, March 31. Accessed March 23, 2020. https://www.cbsnews.com/news/transcript-sen-bernie-sanders-on-face-the-nation-march-31-2019/.

Schumer, Chuck. 2020. "A Vote for Judge Amy Coney Barrett Is a Vote to Eliminate Health Care for Millions in the Middle of a Pandemic." Senate Democrats, September 26. Accessed October 14, 2020. https://www.democrats.senate.gov/newsroom/press-releases/schumer-a-vote-for-judge-amy-coney-barrett-is-a-vote-to-eliminate-health-care-for-millions-in-the-middle-of-a-pandemic.

Shalala, Donna. 2019. "My Fight Continues to Save the Affordable Care Act for Miamians." *Miami Herald*, October 10. Accessed April 13, 2020. https://www.miamiherald.com/opinion/op-ed/article236015948.html.

Sullivan, Sean. 2018. "Republicans Abandon the Fight to Repeal and Replace Obama's Health Care Law." *Washington Post*, November 7. Accessed March 23, 2020. https://www.washingtonpost.com/powerpost/republicans-abandon-the-fight-to-repeal-and-replace-obamas-health-care-law/2018/11/07/157d052c-e2d8-11e8-ab2c-b31dcd53ca6b_story.html.

Tillis, Thom. 2019. "Senators Introduce the Protect Act to Ensure Protections and Affordable Coverage for Americans with Pre-Existing Conditions." April 10. Accessed March 8, 2020. https://www.tillis.senate.gov/2019/4/senators-introduce-the-protect-act-to-ensure-protections-and-affordable-coverage-for-americans-with-pre-existing-conditions.

Trump, Donald J. 2020. "Remarks by President Trump on the America First Healthcare Plan." September 24. Accessed March 8, 2021. https://trumpwhitehouse.archives.gov/briefings-statements/remarks-president-trump-america-first-healthcare-plan/.

U.S. Department of Justice. 2019. "Memo re: RE: *Texas v. United States*, No. 19-10011 (5th Cir.)." March 25. Accessed March 8, 2021. https://theincidentaleconomist.com/wordpress/wp-content/uploads/2019/03/letter-from-DOJ.pdf.

U.S. House of Representatives, Ways and Means Committee. 2019. "House Democrats Unveil Legislation to Strengthen Protections for Pre-Existing Conditions and Lower Health Care Costs." Press Release, March 26. Accessed March 8, 2021. https://waysandmeans.house.gov/media-center/press-releases/house-democrats-unveil-legislation-strengthen-protections-pre-existing.

USA Today. 2020. "Read the Full Transcript from the First Presidential Debate between Joe Biden and Donald Trump." September 30. Accessed October 13, 2020. https://www.usatoday.com/story/news/politics/elections/2020/09/30/presidential-debate-read-full-transcript-first-debate/3587462001/.

Wall Street Journal. 2017. "Pre-Existing Confusion." May 1. Accessed March 8, 2020. https://www.wsj.com/articles/pre-existing-confusion-1493680248.

Wise, Justin. 2018. "13-Year-Old with Genetic Condition Defends ObamaCare in Kavanaugh Hearings." The Hill, September 7. https://thehill.com/blogs/blog-briefing-room/news/405654-13-year-old-with-pre-existing-conditions-testifies-against.

Zeballos-Roig, Joseph. 2020. "Trump Was Asked How He Would Protect Health Coverage for Pre-Existing Conditions if Obamacare Was Wiped Out. Here's His Full Answer." Business Insider, March 20. Accessed March 11, 2020. https://markets.businessinsider.com/news/stocks/trumps-protecting-pre-existing-conditions-full-answer-if-obamacare-undone-2020-3-1028974204.

Short-Term, Limited-Duration Health Insurance

At a Glance

Short-term, limited-duration insurance (STLDI) policies offer inexpensive health insurance for individuals who experience a temporary gap in coverage. These plans traditionally provided coverage for less than a year and did not meet the minimum essential coverage (MEC) requirements established by the Affordable Care Act (ACA). The ACA sought to limit the availability of noncompliant health plans that did not cover essential health benefits such as maternity care, mental health, prescription drugs, and prevention and wellness services. In 2016, the Obama administration issued new regulations limiting the maximum term of short-term health insurance plans to 90 days and banned the guaranteed renewal of such policies.

In 2017, however, President Donald Trump issued an executive order directing the secretary of Health and Human Services to expand the availability of STLDI policies. In October 2018, the Departments of the Treasury, Labor, and Health and Human Services published final regulations overturning the Obama administration's actions. The new regulations restored the maximum coverage term for STLDI plans to 12 months and permitted individuals to renew their policies for up to three years. Demand for short-term, limited-duration plans increased substantially after President Trump signed the Tax Cuts and Jobs Act (TCJA; Pub. L. 115-97) in December 2017. This law eliminated the requirement that individuals pay a tax penalty if they could not demonstrate proof of minimum essential coverage. Although the government does not maintain data on enrollment in STLDI plans as it does for individual plans purchased through the health insurance marketplaces, a 2020 congressional report found that sales of short-term plans increased by 600,000 individuals from the 2018 to 2019 plan year (U.S. House of Representatives, Committee on Energy and Commerce 2020).

Democrats strongly oppose efforts to increase the availability of STLDI plans. Because short-term, limited-duration plans do not have to meet MEC requirements that cover prescription drugs, maternity care, or mental health care, Democrats deride these plans as "junk insurance." In addition, Democrats warn that expanding the availability of such plans will leave Americans with preexisting conditions with inadequate coverage. For example, some plans may charge high-risk patients with chronic conditions higher premiums or deny them coverage outright. For Democrats, ensuring all Americans have access to qualified health plans may be more expensive, but it is a cost well worth paying. Democrats favor policies to limit, or eliminate, the availability of STLDI plans to maintain the stability of the individual health insurance market.

Republicans, on the other hand, argue that STLDI plans offer an affordable option for individuals who cannot afford the high premiums of Obamacare marketplace plans and who do not have access to affordable employer-based coverage. Republicans regard regulations that limit the sale of STLDI plans as unwarranted interference in the marketplace, and they say that federal and state regulation of these plans restricts consumer choice by forcing consumers to purchase more comprehensive, and expensive, coverage than they want or need. Republicans argue that the ACA forced Americans to decide between choosing unaffordable insurance or being uninsured. They believe that expanding the availability of STLDI policies provides more affordable health insurance choices for consumers.

According to Many Democrats . . .

- Short-term limited-duration insurance (STLDI) plans offer "junk insurance" that fails to cover many essential health benefits.
- STLDI plans encourage many young and healthy individuals to opt out of more comprehensive coverage, weakening the risk pool in the individual health insurance market.
- Individuals who opt for STLDI plans face higher out-of-pocket costs.
- Government needs to establish rules to protect consumers in the health insurance marketplace.

According to Many Republicans . . .

- Short-term, limited-duration (STLDI) insurance provides an affordable alternative to Obamacare marketplace plans for individuals who do not qualify for federal subsidies.
- Young and healthy individuals should not have to purchase more expensive coverage to subsidize the care of older and sicker subscribers.
- STLDI plans allow individuals to tailor coverage to their health care needs.
- The federal government should promote competition in health insurance markets and empower consumers.

Overview

Short-term, limited-duration insurance (STLDI) fills gaps in coverage for individuals who are between jobs, unable to obtain employer-sponsored health insurance, or who missed the ACA open enrollment period. The National Association of Insurance Commissioners estimated that insurers sold approximately 160,000 STLDI policies to individuals in 2016 (Rao, Nowak, and Eibner 2018). These plans offer bare bones coverage that often excludes benefits required by the ACA, such as maternity care, behavioral and mental health services, substance abuse treatment, and prescription drugs (Gupta and Field 2018). As a result, STLDI plans offer significantly lower premiums for individuals purchasing coverage in the nongroup health insurance market. Consumers who purchased STLDI plans paid an average monthly premium of $124 in 2016, compared to $393 for an unsubsidized individual market plan, for a cost savings of 70 percent (*Federal Register* 2018).

Before the passage of the ACA in 2010, many individual market plans offered limited coverage. Regulations issued by the Department of Health and Human Services (HHS) in 1997 defined an STLDI plan as a policy with a policy period of less than one year. STLDI plans are a poor choice for individuals with chronic health conditions because they are not defined as standard health insurance products. As a result, insurers often charge higher premiums to people based on their gender, age, or medical history; limit covered services; and impose a maximum cap on covered benefits (Lueck 2018). As these plans did not meet the law's definition of minimum essential coverage, individuals who purchased STLDI plans were subject to a penalty from the IRS for failing to meet the individual health insurance mandate.

Prior to 2016, Federal officials defined a "short-term" health plan as a policy with coverage period not exceeding 364 days. The Obama administration expressed concerns that individuals who did not qualify for premium subsidies might substitute STLDI plans for more expensive marketplace coverage (Rau 2016). To discourage this practice, the Obama administration proposed regulations in June 2016 changing the definition of STLDI plans; under the new rule, STLDI plans could not provide coverage for a period longer than three months, and policies were required to inform consumers that the insurance was not qualifying health coverage (*Federal Register* 2018). The National Association of Insurance Commissioners criticized the new limits, arguing that consumers' "options should not be limited to either paying for coverage they cannot afford or exposing themselves to the risk of losing their coverage after three months if they become sick" (Bell 2016).

The election of Donald Trump in November 2016 marked a turning point in federal policy toward STLDI plans. On his first day in office, President Trump issued an executive order directing federal agencies to "encourage the development of a free and open market in interstate commerce for the offering of healthcare services and health insurance, with the goal of achieving and preserving maximum options for patients and consumers" (Trump 2017a). In October 2017, Trump issued another executive order that reaffirmed "promoting competition in healthcare markets" as a principal policy goal for his administration. He declared that "to the extent consistent with law, government rules and guidelines affecting the United States healthcare system should: (i) expand the availability of and access to alternatives to expensive, mandate-laden PPACA insurance" (Trump 2017b).

In August 2018, the Trump administration finalized a rule extending the length of short-term plans to one year, with the possibility of renewal for up to three years. HHS Secretary Alex Azar declared that the decision reflected the fact that "this administration believes in more options, not fewer, for consumers. Expanding short-term insurance is just part of President Trump's larger agenda to improve health-care choice and competition for Americans" (Azar 2018). Writing in the *Wall Street Journal*, Carolyn Bolton argued that "people—especially the young and families in special circumstances—don't want a one-size-fits-all health insurance 'market' that's clunkier than basic cable." Instead, "in an era when there are more than 60 Ben & Jerry's ice cream flavors, customizable soda machines programmed to behave like mixologists, and IKEA solutions for every nook and cranny imaginable, it's about time Americans are again allowed a health insurance option that can better fit their palate and their pocketbook" (Bolton 2018).

Many health providers and patient advocacy groups strongly objected to the administration's new policy. After the new rule took effect in October 2018, more than 25 patient advocacy groups, including the American Cancer Society, the American Heart Association, and the March of Dimes, issued a joint statement opposing the expansion of STLDI plans. The groups argued that "this rule will siphon younger and healthier individuals out of the individual market risk pool, forcing patients with preexisting health conditions to pay far higher costs for the comprehensive coverage they obtain through the insurance marketplaces. It will also expose those younger, healthier individuals to the significant risk that their health plan will fail to cover critically necessary care if they fall ill or develop a serious medical condition" (American Heart Association 2018). These groups also warned that the Trump administration's action "threatens to split and weaken the individual insurance market, which has provided millions of previously uninsured people with access to quality coverage since the [ACA] went into effect" (Sullivan 2018). The American College of Physicians echoed these concerns, declaring that "this regulation will erode essential patient protections and drive up premiums for those buying coverage through the health insurance exchanges" (López 2018).

After the Trump administration issued its final rule on STLDI plans, opponents challenged the new policy in court. The plaintiffs argued that the 2018 final rule violated the ACA and would increase premiums, destabilize health insurance markets, and offers consumers inadequate coverage (Elfin 2019). In July 2019, U.S. District Court Judge Richard Leon dismissed the lawsuit brought by the Association for Community Affiliated Plans and several other mental health and public health advocacy groups. The court found the plaintiffs failed to demonstrate that falling enrollment in ACA-compliant plans was the direct result of the administration's new rule. Judge Leon's ruling opened the door for the Trump administration's efforts to expand the availability of STLDI plans. In September 2020, President Trump declared, "My Administration increased the availability of renewable short-term, limited-duration healthcare plans, providing options that are up to 60 percent cheaper than the least expensive alternatives under the Patient Protection and Affordable Care Act (ACA) and are projected to cover 500,000 individuals who would otherwise be uninsured" (Trump 2020).

An investigation by Democrats on the U.S. House of Representatives Energy and Commerce Committee, however, led them to charge that "the Trump Administration's policy of expanding these dangerous, unregulated plans presents a threat to the health and financial well-being of American families, particularly in light of the current public health emergency" (U.S. House of Representatives, Committee on Energy and Commerce 2020). In addition, the report noted that "STLDI plans systematically discriminate against individuals with pre-existing conditions, and against women," and "offer wholly inadequate protection against catastrophic medical costs."

The demand for STLDI plans remains uncertain. Surveys conducted by the Kaiser Family Foundation revealed that consumers remain worried about both costs and coverage of such policies. For example, while three out of five respondents who purchased insurance in the nongroup market or through the health insurance marketplaces favored comprehensive coverage that "costs more but covers almost every benefit you need" over plans that "cost less but does not cover every benefit you need," more than one in three enrollees preferred cheaper, less comprehensive plans (Kirzinger et al. 2018). Furthermore, more than three-quarters of nongroup enrollees surveyed worried that their "health insurance premiums will increase so much that you won't be able to afford the plan you have now."

These concerns suggest that the demand for less expensive STLDI plans may be considerably higher than the Trump administration's initial estimates. Furthermore, a subsequent poll conducted in November 2018 found that among individuals who were uninsured or who purchased their own coverage, 21 percent would opt to purchase a short-term plan if given the opportunity to do so (Kirzinger, Wu, and Brodie 2018). In a 2019 survey by eHealth, 61 percent of consumers who had purchased STLDI plans cited the affordability of premiums as the primary reason for selecting a plan, and 43 percent said that without an STLDI plan they would not have health insurance coverage (Moffitt 2019).

In 2018, the Trump administration projected that enrollment in STLDI plans would increase by 600,000 in 2019 and up to 1.4 million by 2028 (*Federal Register* 2018). A 2020 investigation by the U.S. House of Representatives Committee on Energy and Commerce concurred with this assessment, noting that "the significant uptick in enrollment in 2019 indicates that these plans represent a significant and growing proportion of the individual market. Additionally, the enrollment data suggests that the Trump Administration's regulatory actions has caused an increase in the availability of STLDI plans" (U.S. House of Representatives, Committee on Energy and Commerce 2020). Other health policy think tanks, however, predict that demand for STLDI policies will be much higher, resulting in significant consequences for enrollment in the health insurance marketplaces. The Urban Institute projected that the elimination of the ACA's individual mandate penalty, coupled with increased flexibility to renew short-term health plans, could increase the number of people without minimum essential coverage by 2.5 million people in 2019. If a significant number of younger and healthier subscribers abandon ACA-compliant individual market plans for cheaper plans, one study estimated that marketplace premiums could rise by 18.2 percent in the 43 states (including the District of Columbia) that permit the sale of STLDI policies (Blumberg, Buettgens, and Wang 2018).

Short-Term Plans Are Not "Junk Insurance"

After Democrats failed to repeal the Trump administration's new rule expanding the availability of short-term health plans in October 2018, Sen. John Kennedy (R-LA) defended the need for the new policies on the Senate floor.

> If you purchase a short-term, limited duration health plan, it oftentimes does not have the same coverage a company is required to offer if it is a health insurance company offering health insurance under the Affordable Care Act. You don't get the same coverage. That doesn't mean you get no coverage. That doesn't mean the short-term, limited-duration plan is junk insurance, because it is not. It is considered major medical insurance, and issues like lifetime limits, annual limits, coverage of preexisting conditions—there are a variety of plans out there offered. If you want to purchase a plan that is still cheaper than you could buy under ObamaCare that covers preexisting conditions, you can. This idea that these short-term, limited-duration health plans are not insurance at all, or so-called junk insurance, is simply a bunch of nonsense. I will give an example. In the last quarter of 2016, a short-term, limited-duration health plan cost an individual about $124 a month. That is a lot of money for a lot of Americans, but it is much better when you compare it to an unsubsidized ObamaCare plan that costs $393 a month. You could save 70 percent by buying a short-term, limited-duration health plan. Again, the problem was that under ObamaCare, you could only buy one of these short-term plans for 3 months. Now you can buy them for much longer. The self-styled betters of Washington, DC, the cultured, cosmopolitan crowd up here who think they know better than everybody else in America, who think they are smarter than all Americans, would do away with short-term, limited-duration health plans if they could because they think the American people are not smart enough to understand what they are buying.

Source

Congressional Record, vol. 164, no. 169 (October 11, 2018): S6793–S6794. Washington, DC: Government Printing Office. Accessed January 30, 2019. https://www.congress.gov/115/crec/2018/10/11/CREC-2018-10-11-pt1-PgS6793-2.pdf.

In October 2018, the Republican-controlled U.S. Senate defeated a proposal introduced by Sen. Tammy Baldwin (D-WI) that would have overturned the Trump administration's expansion of short-term health plans. Baldwin argued that "junk insurance plans can deny health care coverage to people with pre-existing conditions when they need it the most" (Cancryn and Ollstein 2018). The Senate vote ended in a 50–50 tie, falling short of the majority needed to pass.

Nevertheless, the availability and terms of STLDI policies vary from state to state, as state insurance departments retain broad authority to regulate STLDI plans (Palanker, Kona, and Curran 2019). California, Massachusetts, New Jersey, and New York, for example, all restrict the sale of short-term plans (Palanker, Kona, and Curran 2019). States can also require that short-term plans comply with the same protections offered by plans sold through the individual health insurance marketplace. Twenty-two states limit the initial contract duration of short-term plans to less than 12 months as of 2019, but Colorado and California are the only states that require plans to adhere to the ACA's definition of essential health benefits (Palanker, Kona, and Curran 2019). Other states restrict the sale of multiple consecutive short-term term plans (Lucia et al. 2018).

After the Trump administration issued its final rule in August 2018, the California legislature passed Senate Bill 910, prohibiting health insurers "from issuing, selling, renewing, or offering a short-term limited duration health insurance policy, as defined, for health care coverage in this state" after January 1, 2019. This legislation was signed into law by Gov. Jerry Brown in September 2018. In 2018, nine states issued new regulations or passed legislation imposing new limits on the sale of STLDI plans (Palanker, Kona, and Curran 2019).

Democrats on Short-Term, Limited-Duration Health Insurance

For Democrats, the passage of the Affordable Care Act (ACA) was not only an opportunity to expand access to health insurance but also a means to improve the quality of coverage for consumers. From this vantage point, short-term limited-duration insurance policies represent a step backward. Democrats frequently labeled short-term plans as "junk insurance" because they fail to cover the minimum essential coverage standards established by the ACA. As Sen. Tammy Baldwin (D-WI) argued in a speech on the Senate floor, "These plans are cheap for a reason. They do not have to provide essential health benefits like hospitalization, prescription drugs and maternity care" (Kilgore 2018). As Reps. Diana DeGette (D-CO), Frank Pallone (D-NJ), and Anna Eshoo (D-CA) declared, "The Trump Administration's policy to expand unregulated and misleading plans is a threat to the health and financial well-being of American families, particularly during the COVID-19 crisis." They contended that "these plans are a bad deal for consumers and oftentimes leave patients saddled with thousands of dollars in medical debt" (DeGette 2020).

"Junk Insurance" Plans Deny Coverage to People with Preexisting Conditions

After the Trump administration issued a rule extending the duration and renewability of short-term health plans, Sen. Tammy Baldwin (D-WI) argued the new policy would discriminate against vulnerable patients.

> We can't go back to the days when insurance companies wrote the rules, just as we cannot allow the Trump administration to rewrite the rules on guaranteed healthcare protections that millions of Americans depend on. More than 20 of the leading healthcare organizations in America, representing our Nation's physicians, patients, medical students, and other health experts, are supporting this resolution to overturn the Trump administration's expansion of junk insurance plans. They are doing so because these junk plans will reduce access to quality coverage for millions and increase costs. These junk plans will charge people more for coverage based on their preexisting conditions or deny them coverage outright. These junk plans will leave cancer patients and survivors with higher premiums and fewer insurance options. These junk plans will force premium increases on older Americans. I have heard my colleagues on the other side of the aisle say that they are committed to protecting people with preexisting conditions. Now is your chance to prove it. Anyone who says they support coverage for people with preexisting conditions should support this resolution to overturn the Trump administration's expansion of these junk insurance plans.

Source

Congressional Record, vol. 164, no. 168 (October 10, 2018): S6738–S6739. Washington, DC: Government Printing Office. Accessed October 27, 2018. https://www.congress.gov/crec/2018/10/10/CREC-2018-10-10-pt1-PgS6738.pdf.

In particular, Democrats have voiced objections to the limited coverage and caps on lifetime reimbursements for STLDI plans. As California state senator Ed Hernandez (D) declared, "These short-term policies are dangerous because they subject people to huge healthcare bills, barely cover any services and give people a false sense of security" (Mason and Myers 2018). In 2018, Senator Hernandez sponsored S.B. 910, which banned insurers from selling health insurance plans in California with terms less than 12 months in duration.

Because STLDI plans offer limited coverage, Democrats argue that individuals who become sick will incur much higher out-of-pocket costs when they use services. Rep. Nancy Pelosi (D-CA) warned that "many Americans who enroll in these GOP junk health coverage plans will end up being hit by crushing medical bills, finding that they have been paying for coverage that doesn't cover much at all" (Pelosi 2018). Democrats are particularly concerned about the impact of STLDI policies on patients with chronic illnesses or who live with other preexisting conditions. In a letter to Health and Human Services Secretary Alex Azar, several

Democratic representatives and senators charged that the Trump administration's new rule "would take us back to the days when consumers could be denied coverage or charged more based on age, gender, or health status and when they had no guarantee of coverage for basic benefits" (House Energy and Commerce Committee 2018). Sen. Richard Blumenthal (D-CT) echoed these concerns, warning that STLDI plans "are like Swiss cheese with more holes than cheese. They offer no protection for those with pre-existing conditions like heart disease, diabetes, Parkinson's, pregnancy, cancer" (Hallenbeck 2018). Sen. Ron Wyden (D-OR) dismissed the Trump administration's efforts to expand access to STLDI plans, arguing that "these policies are not going to be worth the paper they're written on" (Frieden 2018).

Democrats also believe that expanding access to STLDI policies will increase premiums for consumers who purchase ACA-compliant plans through the health insurance marketplaces. Several Democratic members of the House Energy and Commerce Committee criticized the Trump administration's new rule, warning that "widespread marketing of these bare bones, junk plans will further destabilize health insurance markets, and will lead to higher premiums for everyone" (Goldstein 2018). Democrats contend that by encouraging younger and healthier individuals to purchase less expensive coverage, the Trump administration is guaranteeing that the remaining customers in the individual market will be older and sicker, driving premiums higher year after year.

This growth in STLDI policies gave new urgency to Democratic calls for new rules to protect consumers in the health insurance marketplace from deceptive practices and false advertising. California became the first state in the nation to issue a ban on STLDI policies in 2018. Sen. Ed Hernandez, the sponsor of S.B. 910, justified the need for government action, arguing, "These plans can bankrupt people. They don't have the protections of the Affordable Care Act. They're junk. It's a huge threat" (Hart 2018).

Republicans on Short-Term, Limited-Duration Health Insurance

According to Republicans, short-term health plans offer affordable alternatives to more expensive ACA-compliant plans in the individual marketplace. "Most Republicans believe that government shouldn't decide what good health insurance looks like. They posit that if I want to buy a 'skinny' health insurance plans that doesn't cover medications or outpatient care (so I can use that money to pay for other needs) I should be able to do that" (Jha 2018). In 2018, for example, STLDI plans offered coverage that was 59 percent cheaper than plans offered through the health care marketplaces for individuals who do not qualify for premium subsidies (Ingram 2018). STLDI plans cost approximately $124 per month, compared to $393 per month for an unsubsidized ACA-compliant plan (Centers for Medicare and Medicaid Services 2018).

The Trump administration continues to advocate for the repeal of the Affordable Care Act (ACA), but in the interim, officials "are looking to do everything we can to take incremental steps that will make insurance coverage of any type more affordable" (Pear 2018). Health and Human Services Secretary Alex Azar observed that "repealing the [individual] mandate and expanding short-term plans mean that millions of middle-class Americans who couldn't afford health insurance will now be able to do so" (Azar 2018). Seema Verma, the Trump administration's top official for the Centers for Medicare and Medicaid Services (CMS), declared that "in a market that is experiencing double-digit rate increases, allowing short-term, limited-duration insurance to cover longer periods gives Americans options and could be the difference between someone getting coverage or going without coverage at all" (Department of Health and Human Services Press Office 2018). Sen. John Kennedy (R-LA) echoed this point in his defense of STLDI plans on the Senate floor in October 2018: "By making these short-term, limited-duration health plans for a longer period of time, we are giving people the flexibility to extend them. The Trump administration, in my judgement, is making sure Americans have access to a reliable, affordable health care option" (Kennedy 2018).

Republicans also believe that government should not force younger and healthier individuals to subsidize the care of older and sicker subscribers by purchasing more comprehensive coverage than they want or need. Sen. Roy Blunt (R-MO) argued that the expansion of STLDI policies will "give people more flexibility to choose coverage options that are best for them, without having to pay for benefits they will never use" (Blunt 2018). Doug Badger, a health policy analyst at the Galen Institute, a conservative health policy think tank, noted, "People in their twenties and thirties are asked to pay unfairly high premiums to subsidize those in their fifties and sixties, who purchase plans at unfairly low rates." In contrast, Badger argued, STLDI plans "offer the opportunity for young people to purchase insurance at a rate that accurately reflects their insurance risks" (Bateman 2018). As a result of the Trump administration's action, "for the first time since the enactment of Obamacare," wrote John Goodman, a conservative health economist, "people will be able to buy insurance that meets individual and family needs rather than the needs of politicians and bureaucrats. They will also be able to pay actuarially fair premiums" (Goodman 2018).

Republicans endorse the expansion of STLDI policies because they offer consumers more choices in the individual insurance marketplace. As House Speaker Paul Ryan (R-WI) declared in 2017, "Republicans have long said that we have to empower patients as consumers to spur competition and bring down costs" (Ryan 2017). Indeed, Republicans cite STLDI alternatives as a key to lowering health insurance costs. As Sen. John Kennedy (R-LA) argued, Americans "watched their health insurance premiums rise through the roof as a result of the Affordable Care Act, and many of them have sought out this alternative, a short-term limited-duration plan, and said Hey, we know it doesn't cover as much as some policies, but it is a heck of a lot cheaper, and we would like to buy it and try it for a while" (Kennedy 2018). In short, consumer choice is a key element of a properly functioning market according to most Republicans.

Republicans criticized the Obama administration for "unfairly" restricting the availability of health plans that many consumers valued. In 2017, Sen. Ron Johnson (R-WI) and more than a dozen of his Republican colleagues urged the Trump administration to repeal limits on the availability of STLDI plans. The senators wrote that "short-term, limited duration plans offered consumers a viable health coverage option until an Obama-era regulation went into effect that greatly restricted the availability of these policies. As health insurers continue to leave the Obamacare exchanges, consumers need more, not fewer, options for health insurance. Reversing this regulation will provide consumers with an important option for health coverage" (Johnson 2017). Sen. John Barrasso (R-WY) concurred, arguing that "Republicans know a better solution is to give Americans more options, not fewer. Let people choose the coverage that works best for them. One simple change to the law could give people back their choices and let them finally start to recover from the damage done by Obamacare" (Barrasso 2018).

Republicans emphasize the argument that individuals may choose STLDI plans because of their lower cost or because their benefits are more tailored to their own circumstances. Furthermore, simply making such policies available does not compel consumers to purchase a STLDI plan. As Scott Atlas of the Hoover Institution asked on Fox News, "Why would anyone be against offering such choices to Americans and instead force them to buy coverage they don't want or value for their hard-earned money?" (Atlas 2018). Ultimately, as HHS Secretary Alex Azar observed, competition is the cornerstone of Republican efforts to reshape the U.S. health care system: "Fundamentally this administration believes in more options, not fewer, for consumers. Expanding short-term insurance is just part of President Trump's larger agenda to improve health-care choice and competition for Americans" (Azar 2018).

Robert B. Hackey and Anxhela Hoti

Further Reading

American Heart Association. 2018. "Final Rule on Short-Term Insurance Plans Will Leave Patients with High Costs, Less Coverage." August 1. Accessed February 4, 2019. https://newsroom.heart.org/news/final-rule-on-short-term-insurance-plans-will-leave-patients-with-high-costs-less-coverage.

Armour, Stephanie. 2019. "Judge Backs Non-ACA Compliant Health Plans." *Wall Street Journal*, July 19. Accessed August 22, 2019. https://www.wsj.com/articles/judge-backs-non-aca-compliant-short-term-health-plans-11563556820.

Atlas, Scott. 2018. "Americans Are 'Winning' on Health Care as Trump Administration Chips Away at ObamaCare." Fox News, August 8. Accessed January 31, 2019. https://www.foxnews.com/opinion/americans-are-winning-on-health-care-as-trump-administration-chips-away-at-obamacare.

Azar, Alex M., II. 2018. "Trump Wants to Help the Forgotten People Hurt by Obamacare. Here's How." U.S. Department of Health and Human Services, August 15. Accessed January 31, 2019. https://www.hhs.gov/about/leadership/secretary/op-eds/trump-wants-help-forgotten-people-hurt-obamacare.html.

Barrasso, John. 2018. "A New Escape Hatch from Obamacare." *Washington Examiner*, February 27. Accessed August 29, 2018. https://www.washingtonexaminer.com/john-barrasso-a-new-escape-hatch-from-obamacare.

Bateman, Ashley. 2018. "California Bans Short-Term Limited Duration Health Plans." Accessed January 31, 2019. https://www.heartland.org/news-opinion/news/california-bans-short-term-limited-duration-health-plans.

Bell, Allison. 2016. NAIC Opposes Federal Short-Term Health Limit. ThinkAdvisor, August 16. Accessed January 31, 2019. https://www.thinkadvisor.com/2016/08/16/naic-opposes-federal-short-term-health-limit/?slreturn=20190031101329.

Blumberg, Linda J., Matthew Buettgens, and Robin Wang. 2018. "Updated: The Potential Impact of Short-Term Limited-Duration Policies on Insurance Coverage, Premiums, and Federal Spending." Urban Institute, March. Accessed January 31, 2019. https://www.urban.org/sites/default/files/publication/96781/2001727_updated_finalized.pdf.

Blunt, Roy. 2018. "Sen. Roy Blunt: Short-Term Health Insurance Will Benefit Millions of Americans." Fox News, August 12. Accessed September 17, 2018. https://www.foxnews.com/opinion/sen-roy-blunt-short-term-health-insurance-will-benefit-millions-of-americans.

Bolton, Carolyn. 2018. "A Lost Love and an ObamaCare Alternative." *Wall Street Journal*, August 12. Accessed February 4, 2019. https://www.wsj.com/articles/a-lost-love-and-an-obamacare-alternative-1534110344.

Cancryn, Adam, and Alice Miranda Ollstein. 2018. "Senate Democrats Fail to Block Trump's Short-Term Health Plans." Politico, October 10. Accessed October 11, 2018. https://www.politico.com/story/2018/10/10/senate-health-resolution-fails-838133.

Centers for Medicare and Medicaid Services. 2018. "Fact Sheet: Short-Term, Limited-Duration Insurance Proposed Rule." February 20. Accessed February 4, 2019. https://www.cms.gov/newsroom/fact-sheets/fact-sheet-short-term-limited-duration-insurance-proposed-rule.

DeGette, Diana. 2020. "New Report Finds Millions of Americans Enrolled in 'Junk Health Plans' That Provide No Real Coverage." June 25. Accessed October 16, 2020. https://degette.house.gov/media-center/press-releases/new-report-finds-millions-of-americans-enrolled-in-junk-health-plans.

Department of Health and Human Services Press Office. 2018. "Trump Administration Works to Give Relief to Americans Facing High Premiums, Fewer Choices." Accessed March 2, 2021. https://public3.pagefreezer.com/browse/HHS.gov/31-12-2020T08:51/https://www.hhs.gov/about/news/2018/02/20/trump-administration-works-give-relief-americans-facing-high-premiums-fewer-choices.html.

Elfin, Dana. 2019. 'Show Me the Evidence, Judge Tells Short-Term Health Plan Rule Challengers." Health Care Dive, May 22. Accessed August 22, 2019. https://www.healthcaredive.com/news/show-me-the-evidence-judge-tells-short-term-health-plan-rule-challengers/555168/.

Federal Register. 2018. "Short-Term Limited-Duration Insurance." 83, no. 150 (August 3): 38212–38243. Accessed January 30, 2019. https://www.govinfo.gov/content/pkg/FR-2018-08-03/pdf/2018-16568.pdf.

Frieden, Joyce. 2018. "Short-Term Insurance Plans Will Hurt Patients, Senators Say." MedPage Today, August 16. Accessed December 10, 2018. https://www.medpagetoday.com/publichealthpolicy/healthpolicy/74613.

Goldstein, Amy. 2018. "Short-Term Health Plans Skirting ACA-Required Benefits and Protections to Be Expanded." *Washington Post*, February 20. Accessed February 3, 2019. https://www.washingtonpost.com/national/health-science/short-term-health-plans-skirting-aca-required-benefits-and-protections-to-be-expanded/2018/02/20/9889c7c6-14d3-11e8-92c9-376b4fe57ff7_story.html?utm_term=.7c3ce93512f4.

Goodman, John C. 2018. "Trump Throws a Life Belt to People Who Buy Their Own Health Insurance." *Forbes*, August 6. Accessed February 4, 2019. https://www.forbes.com/sites/johngoodman/2018/08/06/trump-throws-a-life-belt-to-people-who-buy-their-own-health-insurance/#2cee4a575d90.

Gupta, Atul, and Robert Field. 2018. "What's the Impact of Expanding Short-Term Health Plans?" Wharton School, August 6. Accessed February 4, 2019. http://knowledge.wharton.upenn.edu/article/whats-impact-expanding-short-term-health-insurance/.

Hallenbeck, Brian. 2018. "Blumenthal Says New 'Short-Term' Health Plans Would Shortchange Americans." *New London Day*, August 2. Accessed December 10, 2018. https://www.theday.com/article/20180802/NWS01/180809849.

Hart, Angela. 2018. "Ban Health Insurance That Doesn't Cover Pre-Existing Conditions? Jerry Brown to Decide." *Sacramento Bee*, September 4. Accessed February 3, 2019. https://www.sacbee.com/news/politics-government/capitol-alert/article217016050.html.

House Energy and Commerce Committee. 2018. "Bicameral Democratic Committee Leaders Urge Administration to Withdrawn Harmful Short-Term Insurance Rule." April 13. Accessed November 20, 2018. https://democrats-energycommerce.house.gov/newsroom/press-releases/bicameral-democratic-committee-leaders-urge-administration-to-withdraw.

Ingram, Jonathan. 2018. "Short-Term Plans: Affordable Health Care Options for Millions of Americans." Foundation for Government Accountability, October 30. Accessed February 4, 2019. https://thefga.org/wp-content/uploads/2018/10/Short-Term-Plans-memo-DIGITAL-file-10-30-18.pdf.

Jha, Ashish. 2018. "A Year of Living Dangerously with the Affordable Care Act." BMJ Opinion, January 22. Accessed August 22, 2019. https://blogs.bmj.com/bmj/2018/01/22/ashish-jha-a-year-of-living-dangerously-with-the-affordable-care-act/.

Johnson, Ron. 2017. "Johnson Leads Effort for More Consumer Choice in Health Insurance Markets." Accessed October 16, 2020. https://www.ronjohnson.senate.gov/public/index.cfm/2017/6/johnson-leads-effort-for-more-consumer-choice-in-health-insurance-markets.

Kennedy, John. 2018. "Healthcare Insurance Plans." *Congressional Record*, October 11: S6793–S6794. Accessed January 30, 2019. https://www.congress.gov/115/crec/2018/10/11/CREC-2018-10-11-pt1-PgS6793-2.pdf.

Kilgore, Ed. 2018. "Democrats Lose Senate Vote on Trump's Junk Health Plans but Send a Message." October 10. Accessed November 23, 2018. http://nymag.com/intelligencer/2018/10/democrats-lose-vote-on-junk-health-plans-but-send-a-message.html.

Kirzinger, Ashley, Liz Hamel, Cailey Muñana, and Mollyann Brodie. 2018. "Kaiser Health Tracking Poll—March 2018: Non-Group Enrollees." Kaiser Family Foundation, April 3. Accessed February 4, 2019. https://www.kff.org/health-reform/poll-finding/kaiser-health-tracking-poll-march-2018-non-group-enrollees/.

Kirzinger, Ashley, Bryan Wu, and Mollyann Brodie. 2018. "KFF Health Tracking Poll—November 2018: Priorities for New Congress and the Future of the ACA and Medicaid Expansion." Kaiser Family Foundation, November 28. Accessed November 29, 2018. https://www.kff.org/health-reform/poll-finding/kff-health-tracking-poll-november-2018-priorities-congress-future-aca-medicaid-expansion/.

Levitt, Larry, Rachel Fehr, Gary Claxton, Cynthia Cox, and Karen Pollitz. 2018. "Why Do Short-Term Health Insurance Plans Have Lower Premiums Than Plans That Comply with the ACA?" Kaiser Family Foundation, October. Accessed February 4, 2019. http://files.kff.org/attachment/Issue-Brief-Why-Do-Short-Term-Health-Insurance-Plans-Have-Lower-Premiums-Than-Plans-That-Comply-with-the-ACA.

López, Ana María. 2018. "Internists Say Short-term Plans Will Increase Premiums and Harm Patients." American College of Physicians, August 1. Accessed September 20, 2018. https://www.acponline.org/acp-newsroom/internists-say-short-term-plans-will-increase-premiums-and-harm-patients.

Lucia, Kevin, Justin Giovannelli, Sabrina Corlette, JoAnn Volk, Dania Palanker, Maanasa Kona, and Emily Curran. 2018. "State Regulation of Coverage Options outside of the Affordable Care Act: Limiting the Risk to the Individual Market." Commonwealth Fund, March 29. Accessed November 23, 2018. https://www.commonwealthfund.org/publications/fund-reports/2018/mar/state-regulation-coverage-options-outside-affordable-care-act?redirect_source=/publications/fund-reports/2018/mar/state-regulation-coverage-options-outside-aca.

Lueck, Sarah. 2018. "Key Flaws of Short-Term Health Plans Pose Risks to Consumers." Center on Budget and Policy Priorities, September 20. Accessed November 23, 2018. https://www.cbpp.org/research/health/key-flaws-of-short-term-health-plans-pose-risks-to-consumers.

Mason, Melanie, and John Myers. 2018. "In a Rebuke to Trump, Gov. Jerry Brown Signs Bans on Short-Term Health Plans, Medi-Cal Work Requirements." *Los Angeles Times*, September 22. Accessed February 3, 2019. https://www.latimes.com/politics/essential/la-pol-ca-essential-politics-may-2018-in-a-rebuke-to-trump-gov-jerry-brown-1537647108-htmlstory.html.

Moffitt, Robert. 2019. "Why the Left Is Desperate to Sabotage Trump's Health Care Plans." Heritage Foundation, April 4. Accessed August 22, 2019. https://www.heritage.org/health-care-reform/commentary/why-the-left-desperate-sabotage-trumps-health-care-plans.

Palanker, Dana, Maanasa Kona, and Emily Curran. 2019. "States Step Up to Protect Insurance Markets and Consumers from Short-Term Health Plans." Commonwealth Fund, May 2. Accessed August 22, 2019. https://www.commonwealthfund.org/publications/issue-briefs/2019/may/states-step-up-protect-markets-consumers-short-term-plans.

Pear, Robert. 2018. "'Short Term' Health Insurance? Up to 3 Years under New Trump Policy." *New York Times*, August 1. Accessed September 20, 2018. https://www.nytimes.com/2018/08/01/us/politics/trump-short-term-health-insurance.html.

Pelosi, Nancy. 2018. "Pelosi Statement on Final Trump Administration Rule Unleashing Junk Health Coverage Plans." August 1. Accessed February 4, 2019. https://www.speaker.gov/newsroom/8118/.

Rao, Preethi, Sarah Nowak, and Christine Eibner. 2018. "What Is the Impact on Enrollment and Premiums if the Duration of Short-Term Health Insurance Plans Is Increased?" Commonwealth Fund, June 5. Accessed November 23, 2018. https://www.commonwealthfund

.org/publications/fund-reports/2018/jun/what-impact-enrollment-and-premiums-if-duration-short-term.

Rau, Jordan. 2016. "HHS Announces Plans to Curtail Consumers' Use of Short-Term Insurance Policies." Kaiser Health News, June 8. Accessed February 4, 2019. https://khn.org/news/hhs-announces-plans-to-curtail-consumers-use-of-short-term-insurance-policies/.

Ryan, Paul. 2017. "Our Health Care Plan for America: Paul Ryan." *USA Today*, March 8. Accessed November 23, 2018. https://www.usatoday.com/story/opinion/2017/03/07/health-care-obamacare-replacement-paul-ryan-column/98858696/.

Sullivan, Peter. 2018. "Senate Defeats Measure to Overturn Trump Expansion of Non-ObamaCare Plans." The Hill, October 10. Accessed October 11, 2018. https://thehill.com/policy/healthcare/410775-senate-defeats-measure-to-overturn-trump-expansion-of-non-obamacare-plans.

Trump, Donald J. 2017a. "Executive Order 13765: Minimizing the Economic Burden of the Patient Protection and Affordable Care Act Pending Repeal." *Federal Register*, January 24. Accessed March 2, 2021. https://www.federalregister.gov/documents/2017/01/24/2017-01799/minimizing-the-economic-burden-of-the-patient-protection-and-affordable-care-act-pending-repeal.

Trump, Donald J. 2017b. "Executive Order 13813: Promoting Healthcare Choice and Competition Across the United States." *Federal Register*, October 17. Accessed March 2, 2021. https://www.federalregister.gov/documents/2017/10/17/2017-22677/promoting-healthcare-choice-and-competition-across-the-united-states.

Trump, Donald J. 2020. "Executive Order 13951: An America-First Healthcare Plan." *Federal Register*. September 24. Accessed March 2, 2021. https://www.federalregister.gov/documents/2020/10/01/2020-21914/an-america-first-healthcare-plan.

U.S. House of Representatives, Committee on Energy and Commerce. 2020. "Shortchanged: How the Trump Administration's Expansion of Junk Short-Term Health Insurance Plans Is Putting Americans at Risk." Accessed October 16, 2020. https://degette.house.gov/sites/degette.house.gov/files/STLDI%20Report%2006%2025%2020%20FINAL_.pdf.

Single-Payer Health Insurance

At a Glance

In the months before the coronavirus pandemic reshaped the landscape of American politics, a heated debate over Medicare for All dominated the 2020 Democratic presidential primaries. By 2019, many of the contenders for the Democratic presidential nomination had endorsed Medicare for All, which is an example of a single-payer health care system. In a single-payer system, government enrolls all individuals in a publicly administered health plan financed through taxpayer contributions. Public officials are responsible for defining benefits and covered services, enrolling eligible individuals, and reimbursing providers for care (Congressional Budget Office 2019). Single-payer models offer all citizens access to health insurance regardless of age, employment status, or income. Private insurance, if it is permitted, is limited to services not covered by the public plan.

The contemporary debate over Medicare for All is not new. Sen. Ted Kennedy (D-MA) first championed the idea of a Canadian-style single-payer health care system in the early 1970s. In the United States, numerous proposals to create such a system have appeared at both the federal and state levels over the past several decades.

Many, but not all, Democrats view a single-payer health system—whether Medicare for All or a similar program—as the next logical step in health care reform. By 2018, support for single-payer reform had emerged as a litmus test for progressive Democrats; 225 Democrats running for the House of Representatives endorsed Medicare for All during the 2018 election cycle (Pipes 2018). However, Medicare for All did not prove to be a winning issue for most Democrats. During the 2018 midterm elections Democratic candidates who supported Medicare for All won less than half (45 percent) of their races. Notably, 72 percent of Democratic candidates who declined to endorse Medicare for All won in 2018 (Abramowitz 2019). Nevertheless, progressive supporters of Medicare for All and state-level single-payer initiatives tout the potential of such an approach to reduce administrative costs and lower out-of-pocket health care spending for individuals and families. Democratic supporters of single-payer solutions, such as Sens. Bernie Sanders (I-VT) and Elizabeth Warren (D-MA), emerged as leading challengers for the party's 2020 presidential nomination, although the party eventually coalesced around Joe Biden, the senator from Delaware who served as vice president during President Obama's two terms in office. Surveys conducted during the 2019 Democratic primary campaign found that a majority (55 percent) of Democrats preferred a presidential candidate who would "build on the existing Affordable Care Act." Only 40 percent of Democrats favored candidates who wanted to replace the Affordable Care Act (ACA) with a Medicare for All plan (Kaiser Family Foundation 2020). Biden declined to endorse Medicare for All during the campaign.

In contrast, Republicans have vigorously opposed proposals to create a single-payer insurance plan, frequently describing such proposals as a "government takeover" of the health care system in recent decades. Republicans charge that a single-payer system will erode the quality of patient care, limit patient choice, and inevitably lead to rationing. In addition, Republicans argued that a single-payer national health insurance system would be unaffordable and would require massive tax increases that will cripple the U.S. economy and place an unbearable burden on American workers and families. Finally, Republicans believe that such a system undermines core American values. They argue that "socialized medicine" is incompatible with Americans' long-standing belief in limited government and the power of the free market. More than 80 percent of Republicans favor a "system based on private insurance" rather than a government-run health care system (Jones 2019). Furthermore, two-thirds of Republicans disagree that "it is the responsibility of the federal government to make sure all Americans have health care coverage" (Newport 2018).

According to Many Democrats . . .

- A single-payer health care system will control the cost of health care for businesses, individuals, and the government.
- Health care is a right that should be available to all Americans.
- Single-payer health insurance, such as Medicare for All, will ensure a more equitable health care system and improve health outcomes.

According to Many Republicans . . .

- Single-payer health insurance is unaffordable and will bankrupt the U.S. economy.
- Most Americans prefer a choice of insurers and oppose the abolition of private health insurance.
- A single-payer approach, such as Medicare for All, is a government takeover of the health care system that will result in hospital closures, rationing of care, waiting lists, and diminished choice for patients.

Overview

Government-funded universal health insurance—commonly known today as Medicare for All—has a long history in U.S. health policy debates. In the 1940s, Harry S. Truman became the first president to actively campaign for a government-funded health insurance system. Truman's plan offered limited coverage for inpatient hospital care; drugs and outpatient care such as physician visits were not included. Nevertheless, opponents—including business groups, insurers, and the medical profession—quickly assailed the proposal as an unaffordable and un-American takeover of American medicine that threatened the doctor-patient relationship (Hackey 1997). In the ideologically charged environment of the late 1940s and early 1950s, debates over "socialized medicine" faced united Republican opposition.

The election of Republican Dwight D. Eisenhower to the presidency in 1952 effectively ended the prospects for national health insurance during this era. Instead, supporters of comprehensive health reform embraced a more incremental plan to build upon, rather than replace, the existing private health insurance system (Marmor 1970). Since older Americans used more health care services and had less access to employer-based health insurance coverage, "Medicare" proposals introduced by Rep. Aime Forand (D-RI) in the late 1950s and early 1960s focused attention on expanding public coverage to persons over the age of 65. Eight years after it was first introduced, Medicare was enacted in 1965 to provide hospital insurance (Part A) for all Americans over the age of 65; it also included optional coverage for outpatient services (Part B), such as physician services, laboratory tests, and other ambulatory services. The debate over Medicare was defined by vigorous disagreements about the role of government in financing health care. Some Republicans charged it would lead to "socialized medicine." Despite this criticism, the law passed with overwhelming bipartisan support. The bill passed the House by a margin of 313–115, even though 48 Democrats and 68 Republicans opposed it. In the Senate, Medicare passed by a margin of 68–21 (11 senators abstained from the final vote); 13 Republicans joined Democrats to pass the bill (Social Security Administration 2020).

The term 'Medicare for All' first appeared in 1970s in legislation proposed by Sen. Jacob Javits (R-NY). "Although we spend more money than any other country in the world on health care," Javits said, "the quality of care remains uneven, and for many particularly the poor—it is abysmally low, if not non-existent" (Rosenbaum 2020, 103). A year later, Sen. Edward M. "Ted" Kennedy (D-MA) introduced the Health Security Act (S. 3) to create a Canadian-style single-payer health system financed through payroll taxes. Kennedy held hearings around the nation to drum up support for his proposal, but the plan faced staunch opposition from Republicans and many Democrats. Although Kennedy succeeded in placing single-payer health reform on the public agenda, Congress did not act on the bill. In 1974, Kennedy joined with Rep. Wilbur Mills—the architect of Medicare—to cosponsor a new proposal to create a compulsory system of universal coverage financed through payroll taxes and general revenues. Once again, the proposal failed to gain traction in Congress.

Congress considered multiple proposals for national health insurance during the 1970s, but none won over a majority of congressional Democrats. President Richard Nixon (R) offered a bipartisan path to national health insurance during his final year in office, but progress on health care reform took a back seat to the ongoing Watergate investigation. During the Carter administration, Democrats remained divided over whether to prioritize cost containment or universal coverage (Blumenthal and Morone 2009).

Beginning in the 1980s, physicians David Himmelstein and Steffie Woolhandler published a series of articles documenting the high administrative cost of private health insurance in the United States compared to Canada. Writing on behalf of Physicians for a National Health Program, Himmelstein and Woolhandler published a proposal for "a national health program for the United States" in 1989 in the *New England Journal of Medicine*. The proposal would "fully cover everyone under a single, comprehensive public insurance program" (Himmelstein and Woolhandler 1989). As they noted in a subsequent article, "A large sum might be saved in the United States if administrative costs could be trimmed by implementing a Canadian-style health care system" (Woolhandler and Himmelstein 2003). Their proposal attracted the attention of other health care analysts. As Victor Fuchs, a health economist at Stanford University observed, "A single-payer system would undoubtably lower administrative expenses." In the current U.S. health care system, Fuchs noted, "hospitals, physicians, and other entities and individuals that provide health care must employ armies of 'back office' personnel to bill and collect for that care" (Fuchs 2018.

The early 1990s were characterized by a renewed optimism about the possibility of achieving universal coverage. The election of Harris Wofford—a political novice who won a Senate seat in a 1991 special election in Pennsylvania by focusing on problems with American health care—raised the profile of health care reform as a political issue. The issue dominated the 1992 presidential campaign. Every candidate, Democrats and Republicans alike, offered competing plans for health care reform, which was now seen as a winning issue to woo middle-class voters. Rising health care costs and the growing number of uninsured Americans led prominent Democrats in Congress to proclaim that the time for comprehensive health care reform had finally arrived (Hackey 1993).

In 1993, Sen. Paul Wellstone (D-MN) introduced the American Health Security Act (S. 491), which proposed to create a single-payer health system in which the federal government collected funds through taxes and distributed the revenues to the states, who would administer the program and establish their own health budgets (Wellstone and Shaffer 1993). The Clinton administration, however, sought to build bipartisan support for reform by fusing market-based and regulatory proposals. President Clinton's proposed Health Security Act embraced a 'managed competition' strategy that built upon existing private health insurance rather than seeking to replace the existing health insurance system. In 1994, however, the administration's health care reform proposal died in Congress without ever coming up for a vote. Despite having a majority in both the House and Senate, Democrats were unable to reconcile several competing reform proposals, and none gained a majority. Insurers, business groups, and the pharmaceutical industry unleashed a barrage of attacks on Democratic reform plans. Later that year, Republicans regained control over the House of Representatives for the first time in four decades, effectively ending the prospects for comprehensive national health care reform.

After the demise of national health care reform in the 1990s, proponents of a single-payer health care system shifted their focus to the state level. In the absence of federal action, several states considered single-payer reforms. None succeeded. The experiences of California, Colorado, New York, and Vermont underscore the challenges facing proponents of single-payer health insurance reform.

The California Physicians' Alliance—a state chapter of Physicians for a National Health Program—organized a grassroots signature campaign for a single-payer health initiative in 1994. Organizers collected more than one million signatures in one hundred days to secure a place on the November ballot; it was the largest grassroots campaign of fundraising and signature gathering in California history (Farey and Lingappa 1996). The ballot initiative, formally known as Proposition 186, sought to create a taxpayer-funded universal health insurance system. Any person who "lived in California and intended to stay" would qualify for coverage and receive a "health security card" that entitled them to a full range of health care services. To finance the new benefits, Proposition 186 increased income, payroll, and tobacco taxes and capped payments to health providers (Farey and Lingappa 1996).

Businesses, health insurers, and physicians framed the debate about Proposition 186 in terms of affordability; the proposal required a $40 billion tax increase—the largest in state history (Farey and Lingappa 1996). Hospitals and health insurers—joined by the National Federation for Independent Business and local chambers of commerce—organized a coalition known as Taxpayers against the Government Takeover to oppose the ballot initiative. The coalition mounted a multipronged media assault on single-payer through print, radio, and television. Ads warned voters that Proposition 186 "will force most of us to give up our private coverage and push us into a government health bureaucracy controlled by an elected politician, not a doctor or nurse. This type of government takeover is bad medicine for California" (Danelski et al. 1995). Similar themes of "big government," personal liberty, and loss of consumer choice reappeared in subsequent debates over single-payer health care reform at both the state and federal levels over the next two decades. Ultimately, voters soundly rejected Proposition 186. Nearly three-quarters of Californians (73 percent) voted against the proposed single-payer system (Farey and Lingappa 1996). Despite the resounding defeat of Proposition 186, single-payer advocates continued to press for comprehensive reform in California. In 2006, a bill (SB 840) to create a single-payer health care system passed the legislature but was later vetoed by Gov. Arnold Schwarzenegger (R). After the passage of the Affordable Care Act (ACA) in 2010, California policy makers focused on a series of incremental reforms by expanding Medicaid and implementing a new health insurance marketplace.

Colorado also sought to enact a single-payer health care program through a ballot initiative in 2016. Amendment 69, the Colorado Care System Initiative, proposed a new publicly funded health insurance system that would enroll all residents and ban the sale of private insurance. As in California, insurers mounted an organized campaign to oppose the amendment and outspent proponents by a 4 to 1 ratio (Matthews 2017). As political observers noted, "It took the opposition three seconds to call it a tax and supporters three minutes to explain how it was simply a different way of payment that would save them a whole lot of money" (Matthews 2017). Polls conducted before the election revealed that while more than 60 percent of Democrats supported Amendment 69, more than 60 percent of independent and Republican voters opposed the measure (Stapleton, Adler, and Sohkey 2016). Concerns about higher taxes and the affordability of the proposed plan ultimately soured the public against the proposal; 79 percent of Colorado voters opposed the initiative in the November 2016 election.

In New York, progressive legislators first introduced a proposal to establish a single-payer health care system, known as the New York Health Act (NYHA), in the early 1990s (Lipsitz 2019). The NYHA promised to expand coverage for all residents, regardless of immigration status, and was to be funded through a graduated income tax (Campaign for New York Health 2018). For more than two decades, the legislation gained little traction in the state legislature. Beginning in 2015, however, the NYHA passed in the state Assembly before ultimately dying in the Senate; the bill also passed the Assembly in 2016, 2017, and 2018. When Democrats regained control of both chambers of the legislature in 2018, single-payer supporters believed that the time was finally ripe to enact universal coverage, but the bill failed to move past the committee level in the 2019–20 legislative session.

Supporters of the NYHA were unable to move it forward because it aroused intense opposition from business groups, insurers, and health providers, who organized a coalition called Realities of Single-Payer to oppose the plan (Lipsitz 2019). Each group viewed the NYHA as an existential threat to its current business model. Hospitals described the proposal as "irresponsible" and unaffordable (Young 2019). The proposal also failed to win support from key public-sector unions in the state who had negotiated generous health benefits for their members (Wall Street Journal 2019c). A study by the RAND Corporation estimated that the proposal would require $139 billion in state funding by 2022, with the largest burden falling on upper-income taxpayers (Liu et al. 2018). As the Business Council of New York State noted, "The RAND report confirms what we have been saying for years, a single-payer system would result in the largest tax increase in New York history and cripple an industry that employs tens of thousands across the state" (Business Council of New York State 2018). Budget forecasts from the nonpartisan RAND corporation—a public policy think tank—projected that the cost of the NYHA would exceed the state's total projected tax revenue for the 2022 fiscal year (Vielkind 2019).

Meanwhile, Vermont actively explored the creation of a single-payer health care system from 2010 to 2014—in the process becoming a "beacon for a single-payer health care system in America"—when Gov. Peter Shumlin (D) signed Act 48 into law (Wheaton 2014b). Act 48, also known as Green Mountain Care, was not a true single-payer plan. It exempted self-insured employers and Medicare enrollees (Wheaton 2014a). Advocates celebrated Vermont's plan as proof that states could take the lead on comprehensive health care reform. However, after nearly losing his bid for reelection in 2014, Shumlin abandoned his commitment to a single-payer plan. Act 48's cost, both fiscal and political, made it a political nonstarter. Actuaries estimated implementing Green Mountain Care would increase the state budget by 45 percent and require legislators to raise both income taxes and payroll taxes for employers.

Beginning in 2003, Rep. John Conyers (D-MI) introduced legislation—the United States National Health Insurance Act (also known as the Expanded and Improved Medicare for All Act)—in each Congress until his retirement in 2016. The bill proposed to create a single-payer health care system that provided all individuals residing in the United States with comprehensive, publicly funded health insurance that covered primary care, preventive services, prescription drugs, and mental health services (H.R. 676 2003). Conyers bill, which banned for-profit providers from participating in the new system and also prohibited the sale of private health insurance coverage, never received a hearing or a vote. Subsequent versions of the bill attracted more Democratic cosponsors over time, but single-payer proposals were marginalized during the extensive congressional debate over health care reform in 2009–2010. After the passage of the ACA in 2010, progressive Democrats continued to reintroduce versions of Conyers bill in each subsequent Congress. Single-payer health insurance returned to the forefront of the national debate about health care reform in 2016. Sen. Bernie Sanders (I-VT) made Medicare for All—often dubbed "Bernie Care"—the centerpiece of his presidential bid. Sanders's plan also proposed to establish the federal government as the sole payer for health care services and eliminated the sale of private health insurance plans.

Hospitals, private insurers, and medical device manufacturers all supported the passage of the ACA in 2010 because it promised new customers and boosted demand for their services without significant price controls. In contrast, a single-payer health care system poses a significant economic threat to providers' profits—and in the case of health insurers, to their continued existence. In 2018, health insurers and other industry groups banded together to create the

Partnership for America's Health Care Future (PAHCF). The new coalition organized a broad-based campaign to challenge Medicare for All and other state-level single-payer initiatives. Echoing past opposition to national health insurance in the 1990s, PAHCF warned that Medicare for All would lead to higher taxes, interfere with the practice of medicine, and cede control over health care to government bureaucrats (Pear 2019).

The latest chapter in the battle for Medicare for All began in 2019. Rep. Pramila Jayapal (D-WA) introduced H.R. 1384, the Medicare for All Act of 2019, in the House. It was cosponsored by more than 100 fellow Democrats. And Sen. Bernie Sanders (I-VT) introduced a companion bill in the Senate (S.1129) that included 15 Democratic senators as cosponsors. Both sought to establish a national health insurance program administered by the Department of Health and Human Services that would cover all U.S. residents. In addition, the Medicare for All legislation prohibited the sale of private health insurance policies that duplicated covered services. Patients would no longer be responsible for copayments, coinsurance, or deductibles when using covered services. Because the plan would be fully funded

Medicare for All Puts People over Profits

On February 26, 2019, Rep. Pramila Jayapal (D-WA) introduced the Medicare for All Act of 2019. Joined by over 100 House Democrats as cosponsors, Jayapal declared that nearly five decades after Congress first considered legislation to create a single-payer health care system, the time was finally right for Medicare for All.

> Today in America, 30 million people are uninsured. 40 million are underinsured. We have the most expensive healthcare system in the world and yet our outcomes are the worst of all industrialized countries. I and the more than 100 co-sponsors of this bill refuse to allow this to continue. It's time to put people's health over profit. Our bill will cover everyone. Not just those who are fortunate enough to have employer-sponsored insurance. Not just children. Not just seniors. Not just those who are healthy. Everyone. Because healthcare is a human right. We will need every single person in the country to help us, to stand with us, to organize and to fight for this. . . . Because the industry lobby is going to pour hundreds of millions of dollars into killing this bill, saying it costs too much, scaring you into thinking you're giving up something, pitting the healthy against the sick and the young against the old. It's time to ensure that healthcare is a right and not a privilege, guaranteed to every single person in our country. It is time for Medicare for All.

Source

Jayapal, Pramila. 2019. "Jayapal, Dingell and more than 100 Co-Sponsors Introduce Medicare For All Act of 2019." Press Release, February 28, 2019. Accessed March 7, 2021. https://jayapal.house.gov/2019/02/28/jayapal-dingell-and-more-than-100-co-sponsors-introduce-medicare-for-all-act-of-2019/.

by tax revenue, patients would also no longer pay separate premiums for coverage. The new public plan would cover all medically necessary services, including hospital services, prescription drugs, mental health and substance abuse treatment, dental and vision services, and long-term care (U.S. Senate 2019).

Four Democratic presidential candidates endorsed the Senate version of the Medicare for All bill during the 2020 campaign: Sens. Cory Booker (D-NJ), Kirsten Gillibrand (D-NY), Kamala Harris (D-CA), and Bernie Sanders (I-VT). Sen. Elizabeth Warren developed her own plan during the 2020 presidential primary season but also cosponsored Sanders's bill in the Senate. Despite differences between the time line and projected cost of their respective plans, Warren and Sanders both proposed to enroll all Americans in one government-sponsored health insurance plan. "We don't need to raise taxes on the middle class by one penny to finance Medicare for All," Warren declared. "The very wealthy and big corporations will see their costs go up, but middle-class families will see their costs go down" (Jamerson and Parti 2019). Democrats touted the benefits of Medicare for All for working- and middle-class families. Under a single-payer model, individuals and families would no longer depend on their employers for access to affordable health insurance, and cost sharing and premiums would be eliminated, resulting in significant savings for millions of Americans.

Until the COVID-19 pandemic upended the focus of the 2020 presidential campaign, candidates' positions on Medicare for All defined a crowded Democratic primary field. Moderate Democrats, including former Vice President Joe Biden, former Colorado Governor John Hickenlooper, and Mayor Pete Buttigieg, opposed Medicare for All in favor of incremental reforms that built upon the ACA. The Biden campaign dismissed Warren's plans to pay for Medicare for All by raising taxes on corporations and upper-income individuals as an exercise in "mathematical gymnastics" (Jamerson, Armour, and Rubin 2019). Officials in the Biden campaign also charged that "the Medicare-for-All plans that Senators Warren and Sanders are proposing will not only cost 160 million Americans their private health coverage and force tax increases on the middle class, but it would also kill almost 2 million jobs—and that's according to one of Sen. Warren's own policy advisors" (Rubin 2019). House Speaker Nancy Pelosi (D-CA) declared, "I'm not a big fan of Medicare-for-All," and expressed concerns about the "comfort level that some people have with their current private insurance" as an election issue (Marcus 2019).

Pelosi's observation reflected perhaps the most significant challenge to enacting a single-payer health insurance bill. A single-payer system would directly impact more than 200 million Americans currently enrolled in private health insurance plans, most of which are provided by employers (Galston 2019). As Cass Sunstein, a former Obama administration official and a professor at Harvard Law School, noted, "Right now 158 million Americans get their health insurance through an employer and an additional 14 million obtain private insurance through the individual market. A shift would immediately create uncertainty for about 172 million people—and the uncertainty would involve something of fundamental importance to their daily lives. Many of those millions much like their current plans" (Sunstein 2019). The public, however, remains unclear on this foundational point. Surveys conducted by the Kaiser Family Foundation revealed that two-thirds of those who favored Medicare for All believed that it would not affect their current health insurance coverage (Galston 2019). Critics also argued that the title of the new law —Medicare for All—was "deeply misleading. It implies that the current Medicare system would be extended to all Americans. In fact, Medicare for All differs from Medicare in fundamental ways—with much broader coverage, no cost sharing, and fewer choices of health plans" (Pozen 2019).

The cost of implementing a single-payer system remains a significant political obstacle. The Urban Institute, a liberal think tank, estimated that a Medicare for All plan would cost an additional $34 trillion during its first decade, or "more than the federal government's total cost over the coming decade for Social Security, Medicare, and Medicaid combined" (Brownstein 2019). The projected cost of the new system is unprecedented. Academic health policy experts raised significant questions. Robert Pozen, the former president of Fidelity Investments and a lecturer at MIT, argued, "However you cut it, Medicare for All would inevitably lead to massive tax increases" (Pozen 2019). Paul Starr, a Princeton University professor who authored a classic analysis of the evolution of the U.S. health care system, noted, "We're talking about changing flows of money on just a huge scale. There's no precedent in American history that compares to this" (Abelson and Sanger-Katz 2019). As Jonathan Oberlander, a health policy expert at the University of North Carolina noted, Medicare for All "faces intense opposition from insurers, the medical care industry, and much of organized medicine. It would trigger fierce resistance from conservatives and the business community and anxiety in many insured Americans fearful about changing coverage and the specter of rationing" (Oberlander 2016).

Hospitals and physicians expressed serious concerns about the fiscal impact of transitioning to Medicare for All. As Zirui Song, a health policy scholar at Harvard Medical School observed, "Physicians and hospitals face the prospect of receiving Medicare prices for all patients they serve." Since private insurers generally pay physicians up to 300 percent more than Medicare for in-network care, and considerably more for out-of-network care, physicians' incomes could fall significantly under a Medicare for All model. In response, physicians could either increase the volume of services delivered by seeing more patients or "upcode" billing to maximize reimbursement for covered services (Song 2019).

Physicians remain divided on the issue of Medicare for All. For decades, the medical profession strongly opposed proposals for "compulsory" health insurance, which it saw as a threat to doctors' financial well-being and professional autonomy. In recent years, physicians embraced a more liberal stance; by 2018, 80 percent of physicians' campaign contributions were going to Democratic candidates (Abrams

2019). Although the American Academy of Family Medicine first endorsed "health care for all" in the late 1980s, the American Medical Association (AMA), the largest and most influential organization in the profession, continues to oppose single-payer health care—although not overwhelmingly. At its 2019 annual meeting, the AMA's House of Delegates rejected single-payer reform by a margin of 53 percent to 47 percent. However, progressive physicians scored a victory in 2019 when they persuaded the AMA to withdraw from the PAHCF, a coalition of drug companies, hospitals, and insurers opposed to Medicare for All (Abrams 2019). Meanwhile, membership in the Physicians for a National Health Program, a single-payer advocacy group, reached an all-time high, drawing upon growing interest among medical students (Abrams 2019).

Hospital industry groups warned that "a proposal to create a government-run, Medicare-like health plan on the individual exchange could create the largest ever cut to hospitals—nearly $800 billion" (American Hospital Association 2019). The Federation of American Hospitals, an association of for-profit hospitals, declared that "hospitals oppose legislation that would needlessly upend coverage for hundreds of millions of Americans" (Federation of American Hospitals 2019). The American Hospital Association (AHA)—the nation's leading association of non-profit hospitals—also viewed Medicare for All as a threat to both providers and patients. "While the AHA shares the objective of achieving health coverage for all Americans, we do not agree that a government-run, single-payer model is right for this country. Such an approach would upend a system that is working for the vast majority of Americans and throw into chaos one of the largest sectors of the U.S. economy" (American Hospital Association 2019). Historically, hospitals have shifted costs 40 percent more than average. Indeed, "a Medicare for All plan that extends the current Medicare fee schedule to all patients would therefore lead to a marked decline in revenue from formerly privately insured patients and a small decrease in revenue from formerly Medicaid covered patients." The authors estimated that hospitals could lose more than 15 percent of their revenue annually, totaling more than $151 billion (Schulman and Milstein 2019). The PAHCF argued that "instead of scrapping the whole health care system we should focus on improving what's working and fixing what's broken" (Armour and Peterson 2019).

Americans express mixed support for the concept of a single-payer health care system. Over the past decade, public support for a government-run health care system increased. Nevertheless, a majority of Americans polled by Gallup in 2019 preferred "a healthcare system based on private insurance over a government-run system. Support for a government-run system averaged 36 percent from 2010 to 2014 but has been 40 percent or higher each of the past five years" (Jones 2019). A 2017 Politico/Morning Consult poll found that nearly half (49 percent) of voters favored "a single-payer health care system where all Americans would get their insurance from one government plan"; 35 percent of voters opposed such a plan (Shepard 2017). The Kaiser Family Foundation polls found growing support for the concept of insuring all Americans through a single public plan over the past two decades. From 1998 to 2004, an average of 40 percent of respondents endorsed this approach, but by 2016, fully half of the public (50 percent) expressed support for a single-payer solution (Kaiser Family Foundation 2020). The language used in polling questions has a significant impact on public support for single-payer; questions that mention "Medicare for All" elicit higher favorability than those that describe the system as a "government health plan" (Newport 2016).

The growing popularity of single-payer proposals was particularly evident among Democrats. In April 2017, for example, one poll found that "54 percent of Democrats supported the notion. Five months later, that same polling organization found that support had jumped by 13 points to 67 percent" (Shepard 2017). Nevertheless, public support for single-payer health care reform is conditional. A plan that would "require most Americans to pay more in taxes" or "eliminate private health insurance companies" won support from only 37 percent of respondents, while any proposal that could "lead to delays in people getting some medical tests and treatments"—a frequent charge leveled against Medicare for All by critics—was opposed by 70 percent of the public (Kaiser Family Foundation 2020). Notably, a majority of Medicare for All supporters (55 percent) believed that "they and their family would be able to keep their current health insurance" (Kaiser Family Foundation 2020).

In fact, Medicare for All proposals would ban the sale of private health insurance policies. While the public remains divided on the desirability of a single-payer health insurance plan, a majority (54 percent) of Americans "believe the federal government has a responsibility to ensure that all Americans have health care coverage" (Jones 2019). Single-payer proposals offer one path to universal coverage, but as health economist Victor Fuchs observed, the United States could also achieve universal coverage by expanding subsidies to purchase private insurance and by strengthening the individual mandate to purchase coverage (Fuchs 2018).

Democrats on Single-Payer Health Insurance

Democratic support for a single-payer national health insurance plan is deeply rooted. In the 1940s, President Harry S. Truman became the first president to endorse a compulsory government-run health care system funded through payroll taxes (Oberlander 2016). However, Truman's plan died in the face of withering opposition from business groups, insurers, the medical profession, and congressional Republicans. Opponents attacked the proposal as a threat to personal liberty that would destroy the doctor-patient relationship and erode the quality of care for all Americans (Hackey 1997). After 1965, though, when Democrats led the way in passing Medicare and Medicaid, many members of the party interpreted those legislative triumphs as the first steps in a march toward universal coverage (Oberlander 2016).

In 1971, Sen. Edward "Ted" Kennedy (D-MA) introduced the Health Security Act, a bill that called for a universal single-payer national health insurance plan financed by payroll taxes (Evans and Schiff 2010). Kennedy used his leadership role in the U.S. Senate to raise awareness of the need for comprehensive health care reform by hosting hearings around the nation. The committee's report, "The Health Care Crisis in America," provided a blueprint for reform and a call to action (Evans and Schiff 2010). Kennedy's frustration with the Carter administration's incremental approach to health reform provided the spark for his unsuccessful presidential bid in 1980 (Evans and Schiff 2010). Over the next four decades, Kennedy pressed on with a tireless campaign for national health insurance. Speaking before the 2008 Democratic National Convention, the frail but still formidable senator declared, "This is the cause of my life. . . . We will break the old gridlock and guarantee that every American—north, south, east, west, young, old—will have decent, quality health care as a fundamental right and not a privilege" (Evans and Schiff 2010).

The most recent chapter in the debate over single-payer health care began in 2016, when Sen. Bernie Sanders (I-VT) made a "Medicare for All" single-payer plan a cornerstone of his 2016 presidential campaign. Although Sanders's call for single-payer reform was popular on the campaign trail, fellow Democrats in Congress remained cool to the idea; Sanders's bill failed to attract any cosponsors in 2016. Hillary Clinton refused to embrace Medicare for All, arguing that "people who have health emergencies can't wait for us to have a theoretical debate about some better idea that will never, ever come to pass" (Condon 2016). In subsequent years, Democrats followed Sanders's lead and moved leftward. By 2018, a "Medicare for All" caucus in Congress claimed more than 70 Democrats as members (Armour 2018). In February 2019, Reps. Pramila Jayapal (D-WA) and Debbie Dingell (D-MI) introduced the Medicare for All Act. Their bill, H.R 1384, was cosponsored by118 fellow House Democrats. A similar bill introduced in the Senate (S. 1129) by Sen. Bernie Sanders (I-VT) garnered support from 15 Senate Democrats. The bill's cosponsors included several 2020 presidential candidates, including Sens. Kamala Harris (D-CA), Kirsten Gillibrand (D-NY), and Cory Booker (D-NJ).

The 2020 presidential campaign exposed a significant division within the Democratic party about the future of health care reform. The progressive wing of the party—led by Rep. Alexandria Ocasio-Cortez (D-NY) and Sens. Ed Markey (D-MA), Elizabeth Warren (D-MA), and Bernie Sanders (I-VT), viewed Medicare for All as the next logical step in health care reform. As Ocasio-Cortez declared in 2018, "Medicare for All is a generational investment not a short-term band-aid, and it is a profound decision about who we want to be and how we want to act as a nation" (Re 2018). However, many moderate Democrats expressed skepticism that a single-payer system is politically attainable, and they argued that the party should build on the foundation established by the Affordable Care Act (ACA), also known as Obamacare. Moderates, such as former Vice President Joe Biden, the party's eventual nominee, questioned the financial and political viability of Medicare for All. During the March 2020 Democratic debate, Biden was asked whether he would veto Medicare for All if it passed during his administration. He replied, "I would veto anything that delays providing the security and the certainty of health care being available now." In addition, Biden noted, "You got to look at the cost. I want to know—how did they find $35 trillion? What is that doing? Is it going to significantly raise taxes on the middle class, which it will?" (Higgins 2020).

Democratic supporters of Medicare for All argue that single-payer reform represents the best path to make health care more affordable for businesses and families. Democrats often cite the gnawing fear of financial ruin and the constant worries about the adequacy of coverage, or losing coverage altogether, as a rationale for enacting Medicare for All. As Warren observed, "People who file for bankruptcy looked a lot like my family. The overwhelming majority had once been solidly middle class—and about half had filed for bankruptcy in the aftermath of a serious medical problem. . . . No American should ever die or go bankrupt because of health care costs" (Warren 2018). In addition, "a single-payer system would lift the significant financial burden from businesses that currently fund the healthcare insurance for their employees and would largely eliminate the financial burden of illness, a leading cause of bankruptcy, and debt sent into collection," said Rep. Keith Ellison (D-MN). "Medical debt is one of the leading causes of personal bankruptcy in the United States. If we were to set up a system that was focused more on health and wellness where we all could pay and then we can all benefit, it would make our society stronger, better financially and physically" (Ellison 2018).

Progressive Democrats dismissed opponents' claims that Medicare for All would be unaffordable. Sanders insisted that the additional cost of a single-payer system in terms of higher taxes "will be more than offset by the money you are saving with the elimination of private insurance costs" (Krieg and Luhby 2017). In addition, Warren argued, "Medicare for All will save money by bringing down the staggering administrative costs for insurers in our current system. As the experts I asked to evaluate my plan noted, private insurers had administrative costs of 12 percent of premiums collected in 2017, while Medicare kept its administrative costs to 2.3 percent" (Warren 2018.) In this view, while additional taxes would be required to pay for Medicare for All, individuals would no longer pay premiums or cost sharing for health care services, and so they would actually benefit financially overall. As New York state Assembly member Richard Gottfried noted, "What you ought to care about is how much money leaves your wallet. . . . Under the [New York Health Act], less money will leave your wallet" (Lipsitz 2019). Warren, meanwhile, declared that "over the next ten years, individuals will spend $11 trillion on health care in the form of premiums, deductibles, copays and out of pocket costs. Under my Medicare for All plan that amount will drop from $11 trillion to practically zero" (Warren 2019). In addition, Warren argued that Medicare for All would be a boon for businesses as well because "every company paying for health care today will pay less than they would have if they were still offering their employees comparable private insurance" (Warren 2019).

All Democrats regard health care as a basic right that should be available to all. Progressive Democrats, however, argue that Medicare for All will finally enable the party to realize its long-standing goal of providing affordable health care for all Americans. On the campaign trail in 2016, Sen. Bernie Sanders (I-VT) argued, "Universal health care is an idea that has been supported in the United States by Democratic presidents going back to Franklin Roosevelt and Harry Truman. . . . It is time for our country to join every other major industrialized nation on earth and guarantee health care to all citizens as a right, not a privilege" (DeBenedetti 2016). Sen. Kamala Harris (D-CA) described Medicare for All as an important step toward a more just society: "Medicare for All stands for the proposition that all Americans from the day of their birth, throughout their lives, will have access to health care" (Krieg and Luhby 2017). Rep. Ro Khanna (D-CA) declared, "If we believe that healthcare is a basic right, then it is long past time to have Medicare for All. Every American should be guaranteed decent, basic healthcare from the day they are born. This is not a political issue. This is a moral issue. It is an issue of human decency" (Khanna 2018).

By eliminating financial barriers to care, Democrats also contend that Medicare for All will reduce health disparities and promote a more equitable society. In particular, Democrats argue that a single-payer system would have a particularly significant impact on low-income families, the unemployed, the uninsured, and underserved communities. "Medicare for All would actually help reduce income inequality," asserted Ellison. "One of the problems of the society we live in now is that we have really historic record inequality. . . . [But] a single-payer system can also help level the playing field and help working people make a better go at this economy. Medicare for All would make sure that everyone would have the same access and level of care, regardless of their income, their job, or the community that they live in" (Ellison 2018). Warren went so far as to claim that "Medicare for all would mark one of the greatest federal expansions of middle class wealth in our history. And if Medicare for All can be financed without any new taxes on the middle class, and instead by asking giant corporations, the wealthy, and the well-connected to pay their fair share, that's exactly what we should do" (Warren 2019). According to Sen Bernie Sanders, "Our current dysfunctional health care system is designed to make huge profits for insurance companies and drug companies, rather than provide quality care for every man, woman and child" (Sanders 2018a). The end result of Medicare for All, according to Sanders, will be a more just and equitable system for *all* Americans, not just the uninsured and underserved.

Most Democrats favor an expanded role for government to address important social problems. A 2020 poll by the Pew Research Center found that 79 percent of registered Democrats believed government "should do more to solve problems," and 78 percent agreed that "government regulation of business is necessary to protect the public interest" (Pew Research Center 2020). A majority (74 percent) of Democrats also favored "a single national health insurance program run by the government, sometimes called 'Medicare for all,' that would replace private insurance" (Pew Research Center 2020). Democrats display a strong commitment to improving access to health care. Since 2006, polls conducted by the Kaiser Family Foundation have found that more than 90 percent of Democrats supported "the federal government doing more to help provide health insurance for more Americans" (Kaiser Family Foundation 2020). Over the past two decades, Gallup polls also showed high levels of support for universal coverage; 80 percent of Democrats polled between 2015 and 2019 agreed that "the federal government has a responsibility to ensure all Americans have health care coverage" (Jones 2019).

Republicans on Single-Payer Health Insurance

Republicans reject single-payer health insurance proposals such as Medicare for All as both unaffordable and inconsistent with American values. Seema Verma, the administrator of the Centers for Medicare and Medicaid Services (CMS) under the Trump administration, described Medicare for All as the "greatest threat to the American health care system" (Verma 2019). Rather than a one-size-fits-all approach, Republicans prefer free market prescriptions that they say do a better job of controlling costs, increasing access to health care, and improving the quality of health care. Thus, Republicans endorse proposals to increase price transparency for hospitals and other health providers, offer consumers more affordable health insurance options, and foster competition across state lines to lower costs and improve quality. Republicans regard Medicare for All as a hostile government takeover of American medicine by federal bureaucrats. In this view, "socialized medicine" will require historic tax increases, undermine innovation and choice, and limit Americans' access to medically necessary services. For Republicans, the cure prescribed by single-payer advocates is worse than the disease.

Republicans contend that the cost of a publicly funded single-payer health care system will place a heavy and unsustainable burden on taxpayers. "The costs of implementing [a single-payer system] would be astronomical," insisted Senate Majority Leader Mitch McConnell (R-KY). "The taxes required to pay for it would be sky-high" (McConnell 2017). Verma offered a similar warning: "Spending on a single-payer government-run healthcare system at the federal level will crowd out other priorities, from national defense to infrastructure to spending on education" (Verma 2018). Scott Atlas, a health policy analyst at the Hoover Institution who later served as an adviser to President Donald Trump during the COVID pandemic, concurred with this diagnosis. He warned that Medicare for All "would cost more than $32 billion over its first decade. Doubling federal income and corporate taxes wouldn't be enough to pay for it" (Atlas 2018). Sen. John Barrasso (R-WY) worried that "this single-payer plan means major tax hikes to cover massive costs. It means much longer lines for lower quality care. And it means the elimination of private health insurance for Americans" (Barrasso 2019). Republican lawmakers were not the only ones to voice doubts about Medicare for All and other single-payer plans. The *Wall Street Journal*'s editorial board, for example, asserted that "honest private estimates suggest it would take at least a doubling of individual and corporate taxes [to fund Medicare for All]. . . . But the real savings would have to come from where the money is: cutting payments to doctors and restricting care" (*Wall Street Journal* 2019b).

Republicans believe that a government "takeover" of health care will endanger the fiscal health of hospitals and other health providers and end patients' ability to choose their insurance plans. In particular, Republicans object to proposals that would abolish private health insurance plans. They argue that most Americans are satisfied with their current insurance coverage and prefer choice—which Medicare for All would eliminate. McConnell, for example, described Medicare for All as "a massive expansion of a failed idea, a quadrupling down on the failures of Obamacare, a totally government-run system that would rip health insurance plans away from even more Americans and take away even more of their most

Medicare for All Means "Less Freedom, Lower Quality of Care, and Longer Lines"

Sen. John Barrasso (R-WY) spoke on the Senate floor on May 1, 2019, in opposition to Sen. Bernie Sanders's proposed Medicare for All bill. Barrasso, a practicing physician, decried what he described as a "government takeover" of the U.S. health care system.

> I'm just not sure most Americans understand what Medicare for All means and what it would mean for them personally. And maybe some of the presidential candidates don't even want people to know what it means.
>
> Senator Sanders has claimed that Medicare for All is, as he said, quote, "a struggle for the soul of who we are as a nation."
>
> Let's be clear. Americans are facing a critical choice here, a choice between a big government-run health care system and a system that gives Americans access to quality, affordable care that they can choose that is right for them and their families.
>
> That to me is the choice that we're facing. Because Medicare for All essentially means a complete government takeover of all health care in this country. And central planners in Washington, D.C. would then be in control of the health care for all of us.
>
> Medicare for All would enroll every American in a government-run health care system. It will take away America's health care choices.

Source

Barrasso, John. 2019. "Barrasso: 'Medicare for All' Will Mean Higher Costs and Less Choice for Americans." Press Release, May 1, 2019. Accessed March 7, 2021. https://www.barrasso.senate.gov/public/index.cfm/news-releases?ID=A722560B-F1FF-48EF-8746-D5DB8D170A06.

personal health-care decisions" (McConnell 2017). Rep. Kevin McCarthy (R-CA) declared, "If any of you have had health care provided by your employment, or if you're on Medicare now, [Democrats] are pretty much going to end it as we know it. They want one government-run system" (Armour 2018).

Furthermore, Republicans argue that Medicare for All will undermine the fiscal stability of American hospitals and other health providers. President Donald Trump denounced Medicare for All as a "radical" and "dangerous" plan that "would devastate the American healthcare market and lead to higher taxes. The Democrats' disastrous 'Medicare for All' plan distributes healthcare for 'free,' by creating a government monopoly on healthcare markets and setting all prices paid to suppliers. Under this policy, doctors, hospitals, and pharmaceutical companies would have no choice but to accept whatever the government decides to pay for their services. Consumers, likewise, would have no choice but to use government-directed options" (Trump 2018a).

For Republicans, creating a single-payer health care system represents a radical overreach to remake one-sixth of the U.S. economy. As the *Wall Street Journal* argued, "Medicare for All isn't about universal coverage so much as a federal takeover of American health care" (*Wall Street Journal* 2019a). Verma declared that "doubling down on government and mimicking the failed socialist health care systems of Europe that ration and restrict care, where patients face long periods of time for care, is not the answer" (Verma 2019). Verma also raised the prospect of health care rationing if Medicare for All came to pass: "Government-run healthcare means having bureaucrats dictate decisions about your care, . . . even things like how often you have to see your physician in order to receive treatment" (Verma 2019).

Finally, Republicans warned that Medicare for All would threaten the benefits that seniors had paid for, and come to depend on, through the existing Medicare program. As Trump wrote in 2018, "We have seen Democrats across the country uniting around a new legislative proposal that would end Medicare as we know it and take away benefits that seniors have paid for their entire lives" (Trump 2018b). Sen. John Barrasso (R-WY) echoed this theme, claiming that a single-payer system "means the end of the Medicare program that seniors rely upon and so many depend on, on a daily basis" (Barrasso 2019). Republicans also raised the specter of rationing care for vulnerable seniors in an effort to undercut public support for Medicare for All. "By eliminating Medicare as a program for seniors, and outlawing the ability of Americans to enroll in private and employer-based plans, the Democratic plan would inevitably lead to the massive rationing of health care," said Trump in a statement. "Doctors and hospitals would be put out of business. Seniors would lose access to their favorite doctors. There would be long wait lines for appointments and procedures. Previously covered care would effectively be denied" (Trump 2018b).

For Republicans, opposition to Medicare for All—and to single-payer health insurance in general—is rooted in a belief in limited government. An overwhelming majority (76 percent) of Republicans polled by the Pew Research Center in 2020 felt that "government is doing too many things better left to businesses and individuals." A similar proportion (78 percent) opposed "a single national health insurance program run by the government, sometimes called 'Medicare for all,' that would replace private insurance." Notably, 60 percent of Republicans indicated that they strongly opposed such a plan (Pew Research Center 2020). Support for universal coverage has declined significantly among Republicans over the past two decades. Gallup polls conducted between 2001 and 2008 found that, on average, 38 percent of Republicans believed "the federal government has a responsibility to ensure all Americans have health care coverage." From 2015 to 2019, however, only 21 percent of Republicans shared this view (Jones 2019).

Robert B. Hackey and Anne Capozzoli

Further Reading

Abelson, Reed, and Margot Sanger-Katz. 2019. "Medicare for All Would Eliminate Private Insurance." *New York Times*, March 23. Accessed September 4, 2020. https://www.nytimes.com/2019/03/23/health/private-health-insurance-medicare-for-all-bernie-sanders.html.

Abramowitz, Alan. 2019. "Medicare for All a Vote Loser in 2018 U.S. House Elections." UVA Center for Politics, November 14. Accessed October 2, 2020. https://centerforpolitics.org/crystalball/articles/medicare-for-all-a-vote-loser-in-2018-u-s-house-elections/.

Abrams, Abigail. 2019. "A New Generation of Activist Doctors Is Fighting for Medicare for All." *Time*, October 24. Accessed September 4, 2020. https://time.com/5709017/medicare-for-all-doctor-activists/.

American Hospital Association. 2019. "Statement of the American Hospital Association for the Committee on Rules of the U.S. House of Representatives on the 'Medicare for All Act of 2019.'" April 30. Accessed August 25, 2020. https://www.aha.org/system/files/media/file/2019/04/AHAStatementforRulesCommitteeHearingonMforAll-04302019.pdf.

Armour, Stephanie. 2018. "Some Democrats Want Medicare for All. Others Aren't So Sure." *Wall Street Journal*, October 4. Accessed September 20, 2020. https://www.wsj.com/articles/some-democrats-want-medicare-for-all-others-arent-so-sure-1538645400.

Armour, Stephanie. 2019. "Medicare for All Loses Support amid Lack of Detail on Costs to Voters." *Wall Street Journal*, October 17. Accessed August 28, 2020. https://www.wsj.com/articles/medicare-for-all-loses-support-amid-lack-of-detail-on-costs-to-voters-11571338349.

Armour, Stephanie, and Kristina Peterson. 2019. "House Democrats Reveal Plan for Medicare for All." *Wall Street Journal*, February 26. Accessed March 11, 2021. https://www.wsj.com/articles/house-democrats-reveal-plan-for-medicare-for-all-11551219200.

Atlas, Scott. 2018. "The False Promise of 'Medicare for All.'" *Wall Street Journal*, November 12. Accessed September 20, 2020. https://www.wsj.com/articles/the-false-promise-of-medicare-for-all-1542066511.

Barrasso, John. 2019. "Under One-Size-Fits-All Health Care, Americans Will Pay More and Wait Longer for Worse Care." May 8. Accessed August 25, 2020. https://www.barrasso.senate.gov/public/index.cfm/news-releases?ID=E1C4AD95-D0A4-43C8-91D4-E1ACB42A7218.

Blumenthal, David, and James Morone. 2009. *The Heart of Power: Health and Politics in the Oval Office*. Berkeley: University of California Press.

Brownstein, Ronald. 2019. "The Eye-Popping Cost of Medicare for All." *The Atlantic*, October 16. Accessed August 25, 2020. https://www.theatlantic.com/politics/archive/2019/10/high-cost-warren-and-sanderss-single-payer-plan/600166/.

Business Council of New York State. 2018. "Business Council Reacts to RAND Report on Single-Payer." August 1. Accessed August 29, 2020. https://www.bcnys.org/news/business-council-reacts-rand-report-single-payer.

Campaign for New York Health. 2018. "Guaranteed Healthcare for All New Yorkers." Accessed September 26, 2020. https://www.nyhcampaign.org/learn.

Condon, Stephanie. 2016. "Hillary Clinton: Single-Payer Health Care Will 'Never, Ever' Happen." CBS News, January 29. Accessed September 13, 2020. https://www.cbsnews.com/news/hillary-clinton-single-payer-health-care-will-never-ever-happen/.

Congressional Budget Office. 2019. "Key Design Components and Considerations for Establishing a Single-Payer Health Care System." Accessed March 13, 2021. https://www.cbo.gov/system/files/2019-05/55150-singlepayer.pdf.

Danelski, Ann, Drew Altman, Jan Eldred, Matt James, and Diane Rowland. 1995. "The California Single-Payer Debate: The Defeat of Proposition 186." Kaiser Family Foundation, July 30. Accessed August 28, 2020. https://www.kff.org/health-costs/report/the-california-single-payer-debate-the-defeat/.

DeBenedetti, Gabriel. 2016. "Sanders, Clinton Clash over His New 'Medicare for All' Plan." Politico, January 17. Accessed September 20, 2020. https://www.politico.com/story/2016/01/bernie-sanders-health-plan-217906.

Ellison, Keith. 2018. "Medicare for All." *Congressional Record* 164, no. 8 (April 26): H3692. Accessed August 25, 2020. https://www.congress.gov/congressional-record/2018/04/26/house-section/article/H3692-1.

Evans, Jennifer, and Jaclyn Schiff. 2010. "A Timeline of Kennedy's Health Care Achievements and Disappointments." Kaiser Health News, September 17. Accessed August 25, 2020. https://khn.org/news/kennedy-health-care-timeline/.

Farey, Krista, and Vishwanath Lingappa. 1996. "California's Proposition 186: Lessons from a Single-Payer Health Care Reform Ballot Initiative Campaign." *Journal of Public Health Policy* 17, no. 2: 133–152. Accessed August 29, 2020. https://www.jstor.org/stable/3342694.

Federation of American Hospitals. 2019. "FAH Leader Reacts to Medicare for All Bill." FAH Hospital Policy Blog, February 27. Accessed March 13, 2021. https://www.fah.org/blog/fah-leader-reacts-to-medicare-for-all-bill.

Fuchs, Victor. 2018. "Is Single-Payer the Answer for the U.S. Health Care System?" *JAMA* 319, no. 1: 15–16. Accessed September 30, 2020. https://jamanetwork.com/journals/jama/fullarticle/2666630.

Galston, William. 2019. "Medicare for All Is a Trap." *Wall Street Journal*, February 12. Accessed March 20, 2021. https://www.wsj.com/articles/medicare-for-all-is-a-trap-11550015354.

Hackey, Robert. 1993. "The Illogic of Health Care Reform: Policy Dilemmas for the 1990s." *Polity* 26, no. 2: 233–257.

Hackey, Robert. 1997. "Symbolic Politics and Health Care Reform in the 1940s and 1990s." In *Cultural Strategies of Agenda Denial*, edited by Roger Cobb and Marc Ross, 141–157. Accessed February 20, 2021. https://kansaspress.ku.edu/978-0-7006-0856-0.html.

Hellmann, Jessie. 2019. "'Medicare for All' Complicates Democrats Pitch to Retake Senate." The Hill, August 8. Accessed September 16, 2020. https://thehill.com/policy/healthcare/456574-medicare-for-all-divide-complicates-democrats-pitch-to-retake-senate.

Higgins, Tucker. 2020. "Biden Suggests He Would Veto 'Medicare for All' over Its Price Tag." CNBC, March 10. Accessed September 26, 2020. https://www.cnbc.com/2020/03/10/biden-says-he-wouldd-veto-medicare-for-all-as-coronavirus-focuses-attention-on-health.html.

Himmelstein, David, and Steffie Woolhandler. 1989. "A National Health Program for the United States." *New England Journal of Medicine* 320: 102–108. Accessed October 2, 2020. http://www.pnhp.org/publications/NEJM1_12_89.htm.

H.R. 676. 2003. "Expanded and Improved Medicare for All Act." U.S. House of Representatives, 108th Congress. Accessed September 20, 2020. https://www.congress.gov/bill/108th-congress/house-bill/676?q=%7B%22search%22%3A%5B%22united+states+national+health+insurance+act+2003%22%5D%7D&r=3&s=5.

Jamerson, Joshua, Stephanie Armour, and Richard Rubin. 2019. "Warren Would Tax the Wealthy, Companies to Pay for Medicare for All." *Wall Street Journal*, November 1. Accessed August 28, 2020. https://www.wsj.com/articles/warren-to-tax-wealthy-americans-companies-to-pay-for-medicare-for-all-11572614846.

Jamerson, Joshua, and Tarini Parti. 2019. "Democrats Push Elizabeth Warren for Plan to Pay for Medicare for All." *Wall Street Journal*, October 13. Accessed August 28, 2020. https://www.wsj.com/articles/democrats-push-elizabeth-warren-for-plan-to-pay-for-medicare-for-all-11570982403.

Jones, Jeffrey. 2019. "Americans Still Favor Private Healthcare System." Gallup, December 4. Accessed September 30, 2020. https://news.gallup.com/poll/268985/americans-favor-private-healthcare-system.aspx.

Kaiser Family Foundation. 2020. "Public Opinion on Single-Payer, National Health Plans, and Expanding Access to Medicare Coverage." May 27. Accessed August 25, 2020. https://www.kff.org/slideshow/public-opinion-on-single-payer-national-health-plans-and-expanding-access-to-medicare-coverage/.

Khanna, Ro. 2018. "Medicare for All." *Congressional Record* 164, no. 68 (April 26): H3692–H3695. Accessed August 29, 2020. https://www.congress.gov/congressional-record/2018/4/26/house-section/article/h3692-1?q=%7B%22search%22%3A%5B%22medicare+for+all%22%5D%7D&r=3.

Krieg, Gregory, and Tammy Luhby. 2017. "Inside Sanders' New 'Medicare for All' Bill." CNN, September 13. Accessed September 26, 2020. https://www.cnn.com/2017/09/13/politics/bernie-sanders-medicare-for-all-plan-details/index.html.

Lipsitz, Raina. 2019. "What Happened to New York's Plans for Single-Payer Health Care?" *The Nation*, May 2. Accessed September 16, 2020. https://www.thenation.com/article/archive/single-payer-new-york-health-act/.

Liu, Jodi, Chapin White, Sarah A. Nowak, Asa Wilks, Jamie Ryan, and Christine Eibner. 2018. *An Assessment of the New York Health Act: A Single-Payer Option for New York State*. Santa Monica, CA: RAND Corporation. Accessed September 16, 2020. https://www.rand.org/content/dam/rand/pubs/research_reports/RR2400/RR2424/RAND_RR2424.pdf.

Marcus, Ruth. 2019. "When It Comes to Medicare-for-All, Listen to Nancy Pelosi." *Washington Post*, November 4. Accessed August 29, 2020. https://www.washingtonpost

.com/opinions/warrens-health-care-plan-is-festooned-with-magic-asterisks/2019/11/04/7fe10b12-ff46-11e9-9518-1e76abc088b6_story.html.

Marmor, Theodore. 1970. *The Politics of Medicare*. New York: Aldine de Gruyter.

Matthews, Dylan. 2017. "Single-Payer Health Care Failed Miserably in Colorado Last Year. Here's Why." Vox, September 14. Accessed August 29, 2020. https://www.vox.com/policy-and-politics/2017/9/14/16296132/colorado-single-payer-ballot-initiative-failure.

McConnell, Mitch. 2017. "McConnell on Obamacare: The American People Deserve a Better Way Forward." September 26. Accessed August 28, 2020. https://www.mcconnell.senate.gov/public/index.cfm/pressreleases?ID=62BC3330-7DCC-4C42-98E3-22595403850B.

Newport, Frank. 2016. "American Public Opinion and Sanders' Proposal for Single-Payer Health System." Gallup, March 11. Accessed October 1, 2020. https://news.gallup.com/opinion/polling-matters/189902/american-public-opinion-sanders-proposal-single-payer-healthcare-system.aspx.

Newport, Frank. 2018. "Government Favored to Ensure Healthcare, but Not Deliver It." Gallup, December 3. Accessed October 2, 2020. https://news.gallup.com/poll/245105/government-favored-ensure-healthcare-not-deliver.aspx.

Oberlander, Jonathan. 2016. "The Virtues and Vices of Single-Payer Health Care." *New England Journal of Medicine* 374, no. 15: 1401–1403. Accessed September 26, 2020. https://www.nejm.org/doi/full/10.1056/NEJMp1602009.

Pear, Robert. 2019. "Health Care and Insurance Industries Mobilize to Kill 'Medicare for All.'" *New York Times*, February 23. Accessed September 26, 2020. https://www.nytimes.com/2019/02/23/us/politics/medicare-for-all-lobbyists.html.

Pew Research Center. 2020. "As Voting Begins, Democrats Are Upbeat about the 2020 Field, Divided in Their Preferences." Accessed March 11, 2021. https://www.pewresearch.org/politics/2020/01/30/political-values-and-democratic-candidate-support/.

Pipes, Sally. 2018. "The Future of Health Care Is on the 2018 Ballot." *Washington Examiner*, November 4. Accessed October 1, 2020. https://www.washingtonexaminer.com/opinion/the-future-of-healthcare-is-on-the-2018-ballot.

Pozen, Robert. 2019. "'Medicare for All' Isn't Medicare." *Wall Street Journal*, May 1. Accessed March 13, 2021. https://www.wsj.com/articles/medicare-for-all-isnt-medicare-11556750380.

Re, Gregg. 2018. "Ocasio-Cortez: 'Medicare for All' Would Save 'Very Large Amount of Money,' despite Studies Showing $30T Cost." Fox News, September 16. Accessed August 25, 2020. https://www.foxnews.com/politics/ocasio-cortez-medicare-for-all-would-save-very-large-amount-of-money-despite-studies-showing-30t-cost.

Rosenbaum, Lisa. 2020. "Costs, Benefits, and Sacred Values." *New England Journal of Medicine* 382: 101–104. Accessed September 18, 2020. https://www.nejm.org/doi/full/10.1056/NEJMp1916615.

Rubin, Jennifer. 2019. "Jobs Disappear under Medicare for All." *Washington Post*, November 26. Accessed August 29, 2020. https://www.washingtonpost.com/opinions/2019/11/26/more-bad-news-medicare-for-all/.

Sanders, Bernie. 2016. "Health Care as a Human Right—Medicare For All." Accessed September 26, 2020. https://berniesanders.com/issues/medicare-for-all/.

Sanders, Bernie. 2018a. "Sanders Responds to Trump's Lies on Medicare for All." October 10. Accessed March 11, 2021. https://www.sanders.senate.gov/press-releases/sanders-responds-to-trumps-lies-on-medicare-for-all/.

Sanders, Bernie. 2018b. "Trump Lies about 'Medicare for All' and He's Made Health Care Worse." *USA Today*, October 11. Accessed September 13, 2020. https://www.usatoday.com/story/opinion/2018/10/11/bernie-sanders-donald-trump-lies-medicare-all-health-care-column/1594863002/.

Schulman, Kevin, and Arnold Milstein. 2019. "The Implications of 'Medicare for All' for US Hospitals." *JAMA* 321, no. 17: 1661–1662. Accessed September 13, 2020. https://jamanetwork.com/journals/jama/fullarticle/2730485.

Shepard, Steven. 2017. "Poll: Plurality Supports Single-Payer Health Care." Politico, September 20. Accessed September 13, 2020. https://www.politico.com/story/2017/09/20/single-payer-health-care-poll-242907.

Social Security Administration. 2020. "Vote Tallies for Passage of Medicare in 1965 Actions in Congress." Accessed November 1, 2020. https://www.ssa.gov/history/tally65.html.

Song, Zirui. 2019. "The Pricing of Care under Medicare for All: Implications and Policy Choices." *JAMA* 322, no. 5: 395–396. Accessed September 30, 2020. https://jamanetwork.com/journals/jama/fullarticle/2737591.

Stapleton, Carey, E. Scott Adler, and Anand Sohkey. 2016. "The 2016 Colorado Political Climate Study." University of Colorado Boulder. Accessed August 29, 2020. https://projects.fivethirtyeight.com/polls/20161102_CO_1.pdf.

Sunstein, Cass. 2019. "It's Not Cowardly to Worry about Medicare for All." *Twin Cities Pioneer Press*, August 11. Accessed September 13, 2020. https://www.twincities.com/2019/08/11/cass-sunstein-its-not-cowardly-to-worry-about-medicare-for-all/.

Trump, Donald. 2018a. "Congressional Democrats Want to Take Money from Hardworking Americans to Fund Failed Socialist Policies." October 23. Accessed March 11, 2021. https://trumpwhitehouse.archives.gov/briefings-statements/congressional-democrats-want-take-money-hardworking-americans-fund-failed-socialist-policies/.

Trump, Donald. 2018b. "Democrats 'Medicare for All' Plan Will Demolish Promises to Seniors. *USA Today*, October 10. Accessed August 25, 2020. https://www.usatoday.com/story/opinion/2018/10/10/donald-trump-democrats-open-borders-medicare-all-single-payer-column/1560533002/.

U.S. Senate. 2019. "S.1129 - Medicare for All Act of 2019." Accessed March 13, 2021. https://www.congress.gov/bill/116th-congress/senate-bill/1129?q=%7B%22search%22%3A%5B%22s+1129%22%5D%7D&s=1&r=3.

Verma, Seema. 2018. "Remarks by Administrator Seema Verma at the America's Health Insurance Plans (AHIP) 2018 National Conference on Medicare." October 16. Accessed March 11, 2021. https://www.cms.gov/newsroom/press-releases/speech-remarks-administrator-seema-verma-americas-health-insurance-plans-ahip-2018-national.

Verma, Seema. 2019. "Remarks by Administrator Seema Verma at the Federation of American Hospitals 2019 Public Policy Conference." March 4. Accessed August 25, 2020. https://www.cms.gov/newsroom/press-releases/speech-remarks-administrator-seema-verma-federation-american-hospitals-2019-public-policy-conference.

Vielkind, Jimmy. 2019. "New York Lawmakers Weigh Single-Payer Health Bill." *Wall Street Journal*, May 28. Accessed September 16, 2020. https://www.wsj.com/articles/new-york-state-lawmakers-weigh-single-payer-health-bill-11559077567.

Wall Street Journal. 2019a. "Bernie's Medicare-for-All Bailout." August 14. Accessed September 4, 2020.https://www.wsj.com/articles/bernies-medicare-for-all-bailout-11565824740.

Wall Street Journal. 2019b. "The Burdens of BernieCare." May 5. Accessed September 13, 2020. https://www.wsj.com/articles/the-burdens-of-berniecare-11557091123.

Wall Street Journal. 2019c. "Public Unions vs. Single-Payer." May 30. Accessed September 4, 2020. https://www.wsj.com/articles/public-unions-vs-single-payer-11559258778.

Warren, Elizabeth. 2018. "Ending the Stranglehold of Health Care Costs on American Families." Accessed September 26, 2020. https://elizabethwarren.com/plans/paying-for-m4a.

Wellstone, Paul, and Ellen Shaffer. 1993. "The American Health Security Act – A Single -Payer Proposal." *New England Journal of Medicine* 328 no. 20: 1489–1493. Accessed March 13, 2021. https://www.nejm.org/doi/full/10.1056/nejm199305203282013.

Wheaton, Sarah. 2014a. "Vermont Bails on Single-Payer Health Care." Politico, December 17. Accessed August 28, 2020. https://www.politico.com/story/2014/12/vermont -peter-shumlin-single-payer-health-care-113653.

Wheaton, Sarah. 2014b. "Why Single-Payer Died in Vermont." Politico, December 20. Accessed August 29, 2020. https://www.politico.com/story/2014/12/single-payer-vermont-113711.

Woolhandler, Steffie, and David Himmelstein. 2003. "Costs of Heath Care Administration in the United States and Canada." *New England Journal of Medicine* 349, no. 8. Accessed October 1, 2020. https://www.nejm.org/doi/full/10.1056/nejmsa022033.

Young, Shannon. 2019. "Lawmakers Face an Uphill Climb on Single-Payer in 2020." Politico, December 30. Accessed September 16, 2020. https://www.politico.com/states /new-york/albany/story/2019/12/30/lawmakers-face-an-uphill-climb-on-single-payer -in-2020-1235558.

Vaccine Mandates

At a Glance

Vaccination represents a fundamental achievement in medicine and public health. While Democrats and Republicans have generally agreed about the effectiveness of vaccines as public health measures, partisan controversy has focused on government-imposed vaccine mandates and what exemptions, if any, should be permitted. In 2020, all 50 states and Washington, DC, had vaccination requirements for schoolchildren, and they all provided for medical exemptions to these state mandates. The District of Columbia and 45 states allow religious exemptions, and 15 states allow philosophical exemptions; however, 5 states—California, Maine, Mississippi, New York, and West Virginia—do not allow nonmedical exemptions to their state vaccination mandates.

Democrats and Republicans hold different positions on whether vaccine mandates constrain individual liberty, consumer freedom, and the parental right to decide what most benefits children. The two parties have also disagreed about what constitutes appropriate levels of government oversight and regulation. Democrats have expressed strong support for extensive vaccine mandates and advocated against allowing exemptions for reasons other than those with medical relevance. In this context, Democrats contend that the public health benefits of vaccination outweigh any challenges that mandates may pose to individual liberty, and, therefore, substantial government oversight and regulation is warranted. Republicans also support vaccination but contend that in some situations nonmedical exemptions from vaccine mandates should be permitted. In this context, Republicans argue that extensive vaccine mandates threaten the personal liberty of consumers and parents. For this reason, Republicans criticize government-imposed vaccine mandates. In recent years, partisan rhetoric has increasingly focused on whether nonmedical exemptions should be permitted, whether governments have the right to impose strict mandates that may infringe upon individual liberty and freedom of choice, and the implications of recent outbreaks of vaccine-preventable diseases for policy decisions.

According to Many Democrats . . .

- Vaccinations are valuable tools in protecting public health and American families.
- The public health benefits delivered by vaccine mandates outweigh the constraints that mandates may pose to individual liberty and freedom of choice, which are not absolute.
- Federal and state governments have a responsibility to enforce vaccine mandates to prevent outbreaks and to protect the health and lives of American citizens.
- Recent outbreaks of vaccine-preventable diseases illustrate the need for stricter vaccine mandates.
- Medical exemptions to vaccine mandates may be permitted, but religious and philosophical exemptions should not be allowed.

According to Many Republicans . . .

- Vaccinations are valuable tools in protecting public health and American families.
- Vaccine mandates infringe on individual liberty and freedom of choice.
- Federal and state governments need to balance their responsibility to protect the health and lives of citizens with the responsibility of ensuring that citizens can preserve individual liberty and freedom of choice.
- Recent outbreaks of vaccine-preventable diseases require policy action, but imposing stricter vaccine mandates may not be the most effective response.
- In addition to medical exemptions, there are scenarios that warrant exemptions from vaccine mandates for religious and philosophical reasons.

Overview

The development of vaccines to prevent the spread of infectious disease has been one of the greatest public health triumphs in modern history. Immunizations administered during childhood and into adolescence dramatically reduced deaths and injuries previously associated with outbreaks of infectious diseases such as measles, polio, and tuberculosis (Siddiqui, Salmon, and Omer 2013). Although some on the political fringe may deny the efficacy of vaccination or trade in conspiracy theories, such claims and beliefs have not found much support among mainstream Democratic or Republican officials or lawmakers. But guided by their respective interpretations of individual liberty and freedom of choice and their preferred policy responses to outbreaks of vaccine-preventable diseases, Democrats and Republicans do differ in how they view vaccine mandates. American conservatives have

Vaccines Are "Safe, Effective, and Life-Saving"

Sen. Patty Murray (D-WA) offered the following comments at the March 5, 2019, Senate HELP hearing, emphasizing the importance of strengthening vaccine education campaigns.

Vaccine coverage rates are declining in certain areas, contributing to the rise in preventable outbreaks. Like in Clark County, Washington, where public health officials continue to respond to a measles outbreak. The immunization rate among children in that community is less than 70 percent—far below what is needed to keep families safe. The result is a true public health emergency—over 70 confirmed cases and counting. And the majority of cases have affected children under ten years old who are unvaccinated.

These outbreaks are a clear sign we have to do more to address vaccine hesitancy and make sure parents have the facts they need to understand the science: vaccines are safe, effective, and life-saving. Parents across the country want to do what is best for their families to keep them safe—which is why they need to be armed with knowledge about the importance of vaccination. And why we need research into vaccine communication tools and strategies to help us better educate people to address vaccine hesitancy, and build vaccine confidence. We also need to understand the roles social media and online misinformation play in spreading dangerous rumors and falsehoods. And we need to better prepare the full spectrum of health care providers—who are often the professionals people trust most—to counter vaccine hesitancy and promote vaccination.

Source

U.S. Senate Committee on Health, Education, Labor, and Pensions. 2019. "Murray Stresses Need to Build Vaccine Confidence, Educate People about How Vaccines Are Safe, Effective, and Life-Saving." March 5, 2019. Accessed February 20, 2021. https://www.help.Senate.gov/ranking/newsroom/press/murray-stresses-need-to-build-vaccine-confidence-educate-people-about-how-vaccines-are-safe-effective-and-life-saving.

traditionally endorsed vaccination while simultaneously advocating for individual liberty and parental freedom of choice. On the other hand, American liberals have emphasized that the public health benefits delivered by vaccine mandates demonstrate the need for stricter vaccination requirements and increased policy action.

This philosophical divide has precedents dating to the 19th century. During that time, many states enacted compulsory smallpox vaccination laws for children and adults. Penalties for refusing immunizations against smallpox included exclusion from school systems for children and substantial fines or quarantine for adults (Colgrove 2016). The 1905 U.S. Supreme Court case *Jacobson v. Massachusetts* upheld the right of state governments to enact compulsory vaccine mandates. The court's decision reflected the widely held belief that preventing outbreaks of vaccine-preventable diseases that threaten public health warranted the forfeiture of individual liberty (Gostin 2005).

The use of coercion to ensure vaccine compliance raises important questions about individual liberty, freedom of choice, and government regulation in the name of public health. By 2019, all states mandated immunization for enrollment in public schools, and all states also allowed medical exemptions to those mandates. However, states vary with respect to which vaccines are mandated. For example, Connecticut, New Jersey, Ohio, and Rhode Island have mandated the influenza vaccine for children in childcare facilities, but Rhode Island and Virginia (and the District of Columbia) are the only states that have mandated the human papillomavirus (HPV) vaccine for secondary school students.

The criteria for religious and philosophical exemptions vary greatly from state to state. The District of Columbia and 45 states permit religious exemptions, and 15 states also include philosophical exemptions (National Conference of State Legislatures 2019). Of the 5 states that do not allow religious exemptions, 2 are traditionally blue states (California and New York), 2 are red states (Mississippi and West Virginia), and 1 is a state that has voted blue during presidential elections since 1992 but alternated parties in the governorship during that time (Maine). States that allow philosophical exemptions have specific provisions and limitations. For example, Virginia only allows personal exemptions for HPV, while Washington allows personal exemptions for all vaccines except the measles, mumps, and rubella (MMR) vaccine. In Arizona, personal exemptions are only valid for enrolled schoolchildren.

The use of religious and philosophical exemptions has become a great source of controversy because of the resurgence of vaccine-preventable diseases once deemed nearly eradicated. Following a 2014 outbreak of measles at Disneyland in California, some municipalities and state governments that once allowed religious and philosophical exemptions began enacting legislation to strictly regulate, if not eliminate, such exemptions. In February 2015, California's Democratic U.S. senators, Barbara Boxer and Dianne Feinstein, drafted a letter to Diana Dooley, the state's Health and Human Services secretary, arguing that "there should be no such thing as a philosophical or personal belief exemption" (Willon and McGreevy 2015). As a result of the 2014 outbreak, California Democratic state senators Richard Pan and Ben Allen coauthored S.B. 277, which required all children enrolled in public and private schools or daycare centers to be immunized against 10 different childhood diseases, including measles. The bill also eliminated religious and philosophical exemptions (S.B. 277).

In June 2015, the California State Senate voted on S.B. 277 largely along party lines. Of the 24 senators who voted for the bill, 22 were Democrats; of the 14 senators who voted against the bill, 12 were Republicans. Democratic state senator Bill Monning framed his support as upholding a social contract among citizens: "You're making a choice not just for your child, not just for your family, but a choice that affects another person's child" (White 2015). On the other hand, Republican state senator Joel Anderson argued the bill violated religious freedom: "So now what I'm getting from this is I have to commit a felony and be sentenced to prison before I can practice my faith" (Koseff 2015). Gov. Jerry Brown (D) signed the bill on June 30, 2015 (California Legislative Information 2015). Brown remarked, "While it's true that no medical intervention is without risk, the evidence shows that immunization powerfully benefits and protects the community" (ABC7 San Francisco 2015). Following implementation, California's school vaccination rate reached its highest level since 2001, and approximately 96 percent of kindergarteners entering school for the 2016–2017 school year had received all the required vaccinations under S.B. 277 (Sun 2017).

Although S.B. 277 proved successful in California, vaccine-preventable disease outbreaks have continued elsewhere around the country in recent years. In 2019, hundreds of cases of measles were confirmed in 26 different states (Belluck and Hassan 2019). Politicians from both sides of the aisle proposed different methods to mitigate the outbreak of a disease once declared eradicated in the United States. For their part, federal regulators also voiced concern with the perceived lack of state action. In February 2019, the commissioner of the U.S. Food and Drug Administration, Dr. Scott Gottlieb, suggested the possibility of federal intervention if state governments refused to narrow their exemption policies. He argued, "Some states are engaging in such wide exemptions that they're creating the opportunity for outbreaks on a scale that is going to have national implications" (Gstalter 2019).

Between 2014 and 2019, public opinion polls demonstrated a growing ideological divide among Democrats and Republicans with respect to vaccine mandates. In one 2015 Pew Research Center poll, 87 percent of Democrats and 89 percent of Republicans overwhelmingly agreed that the MMR vaccine was safe for children (Pew Research Center 2015). In 2017, 90 percent of self-identified liberal respondents supported an MMR vaccine mandate compared to 73 percent of conservative respondents. Conservatives were almost three times more likely than liberals to support the parental right to vaccine exemption (Pew Research Center 2017). By 2019, public polls still indicated general support for vaccine mandates despite a continued downward trend among liberals and conservatives alike: 70 percent of self-identified liberals and 54 percent of conservatives favored vaccine mandates according to one poll (Sheffield 2019). Although a majority of Americans on both sides of the aisle have indicated support for vaccine mandates, partisan differences continue to shape vaccine-related policy making. One 2019 analysis of state vaccine exemption laws determined that while most bills proposed between 2011 and 2017 expanded exemption categories, those that were actually enacted ultimately restricted nonmedical exemptions (Goldstein, Suder, and Purtle 2019).

The COVID-19 pandemic cast partisan debates about vaccination mandates in new light. As COVID-19 became a pressing public health crisis in the United States throughout 2020, public attention turned to whether and when an FDA-approved COVID-19 vaccine would be available to the American public. In May 2020, the Trump administration announced Operation Warp Speed, a public-private partnership charged with developing and distributing a COVID-19 vaccine. Between July and September, however, the percentage of Americans who indicated a willingness to be vaccinated against COVID-19 dropped from 66 percent to 50 percent. During that time, polling data indicated that Democrats were generally more willing to get vaccinated against COVID-19 than Republicans (Saad 2020). Democratic willingness dropped from 78 percent to 53 percent between August 17 and September 30 after President Trump announced on Labor Day that "we're going to have a vaccine very soon, maybe even before a very special date. You know what date I'm talking about" (Phelps 2020). A Pew Research Center poll conducted the week after Trump's statement indicated bipartisan concern that the FDA vaccine approval process would move too fast, with 69 percent of Republicans and 86 percent of Democrats in agreement (Tyson, Johnson, and Funk 2020). In December 2020, the Food and Drug Administration granted the first emergency use authorization to a COVID-19 vaccine. Soon thereafter, states began vaccinating certain priority populations according to each state's eligibility guidelines.

Democrats on Vaccine Mandates

The resurgence of vaccine-preventable diseases in the United States in the early 21st century has elevated Democratic calls for stricter vaccine mandates. Across the United States, Democrats introduced new legislation to enforce stricter vaccine mandates and eliminate certain exemptions, and many Democratic-led states succeeded in turning these bills into laws. In doing so, Democrats maintained that the public health benefits delivered by vaccination mandates outweighed any challenge that these mandates posed to individual liberty and freedom of choice. For Democrats, disease outbreaks of the 2010s illuminated the need for federal and state regulatory agencies to enact stricter requirements and to limit, or even eliminate, nonmedical exemptions.

In 2019, Democrats in Arizona, Colorado, Maine, New Jersey, New York, and Washington sought to bolster vaccine mandates in their respective states. In three of those states—Colorado, Maine, and Washington—stricter mandates moved forward with only Democratic support. In December 2019, the New Jersey State Senate postponed a vote on a bill that would have eliminated religious exemptions to the state's vaccination requirements. Senate President Stephen Sweeney (D) promised to revive the bill: "We're not walking away from it" (Otterman and Tully 2019). In February 2020, legislators in Illinois introduced a bill to eliminate religious exemptions, and legislators in Connecticut voted to approve a similar bill in committee. However, in March, the General Assemblies in both states suspended their 2020 legislative sessions before taking any action on the bills due to the COVID-19 pandemic.

Assemblywoman Lorena Gonzalez (D-CA) offered a fairly representative argument for her party's stance on vaccination exemptions and penalties, stating that if "your personal decision [to go unvaccinated] is going to affect other kids in the community," the state had the right to impose limitations on unvaccinated children (Kluger 2019). In April 2019, the Colorado House of Representatives approved H.B. 1312, which required parents to submit exemption request forms in person. Representative Kyle Mullica (D), who sponsored the bill, justified the measure as a matter a public safety: "It's about creating a safe environment for them where they can't catch a preventable disease" (Garcia 2019). In May 2019, the bill died in the state senate after Democrats temporarily delayed debate on the matter, in part for procedural reasons (Senate Majority Leader Steve Fenberg argued that there was not enough time for sufficient debate) and practical reasons (Gov. Jared Polis had already objected to the bill) (Staver 2019b).

Democrats frequently argue that state governments have a responsibility to enforce vaccine mandates to prevent outbreaks and to protect the health and lives of American citizens. In March 2019, Matt Ritter (D), Connecticut's House Majority Leader, promised that the General Assembly would vote on eliminating religious exemptions for vaccinations for school-aged children within a year. John Elliott, a fellow Democratic state representative, supported Ritter's vow. Elliott asked, "Do we want to wait until we have deaths and large scale outbreaks or do we want to solve the problem before it gets to Connecticut?" (Stuart 2019b). Although the Public Health Committee passed the bill in February 2020, the bill failed to move to the House floor after the COVID-19 pandemic forced the early adjournment of the 2020 legislative session in April 2020 (Carlesso 2020). Ritter promised to eliminate religious exemptions in Connecticut the same month that officials in Rockland County, New York, declared a state of emergency following 100 confirmed cases of measles. Rockland County officials announced that minors who had not received the MMR vaccine against measles would be banned from public places until they received the immunization or until the ban expired in 30 days. Furthermore, the county announced that parents and guardians found in violation of the ban would be held accountable and could face fines up to $500 or six months in jail (Bever 2019).

In May 2019, Connecticut Attorney General William Tong (D) issued a formal opinion to justify narrowing exemptions in the state. As he explained, "There is no serious or reasonable dispute as to the State's broad authority to require and regulate immunizations for children: the law is clear that the State of Connecticut may create, eliminate, or suspend the religious exemption" (Stuart 2019a). In September 2019, Gov. Ned Lamont (D) endorsed narrowing exemptions within the state and encouraged the state legislature to act on the matter. Lamont argued, "Parents will still have a choice regarding the medical decisions for their children, but if you make the choice not to protect your children against preventable diseases then alternate decisions must be made about where to educate your children" (Connecticut's Official State Website 2019).

Democrats have argued that recent outbreaks of vaccine-preventable diseases illuminate the need for stricter vaccine mandates. In Colorado, Democratic state representative Kyle Mullica argued, "We see outbreaks happening all over the country right now. I'd rather be proactive, than reactive on something. We shouldn't have to wait for a kid to die, to declare a state of emergency, before we act on something" (Frank 2019). In May 2019, Gov. Janet Mills (D) of Maine signed into law LD 798, which ended all nonmedical vaccine exemptions. Upon the bill's passage with predominantly Democratic support in the state house and senate, sponsor Ryan Tipping (D) declared that the lawmakers felt that they had little choice but to act: "As we hear more reports of measles and other preventable diseases in Maine and across the country, it has become clear that we must act to ensure the health of our communities" (WMTW 2019). While many states have required vaccination for public school enrollment, Democratic legislators in some states have sought to expand mandates to cover other environments where students from public and private schools may congregate. For example, in June 2019, New York state senator David Carlucci (D) introduced a bill mandating measles vaccinations for all children attending New York summer camps (Hogan 2019).

Democrats have maintained that while medical exemptions to vaccine mandates are permissible for people with health issues that might be exacerbated by vaccination, religious and philosophical exemptions should not be allowed. Despite 166 confirmed cases of measles, a judge lifted the March 2019 Rockland County ban one week later. According to reports, the judge lifted the ban due to the number of confirmed measles cases not meeting the legal requirements for issuing a state of emergency. New York state senator Carlucci responded, "It's very simple: Just remove all nonmedical exemptions. Make it clear and simple to school administrators, make it clear and simple to parents. Cut through the nonsense that's out there and let's govern by science or else, we're going to have a real, real problem on our hands" (CBS News 2019).

By April 2019, 425 cases of measles had prompted New York state legislators to introduce bills eliminating nonmedical exemptions. Senate bill S2994 and state assembly bill A2371 mirrored the legislation that California enacted in 2015 by eliminating all nonmedical exemptions. Democratic state senator Brad Hoylman declared, "New York's religious belief exemption is a personal belief loophole" (Goldblatt and Yellin 2019). Another Democratic assembly member, Jeffrey Dinowitz, argued that religious beliefs did not trump public safety: "I'm not aware of anything in the Torah, the Bible, the Koran or anything else that suggests you should not get vaccinated" (Kleeper 2019). In June 2019, the Democratic-led New York State Senate and Assembly repealed the state's religious exemption, which Gov. Andrew Cuomo (D) then signed into law. Cuomo emphasized that "I understand freedom of religion. . . . I have heard the anti-vaxxers' theory, but I believe both are overwhelmed by the public health risk" (Kleeper 2019).

Unlike Cuomo and Connecticut's Ned Lamont, other Democratic governors, such as Colorado's Jared Polis, have been disinclined to narrow vaccination exemptions in the name of public health. Although Democratic legislators in Colorado sought to strengthen the state's vaccine mandate, Polis opposed eliminating non-medical exemptions. In one March 2019 statement, Polis argued, "Forcing people to receive shots they don't want creates mistrust of government, mistrust of vaccinations, and would ultimately backfire and hurt public health" (Seaman 2019). Polis instead instructed legislators to focus on improving access to vaccination and educating the public about its benefits. Polis defended his approach as a "third way between the government forcing people to get shots, which is counterproductive, and simply allowing these [vaccination] rates to go down, which is counterproductive to public health and will result in people dying" (Staver 2019a).

Republicans on Vaccination Mandates

Republicans have argued that state governments must strike a balance between protecting public health and preserving individual liberty and freedom of choice. Maintaining that exemptions for religious and philosophical reasons are warranted, Republicans contend that because vaccine mandates constrain individual liberty, policy makers should remain cognizant of parental rights when expanding vaccine mandates.

In April 2019, the Washington State Senate passed a bill that eliminated the personal belief exemption for the MMR vaccine. Under the new legislation, medical exemptions for the MMR vaccine would still be permitted, and the bill did not eliminate religious or philosophical exemptions for other required immunizations. Republican state representative Joe Schmick opposed the bill, maintaining that "the parents should be making this call, and they should be the ones to decide" (La Courte 2019).

In May 2019, the Maine State Senate passed a bill eliminating the philosophical exemption while retaining medical and religious exemptions. However, the state house of representatives insisted that the bill eliminate the religious and philosophical exemptions. Republican state representatives argued that eliminating these exemptions violated the principles of religious freedom and freedom of choice. Representative Justin Fecteau (R) remarked, "I feel that starting something and changing the rules halfway through sounds more like a game of Monopoly with a toddler than a sound state policy" (Thistle 2019). Further south, two Republican state senators in Mississippi introduced vaccine exemption bills during the 2019 legislation session despite the fact that the state had not recorded any new cases of measles since the early 1990s. One sponsor promoted his proposed exemption by claiming that it was not the "government's role to tell every parent how to raise their child" (Pittman 2019). Neither bill advanced out of committee, nor did similar efforts during the previous legislative session, but their introduction nevertheless demonstrated the commitment to religious freedom among some American conservatives.

Republicans also argue that state governments need to balance their responsibility to protect the health and lives of citizens with the responsibility of ensuring that the constitutional rights of citizens are preserved. When the vaccine mandate debate reemerged in Colorado in 2019, Democratic state legislators contemplated new legislation that would eliminate the state's philosophical exemption against vaccination. Most members of the state GOP lined up in opposition to the idea. Colorado state representative Shane Sandridge (R) emphasized to his constituents that "we are fighting for your rights. You know what's best for your children" (Garcia 2019). This was not a new position for Colorado Republicans to take. In 2014, they had blocked legislation that would have required parents to obtain permission from a licensed physician if they did not vaccinate their children. At that time, Republican state senator Kevin Lundberg surmised, "This boils down to, does the

Persuasion, Not Force, Is the Appropriate Way to Encourage Vaccination

Sen. Rand Paul (R-KY) offered the following comments at the March 5, 2019, Senate HELP hearing, raising his concern over influenza vaccine mandates.

> Now proponents of mandatory government vaccination argue that parents who refuse to vaccinate their children risk spreading these diseases to the immune-compromised community. There doesn't seem to be enough evidence of this happening to be recorded as a statistic, but it could happen. But if the fear of this is valid, are we to find that next we'll be mandating flu vaccines? Between 12,000 and 56,000 people die from the flu or are said to die from the flu in America, and there's estimated to be a few hundred from measles. So I would guess that those who want to mandate the measles [vaccine] will be after us on the flu next. Yet the current science only allows for "educated guessing" when it comes to the flu vaccine. Each year, before that year's flu strain is known, scientists put their best guess into that year's vaccine. Some years, it's completely wrong; we vaccinate for the wrong strain of flu. Yet five states already mandate flu vaccines. Is it really appropriate to mandate a vaccine that more often than not vaccinates for the wrong flu strain?
>
> As we contemplate forcing parents to choose this or that vaccine, I think it's important to remember that force is not consistent with the American story, nor is force consistent with the liberty our forefathers sought when they came to America. I don't think you have to have one or the other, though. I'm not here to say "don't vaccinate your kids." If this hearing is for persuasion, I'm all for the persuasion. I vaccinated myself. I vaccinated my kids. For myself and my children, I believe that the benefits of vaccines greatly outweigh the risks, but I still do not favor giving up on liberty for a false sense of security.

Source

U.S. Senate Committee on Health, Education, Labor, and Pensions. 2019. "Vaccines Save Lives: What Is Driving Preventable Disease Outbreaks?" March 5, 2019. Accessed February 20, 2021. https://www.help.Senate.gov/hearings/vaccines-save-lives-what-is-driving-preventable-disease-outbreaks.

government force everyone to conform or do we empower everyone to make decisions on their own?" (Riccardi 2015).

Similarly, when the Maine Legislature considered repealing its religious exemption for vaccination in 2019, Republican state senator Brad Farrin insisted that "a vote against this bill isn't a vote against vaccinations, it's a vote in support of parental choice and religious freedoms" (Shepherd 2019). On the other side of the country, the Democratic-majority Oregon House of Representatives passed a 2019 bill to eliminate vaccination exemptions for religious, personal, or philosophical reasons. House bill 3063 passed with a vote of 35–25, with only two Republicans voting in favor. Under the legislation, children who had not received all required immunizations could attend school until a specified deadline, but unvaccinated children would have to be homeschooled or elect to complete online coursework after the deadline. Several Republican state representatives opposed the bill after its passage in the house. Republican state representative Bill Post, for example, urged his colleagues to "say no to forcing families to submit to this one size fits all government meddling in the practice of medicine" (Stracqualursi 2019). Although Democrats held supermajorities in the Oregon House of Representatives and Senate and also occupied the governor's office, senate Democrats abandoned the bill as part of a deal to secure Republican support for school funding in another tax bill. As bill cosponsor Cheri Helt (R) concluded, "It's disappointing that once again the loudest, most extreme voices in our politics prevailed and the sensible-center and thoughtful policy-making lost" (Blumberg 2019).

Republicans have suggested that the resurgence of vaccine-preventable disease outbreaks requires policy action, but they argue that stricter vaccine mandates may not be the most effective response. In February 2019, Arizona legislators endorsed three vaccine-related bills along party lines. Republican state representative Nancy Barto, who sponsored all three bills, argued, "We are here to acknowledge vaccines have a place, but it's every parent's individual right to decide the vaccine's place in the child's life" (Innes 2019). The bills differed from those implemented in other states by expanding rather than narrowing exemption categories, by requiring physicians to offer laboratory tests that measure the level of antibodies in the blood, and by providing parents with vaccine injury guidance.

The year before, Arizona had canceled a pilot vaccine education program at the recommendation of the Governor's Regulatory Review Council, a regulatory body appointed by Gov. Doug Ducey (R) that had received complaints from anti-vaccination parents. Republican state representative Heather Carter, who had helped create the pilot program, expressed disappointment in the decision: "Providing information doesn't take away a parent's choice to seek an exemption. . . . We all want to live in safe and healthy communities" (Innes 2018). Demonstrating an emerging divide among Arizona Republicans, Ducey openly declared that he would refuse to sign any anti-vaccination legislation. As Ducey said, "I'm pro-vaccination and anti-measles" (Forman 2019).

Other Republicans express concerns that narrowing exemptions would take states down a slippery slope toward the elimination of parental freedom to make medical decisions for their children—even while defending vaccination as a public health practice. During a March 2019 U.S. Senate hearing about vaccine-preventable outbreaks, Sen. Rand Paul (R-KY) asserted, "I believe that the benefits of vaccines greatly outweigh the risks, but I still do not favor giving up on liberty for a false sense of security" (Hellmann 2019). When Democratic state representatives in Connecticut announced in April 2019 that they intended to eliminate the state's religious exemption for vaccination, Republican state representative Noreen Kokoruda argued that "anybody who thinks this bill is not just the first step to totally taking parents' rights away and religious exemptions away is wrong" (Stuart 2019c).

Todd M. Olszewski and Amanda McGrath

Further Reading

ABC7 San Francisco. 2015. "Governor Jerry Brown Signs School Vaccination Bill." June 30. Accessed September 19, 2019. https://abc7news.com/politics/governor-jerry-brown-signs-school-vaccination-bill/818476/.

Belluck, Pam, and Adeel Hassan. 2019. "Measles Outbreak Explained: Your Questions Answered." *New York Times*, March 28. Accessed April 11, 2019. https://www.nytimes.com/2019/02/20/us/measles-outbreak.html.

Bever, Lindsey. 2019. "Unvaccinated Children Banned from Public Spaces amid Measles Outbreak in New York Suburb." *Washington Post*, March 27. Accessed May 3, 2019. https://www.washingtonpost.com/health/2019/03/26/unvaccinated-children-banned-public-spaces-amid-measles-outbreak-new-york-suburb/?utm_term=.86e4a7a3ec9b.

Blumberg, Antonia. 2019. "Oregon Democrats Abandon Vaccine Gun Bills in Congress to Republicans." HuffPost, May 14. Accessed September 19, 2019. https://www.huffpost.com/entry/oregon-democrats-kill-vaccine-bill_n_5cdb1df2e4b061f59bf8dcba.

California Legislative Information. 2015. "SB-277 Public Health: Vaccinations." Accessed April 12, 2019. https://leginfo.legislature.ca.gov/faces/billVotesClient.xhtml?bill_id=201520160SB277.

Carlesso, Jenna. 2020. "Proponents of Bill Ending Connecticut's Religious Exemption to Vaccines Eye Special Session for Vote." CT Mirror, May 28. Accessed October 31, 2020. https://ctmirror.org/2020/05/28/proponents-of-bill-ending-connecticuts-religious-exemption-to-vaccines-eye-special-session-for-vote/.

CBS News. 2019. "Rockland County Measles Outbreak: Judge Lifts Ban on Unvaccinated Children, but Not because Outbreak Ended." April 5. Accessed May 3, 2019. https://www.cbsnews.com/news/rockland-county-measles-outbreak-judge-lifts-ban-on-unvaccinated-children-today-2019-04-05/.

Centers for Disease Control and Prevention. 2019. "State Vaccination Requirements." Accessed April 9, 2019. https://www.cdc.gov/vaccines/imz-managers/laws/state-reqs.html.

Cohen, Elizabeth, and John Bonifield. 2019. "FDA Chief: Federal Government Might Step in if States Don't Change Lax Vaccine Laws." CNN, February 20. Accessed April

27, 2019. https://www.cnn.com/2019/02/20/health/vaccine-exemptions-fda-gottlieb/index.html.

Colgrove, James. 2016. "Vaccine Refusal Revisited—The Limits of Public Health Persuasion and Coercion." *New England Journal of Medicine* 375: 1316–1317.

Connecticut's Official State Website. 2019. "Governor Lamont Announces Support for Eliminating Vaccination Exemptions for Children Who Attend Public Schools." September 16. Accessed September 19, 2019. https://portal.ct.gov/Office-of-the-Governor/News/Press-Releases/2019/09-2019/Governor-Lamont-Announces-Support-for-Eliminating-Vaccination-Exemptions.

Forman, Carmen. 2019. "Ducey Declares Arizona 'Pro-Vaccination' State, Vows to Kill Vaccine Exemption Bills." *Arizona Capital Times*, February 27. Accessed September 19, 2019. https://azcapitoltimes.com/news/2019/02/27/ducey-declares-arizona-pro-vaccination-state-vows-to-kill-vaccine-exemption-bills/.

Frank, John. 2019. "A Push to Fix Colorado's Lowest-in-the-Nation Vaccine Rates Has an Unexpected Critic: Jared Polis." *Colorado Sun*, February 21. Accessed April 30, 2019. https://coloradosun.com/2019/02/21/colorado-vaccination-rate-lowest-fix-jared-polis/.

Garcia, Nic. 2019. "Colorado House Advances Vaccination Bill; Polis Insists He Still Wants Changes." *Denver Post*, April 27. Accessed September 18, 2019. https://www.denverpost.com/2019/04/27/colorado-vaccination-bill-vote-measles/.

Goldblatt, Rochel Leah, and Deena Yellin. 2019. "Measles Outbreak: NY Legislators Move to End Religious Exemptions from Vaccines." *Rockland/Westchester Journal News*, April 5. Accessed May 1, 2019. https://www.usatoday.com/story/news/nation/2019/04/05/measles-religious-exemptions-new-york/3373793002/.

Goldstein, Neil, Joanna Suder, and Jonathan Purtle. 2019. "Trends and Characteristics of Proposed and Enacted State Legislation on Childhood Vaccination Exemption, 2011–2017." *American Journal of Public Health* 109, no. 1: 102–107.

Gostin, Lawrence O. 2005. "*Jacobson v Massachusetts* at 100 Years: Police Power and Civil Liberties in Tension." *American Journal of Public Health* 95, no. 4: 576–581.

Gstalter, Morgan. 2019. "FDA Chief Says Feds Might Intervene if States Continue Allowing Vaccine Exemptions." The Hill, February 20. Accessed September 18, 2019. https://thehill.com/policy/healthcare/state-issues/430736-fda-chief-says-feds-might-intervene-if-states-continue-to.

Hellmann, Jessie. 2019. "Paul Says Forced Vaccinations Is 'Giving Up on Liberty for a False Sense of Security.'" The Hill, March 5. Accessed May 1, 2019. https://thehill.com/policy/healthcare/432739-sen-paul-says-forcing-parents-to-vaccinate-their-children-is-giving-up-on.

Hogan, Bernadette. 2019. "Bill Would Mandate Measles Vaccine for Summer Camp Kids." *New York Post*, June 6. Accessed September 19, 2019. https://nypost.com/2019/06/06/bill-would-mandate-measles-vaccine-for-summer-camp-kids/.

Hooks, Christopher. 2019. "An Afternoon with Robert F. Kennedy Jr. and the Texas Anti-Vaccine Movement." *Texas Monthly*, May 4. Accessed May 10, 2019. https://www.texasmonthly.com/politics/an-afternoon-with-robert-f-kennedy-jr-and-the-texas-anti-vaccine-movement/.

Innes, Stephanie. 2018. "Arizona Cancels Vaccine Program after Backlash from Parents Who Don't Vaccinate." *Arizona Republic*, October 18. Accessed September 19, 2019. https://www.azcentral.com/story/news/local/arizona-health/2018/10/18/arizona-course-vaccines-canceled-after-parental-backlash/1149710002/.

Innes, Stephanie. 2019. "Disregarding Health Warnings, Arizona Lawmakers Move Forward on Vaccine Exemptions for Kids." *Arizona Republic*, February 22. Accessed September 19, 2019. https://www.azcentral.com/story/news/local/arizona-health/2019/02/22/disregarding-warnings-arizona-lawmakers-move-forward-vaccine-exemptions/2942680002/.

Kleeper, David. 2019. "New York, Like Maine, End Religious Exemption to Vaccine Mandates." *Portland Press Herald*, June 14. Accessed September 19, 2019. https://www.pressherald.com/2019/06/14/new-york-like-maine-ends-religious-exemption-to-vaccine-mandates/.

Kluger, Jeffrey. 2019. "'They're Chipping Away.' Inside the Grassroots Effort to Fight Mandatory Vaccines." *Time*, June 13. Accessed September 18, 2019. https://time.com/5606250/measles-cases-rise-fighting-vaccines/.

Koerner, Claudia. 2019. "We Asked All of the 2020 Presidential Candidates Their Thoughts on Vaccines. Here's What They Said." Buzzfeed, April 30. Accessed May 1, 2019. https://www.buzzfeednews.com/article/claudiakoerner/2020-presidential-candidates-vaccines-measles-health.

Koseff, Alexei. 2015. "California Senate Approves Vaccination Bill." *Sacramento Bee*, May 14. Accessed September 18, 2019. https://www.sacbee.com/news/politics-government/capitol-alert/article20999688.html.

La Courte, Rachel. 2019 "Washington State Lawmakers Pass Bill Limiting Measles Vaccine Exemptions." *Time*, April 24. Accessed May 10, 2019. http://time.com/5576965/washington-state-measles-vaccine-exemptions/.

McKinley, Jesse. 2019. "Facing Measles Outbreak, N.Y. Lawmakers Want to Let Teenagers Get Vaccines on Their Own." *New York Times*, March 11. Accessed September 18, 2019. https://www.nytimes.com/2019/03/11/nyregion/measles-vaccination-laws-ny.html.

National Conference of State Legislatures. 2019. "States with Religious and Philosophical Exemptions from School Immunization Requirements." Accessed September 18, 2019. http://www.ncsl.org/research/health/school-immunization-exemption-state-laws.aspx.

National Vaccine Information Center. 2018. "California State Vaccination Requirements." Accessed April 11, 2019. https://www.nvic.org/Vaccine-Laws/state-vaccine-requirements/california.aspx.

Ollove, Michael. 2019. "Teens of 'Anti-Vaxxers' Can Get Their Own Vaccines, Some States Say." PEW Charitable Trusts, June 24. Accessed September 18, 2019. https://www.pewtrusts.org/en/research-and-analysis/blogs/stateline/2019/06/24/teens-of-anti-vaxxers-can-get-their-own-vaccines-some-states-say.

Otterman, Sharon, and Tracey Tully. 2019. "Strict Vaccine Law Stumbles in N.J. Legislature." *New York Times*, December 16. Accessed November 1, 2020. https://www.nytimes.com/2019/12/16/nyregion/vaccines-measles-nj-religious-exemptions.html.

Pew Research Center. 2015. "83% Say Measles Vaccine Is Safe for Healthy Children." Accessed September 18, 2019. https://www.people-press.org/2015/02/09/83-percent-say-measles-vaccine-is-safe-for-healthy-children/.

Pew Research Center. 2017. "Vast Majority of Americans Say Benefits of Childhood Vaccines Outweigh Risks." Accessed September 18, 2019. https://www.pewinternet.org/2017/02/02/vast-majority-of-americans-say-benefits-of-childhood-vaccines-outweigh-risks/ps_2017-02-02_vaccines_0-01/.

Phelps, Jordyn. 2020. "Trump Makes Rosy Vaccine Timing Front and Center in Campaign, Predicting It's Possible Before Election Day." ABC News, September 8. Accessed March 9,

2021. https://abcnews.go.com/Politics/trump-makes-rosy-vaccine-timing-front-center-campaign/story?id=72877119.

Pittman, Ashton. 2019. "As Mississippi Evades Measles, Activists Want Vaccine Exemptions." *Jackson Free Press*, May 6. Accessed September 19, 2019. http://www.jacksonfreepress.com/news/2019/may/06/mississippi-evades-measles-activists-want-vaccine-/.

Riccardi, Nicholas. 2015. "Vaccine Skeptics Find Unexpected Allies in Conservative GOP." PBS, February 6. Accessed April 30, 2019. https://www.pbs.org/newshour/health/vaccine-skeptics-find-unexpected-allies-conservative-gop.

Saad, Lydia. 2020. "Americans' Readiness to Get COVID-19 Vaccine Falls to 50%." Gallup, October 12. Accessed November 1, 2020. https://news.gallup.com/poll/321839/readiness-covid-vaccine-falls-past-month.aspx.

S.B. 277. 2015 Reg. Sess. (Cal. 2015). Accessed September 19, 2019. https://leginfo.legislature.ca.gov/faces/billAnalysisClient.xhtml?bill_id=201520160SB277.

Seaman, Jessica. 2019. "Colorado Could Be Next State to Consider Making It Harder for Parents to Opt Kids Out of Vaccines." *Denver Post*, March 4. Accessed September 19, 2019. https://www.denverpost.com/2019/03/04/vaccines-exemptions-opt-out-colorado/.

Sheffield, Matthew. 2019. "Poll Shows Emerging Ideological Divide over Childhood Vaccinations." The Hill, March 14. Accessed September 18, 2019. https://thehill.com/hilltv/what-americas-thinking/434107-polls-show-emerging-ideological-divide-over-childhood.

Shepherd, Michael. 2019. "Old Town Senator Changes Vote, Clearing the Way for Stricter Maine Vaccine Mandate." *Bangor Daily News*, May 14. Accessed September 19, 2019. https://bangordailynews.com/2019/05/14/news/state/old-town-Senator-changes-vote-clearing-the-way-for-stricter-maine-vaccine-mandate/.

Siddiqui, Mariam, Daniel Salmon, and Saad Omer. 2013. "Epidemiology of Vaccine Hesitancy in the United States." *Human Vaccines & Immunotherapeutics* 9, no. 12: 2643–2648.

Staver, Anna. 2019a. "Colorado's Worst-in-the-Nation Measles Vaccination Rate Drops Again." *Denver Post*, June 13. Accessed September 19, 2019. https://www.denverpost.com/2019/06/13/colorado-vaccination-measles-immunization-2019/.

Staver, Anna. 2019b. "Vaccination Bill Dead in Colorado Senate, Sparking Accusations of Putting Politics before Kids' Health." *Denver Post*, May 2. Accessed September 18, 2019. https://www.denverpost.com/2019/05/02/vaccine-vaccination-bill-colorado-Senate/.

Stracqualursi, Veronica. 2019. "Oregon House Passes Bill Removing Religious, Philosophical Exemptions for Vaccines." CNN, May 6. Accessed May 10, 2019. https://www.cnn.com/2019/05/07/politics/oregon-vaccine-bill/index.html.

Stuart, Christine. 2019a. "CT Can Eliminate Religious Exemptions for Child Vaccines, AG Says." *New Haven Register*, May 6. Accessed September 18, 2019. https://www.nhregister.com/local/article/CT-can-eliminate-religious-exemptions-for-child-13823459.php.

Stuart, Christine. 2019b. "CT Dem Leader Seeks to End Religious Exemptions for Children's Vaccines." *New Haven Register*, March 13. Accessed April 30, 2019. https://www.nhregister.com/local/article/Religious-exemptions-for-children-s-vaccines-13685612.php.

Stuart, Christine. 2019c. "Opponents: Parental Rights at Stake in CT Child Vaccination Plan." *New Haven Register*, May 1. Accessed May 10, 2019. https://www.nhregister.com/local/article/Opponents-CT-child-vaccination-plan-first-step-13810107.php.

Sun, Lena H. 2017. "California Vaccination Rate Hits New High after Tougher Immunization Law." *Washington Post*, April 13. Accessed April 12, 2019. https://www.washingtonpost.com/news/to-your-health/wp/2017/04/13/california-vaccination-rate-hits-new-high-after-tougher-immunization-law/.

Thistle, Scott. 2019. "Vaccine Bill Splits Maine House and Senate over Religious Exemption." *Portland Press Herald*, May 9. Accessed March 9, 2021. https://www.pressherald.com/2019/05/09/vaccine-bill-again-splits-maine-house-and-senate-over-religious-exemption/#

Tyson, Alec, Courtney Johnson, and Cary Funk. 2020. "U.S. Public Now Divided over Whether to Get COVID-19 Vaccine." Pew Research Center, September 17. Accessed November 1, 2020. https://www.pewresearch.org/science/2020/09/17/u-s-public-now-divided-over-whether-to-get-covid-19-vaccine/.

U.S. Senate Committee on Health, Education, Labor, and Pensions. 2019a. "Full Committee Hearing—Vaccines Save Lives: What Is Driving Preventable Disease Outbreaks?" March 5. https://www.help.Senate.gov/hearings/vaccines-save-lives-what-is-driving-preventable-disease-outbreaks.

U.S. Senate Committee on Health, Education, Labor, and Pensions. 2019b. "Murray Stresses Need to Build Vaccine Confidence, Educate People about How Vaccines Are Safe, Effective, and Life-Saving." March 5. https://www.help.Senate.gov/ranking/newsroom/press/murray-stresses-need-to-build-vaccine-confidence-educate-people-about-how-vaccines-are-safe-effective-and-life-saving.

White, Jeremy B. 2015. "California Vaccine Bill Clears First Committee." *Sacramento Bee*, April 8. Accessed September 18, 2019. https://www.sacbee.com/news/politics-government/capitol-alert/article17904647.html.

Willon, Phil, and Patrick McGreevy. 2015. "Feinstein, Boxer Urge California to Reconsider Vaccine Exemptions." *Los Angeles Times*, February 4. Accessed April 11, 2019. https://www.latimes.com/local/political/la-me-ln-feinstein-boxer-urge-california-to-restrict-vaccine-exemptions-20150204-story.html.

WMTW. 2019. "Governor Mills Signs Bill Ending Nonmedical Vaccine Exemptions." May 24. Accessed September 19, 2019. https://www.wabi.tv/content/news/Governor-Mills-signs-bill-ending-nonmedical-vaccine-exemptions-510390381.html.

Zipprich, Jennifer, Kathleen Winter, Jill Hacker, Dongxiang Xia, James Watt, and Kathleen Harriman. 2015. "Measles Outbreak—California, December 2014–February 2015." Centers for Disease Control and Prevention, *Morbidity and Mortality Weekly Report* 64, no. 6: 153–154.

Veterans' Health Care

At a Glance

As former Veterans Affairs (VA) Secretary David Shulkin observed, "The mission set forward by President Abraham Lincoln to care for those who have 'borne the battle' is a sacred duty" (Shulkin 2019). As the nation's largest integrated health care delivery system, the VA cared for more than nine million veterans in 2019. The VA health care system includes 170 VA Medical Centers and more than 1,000 outpatient clinics located throughout the U.S. states and territories (U.S. Department of Veterans Affairs 2019b).

Over the past decade, the VA has struggled to fulfill its mission. Concerns about access to care have dogged the VA, and media reports of long delays for appointments eventually brought reform to the forefront of the nation's policy agenda. After investigative journalists exposed "secret" waiting lists at VA hospitals in 2014, policy makers and the public clamored for action. Sen. Tom Coburn (R-OK) charged, "Poor management is costing the department billions of dollars more and compromising veterans' access to medical care" (Devine 2015.

However, even after Congress passed legislation in 2014 that enabled veterans to seek care outside of the VA health care system, concerns about access to care for veterans who lived far from VA facilities or who required prompt access to medical care remained unresolved. In 2018, Congress passed the VA Maintaining Internal Systems and Strengthening Integrated Outside Networks (MISSION) Act, which further expanded veterans' ability to access health care services from private providers. In recent years, however, disputes over the wisdom of increased use of private providers outside of the VA system have escalated. Democrats in particular have painted these efforts as a thinly veiled effort on the part of the Republican party to "privatize" the VA and avoid making the necessary expenditures to upgrade and reform the VA health care system. Republicans have angrily denied these charges, which they say have disrupted the historically bipartisan consensus on veterans' issues.

VA MISSION Act Is a Missed Opportunity

House Minority Leader Nancy Pelosi (D-CA) issued this statement on May 16, 2018, after the House of Representatives passed H.R. 5674, the VA MISSION Act, by a vote of 347–70.

Just as the military pledges to leave no soldier behind on the battlefield, we must leave no veteran behind once they come home. I commend the Committee leaders for working towards a bipartisan, bicameral agreement, but the VA MISSION Act is a missed opportunity.

I salute Ranking Member Tim Walz for his outstanding leadership in ensuring Democratic priorities were included in this legislation. The bill rightly expands caregiver benefits to all eras, replaces the flawed Veterans Choice Program and consolidates the many community care initiatives—but this bill is far from perfect. Without a sustainable source of funding, this bill is fiscally irresponsible and fails to provide a long-term solution to avoid the risk of triggering devastating sequestration and potential budget cuts to critical VA initiatives. The bill also fails to include sufficient guardrails to keep veterans in VA and fulfill the Department's mission at a time of great uncertainty.

This bill opens the doors to VA privatization during a time when the Department has zero leadership. By handing the Trump Administration's ideologues and Koch Brothers the keys to an underfunded VA, Republicans are pushing forth their campaign to dismantle veterans' health care. Over and over again, the GOP has left our veterans behind—slashing Medicaid, gutting SNAP and dismantling vital consumer protections against Wall Street's greed and abuse. Democrats will continue to fight for better health care for our veterans, and to defend VA's mission as the chief coordinator, provider and advocate for our men and women who served.

Source

Pelosi, Nancy. 2019. "Pelosi Statement on Passage of VA MISSION Act." Press Release, May 18, 2018. Accessed February 27, 2021. https://pelosi.house.gov/news/press-releases/pelosi-statement-on-passage-of-va-mission-act.

Democrats support efforts to decrease waiting times for veterans but oppose proposals to increase the use of private doctors and hospitals. They generally believe that the answer is to make greater investments in the VA system to improve its responsiveness and efficiency. Democrats note that the VA is uniquely suited to meet the special health care needs of U.S. veterans. As a fully integrated nationwide system, the VA coordinates primary care, specialty services, and mental and behavioral health care. In contrast, care provided by doctors and hospitals in the wider community can often be fragmented. As a result, Democrats argue that increasing the use of private providers may result in lower-quality services and poorer health care outcomes for veterans.

In addition, Democrats argue that the VA provides high-quality care and that most veterans are satisfied with the quality of care they receive. For Democrats, the solution to the VA's access problems is to strengthen the existing system rather than diverting patients to unfamiliar providers outside of the VA. Finally, Democrats argue that recent GOP proposals to promote veterans' choice of providers are part of a Republican plan to "privatize" the VA. Democrats fear that increasing the use of private providers drains much-needed resources that could be better used to meet the physical and mental health care needs of veterans within the VA system and that such a shift makes veterans more vulnerable to corporate profit-making strategies that do not always make patient health and financial well-being their highest priority.

Republicans support proposals that enable veterans to seek care outside of the VA health care system. Doing so, they argue, will reduce waiting times and improve veterans' ability to access health care services closer to home rather than traveling long distances to VA facilities. Republicans point to ongoing quality problems, such as long waiting times, as a principal justification for expanding the use of private providers. Republicans regard the VA as an institution that underscores the limitations of a sprawling government bureaucracy in which patients must overcome burdensome rules and regulations to access care. Finally, Republicans argue that choice of provider should be available for all veterans, just as it is for Americans with private health coverage. Republicans defend recent proposals such as the VA MISSION Act as a way to enable veterans to choose who provides their health care and where they should receive services.

According to Many Democrats . . .

- Allowing veterans to seek care outside of the VA system will lower the quality of services.
- The VA provides high-quality care to veterans, and most patients are highly satisfied with the health care services they receive.
- Allowing veterans to seek care outside of the VA network is a slippery slope that will lead to the privatization of services over time; additional funding should be used to strengthen the VA.

According to Many Republicans . . .

- Allowing veterans to seek care outside of the VA system will reduce waiting times and allow veterans to obtain the latest treatments and services.
- The VA suffers from chronic quality problems.
- Choice of provider should be available for all veterans; every veteran should be able to select the care (and setting) that best fits his or her needs.

VA MISSION Act Will Give Veterans the Care They Deserve

Sen. Marsha Blackburn (R-TN) spoke on the Senate floor in support of the VA MISSION Act on June 24, 2019.

I join my colleagues today to mark the implementation of an updated and more streamlined health care system for veterans made possible by the VA MISSION Act. Once the new structure is fully in place, members of the military community who have been neglected for far too long will finally get the attention and care they have earned. I say "neglected," because anyone who is familiar with the former VA health care system knows that there was no such thing as "heading to the VA for a quick checkup."

I've heard hundreds of stories from veterans whose experiences with that system would constitute a comedy of errors, if the consequences hadn't taken such a toll on their health and sanity. The reason you hear those stories is because we have asked generations of veterans to put their physical and emotional health in the hands of practitioners whose hands were tied by arbitrary rules and procedures that turned even simple treatments into a logistical nightmare.

But as of this month, we have dealt with many of those roadblocks. The new Community Care Program, which adopted elements of the successful Veteran's Choice Program, will continue to allow veterans to seek care close to home. What was once a cluster of seven programs has been merged into a single system, making the whole process simpler and easier to understand. Options will expand even more with the authorization of local provider agreements, and access to walk-in community clinics.

Source

Blackburn, Marsha. 2019. "VA MISSION Act Will Give Veterans the Care They Deserve." Press Release, February 27, 2021. Accessed March 7, 2021. https://www.blackburn.senate.gov/2019/6/blackburn-va-mission-act-will-give-veterans-care-they-deserve.

Overview

The VA employs its own physicians, nurses, and allied health professionals and operates its own network of hospitals and outpatient clinics. Questions of funding are an ongoing challenge for would-be reformers, as the VA "incurs the high fixed costs of a brick-and-mortar health care system, the largest salaried workforce in the federal government, and a large administration" (Weeks and Auerbach 2014). Today's VA health care system traces its roots to the decade after the Civil War, when homes for disabled veterans opened across the nation. In 1930, President Herbert Hoover reorganized several of the nation's existing veteran's programs, including pension and health care services, into a new independent federal agency—the Veterans' Administration (Kizer, Demakis, and Feussner 2000). After World War II, Congress enacted Public Law 79-293, which established the Department of

Medicine and Surgery within the VA to manage the health care needs of millions of returning veterans. In 1988, the VA was elevated to cabinet-level status, and the Department of Medicine and Surgery was renamed the Veterans Health Administration (Fonseca et al. 1996).

Americans harbor mixed views of the VA. In a 2019 survey, a slight majority of Americans held a favorable view of the VA (52 percent). The VA, however, trailed the Internal Revenue Service (55 percent) in favorability among the public, and more than a third of those polled (38 percent) held an unfavorable view of the VA (Pew Research Center 2019).

The number of veterans in the United States has been declining as older generations of veterans from World War II and Korea reach the end of their lives. In 2000, 26.2 million Americans were military veterans; by 2018, this number had fallen to 18 million. Fewer Americans serve in the military today than in past decades, and many veterans from recent conflicts in Iraq and Afghanistan served multiple tours of duty. In 2018, about 9 percent of veterans—or 1.7 million—are women; as more women serve in the military over time, the proportion of female veterans is projected to rise to 17 percent by 2040 (Vespa 2020). Over the past two decades, the number of women using the VA system tripled, in what one VA consultant described as a "tsunami wave of women veterans" (Kesling 2019). Although roughly 500,000 women now use the VA, the department has been slow to accommodate women's health care needs. Critics also argue that the VA system requires a cultural shift, as one in five women reported harassment while accessing services at VA facilities (Kesling 2019).

Concerns about access to care for veterans are not new. From the 1970s through the early 1990s, concerns about the quality of care in the VA were commonplace. Under the leadership of Dr. Kenneth Kizer in the 1990s, the VA reorganized itself and emerged as a national leader in patient safety, pioneering a national integrated electronic medical record system, bar code technologies to reduce medication errors, and an integrated pharmacy system to automatically refill prescriptions. At the same time, the VA reduced the number of inpatient hospital beds by more than 50 percent and redirecting resources to fund hundreds of outpatient community-based clinics around the nation (Stires 2006). In the 1990s, the VA created new incentives for managers (often equal to 10 percent of their salaries) for meeting performance standards related to quality, patient satisfaction and waiting times, and adherence to care guidelines (Oliver 2007).

The VA is not the principal source of medical care for most U.S. veterans (Auerbach Weeks, and Brantley 2013). Nearly all veterans over the age of 65 are covered by Medicare, and over 75 percent of younger veterans have health insurance coverage beyond the VA system (Auerbach, Weeks, and Brantley 2013). For example, in 2014, "a total of 9.1 million of the 21.6 million U.S. veterans were enrolled in the VHA, but only 5.8 million were actual VHA patients, and these patients relied on the VHA for, on average, less than 50 percent of their health care services" (Giroir and Wilensky 2015). In other words, the use of private providers is the norm, not the exception, for most veterans. Indeed, the VA "private sector providers are often the only practical option for veterans in rural areas or those requiring specialty service not offered by their local VA medical center" (Sheetz and Shulkin 2018). Thus, the principal question facing policy makers and veterans groups is not *whether* veterans should be able to receive care from private-sector providers but *to what extent* the VA should coordinate such care and impose limits on the use of private services that could be offered by the VA itself.

In any health care system with a large patient base, ensuring that patients receive access to timely care is an ongoing challenge. In 2014, news reports revealed that managers and administrators falsified data to hide long waiting times for veterans seeking care at the VA Medical Center in Phoenix, Arizona. A report by the VA's inspector general found the average wait for an initial primary care appointment was 115 days, far longer than the 24 days hospital staff reported (Oppel and Shear 2014). Under VA rules, new appointments must be scheduled within 14 days after a veteran is declared eligible for services, but VA staff maintained a separate waiting list for over 1,700 veterans outside of the VA's national electronic health record system to hide longer waiting times (Zezima 2014). The VA's performance measures encouraged staff to underreport wait times, as this was a key factor in determining end-of-year performance bonuses and salary increases (Oppel and Shear 2014). The inspector general concluded that similar practices were "systemic throughout" the VA health care system (Oppel and Shear 2014).

Although VA Secretary Eric Shinseki decried the report's findings as "indefensible and unacceptable," he submitted his resignation within days of the report's release. Similar incidents were reported in Fort Collins, Colorado, where staff manipulated schedules in an effort to increase physicians' productivity (Zezima 2014). Efforts to address the waiting list scandal and improve the quality of care for veterans became a top priority for the Obama administration and Congress in 2014. As President Barack Obama explained, "We've already taken the first steps to change the way the VA does business. . . . We've reached out to more than 215,000 veterans so far to make sure that we're getting them off wait lists and into clinics both inside and outside the VA system" (Obama 2014).

In response to concerns about waiting times for veterans, Congress enacted H.R. 3230, the Veterans Access, Choice, and Accountability (VACA) Act, in July 2014. VACA passed by overwhelming margins in both the House (420–5) and Senate (91–3) and was signed into law by Obama on August 7, 2014. The new law granted the VA "expansive authority for the next few years to contract with health providers who are not employed by the VA" (Elmendorf 2014). The Obama administration heralded the new Veterans Choice Program as a way to reduce waiting times and improve access to care. President Obama promised, "If you live more than 40 miles from a VA facility, or if VA doctors can't see you within a reasonable amount of time, you'll have the chance to see a doctor outside the VA system" (Obama 2014). In addition to establishing a driving distance requirement, the new

Veterans Choice Program (VCP) allowed veterans who faced a delay of more than 30 days for an appointment or procedure to receive care outside of the VA (U.S. Department of Veterans Affairs 2017).

VA Secretary David Shulkin described the Obama administration's efforts to reform the VA as "arguably the most scrutinized turnaround in contemporary U.S. medicine" (Shulkin 2016, 1003). Shulkin noted that "in the two years since unacceptable VA waiting times came to light, it's become apparent that the VA alone cannot meet all of the health care needs of U.S. veterans" (Shulkin 2016, 1004).

The results of the VCP were mixed. While 1.9 million veterans sought care outside of the VA from 2014 to 2018, veterans continued to experience long wait times (Advisory Board 2018). In addition, two private companies—HealthNet and TriWest Healthcare Alliance—received more than $2 billion in overhead costs to administer the new program. The VA paid the contractors a $295 "service fee" to coordinate medical records and scheduling for each referral to an outside provider (Advisory Board 2018). Sen. Jon Tester (D-MT) fumed at the cost of administering the program. He argued, "The VA has an obligation to taxpayers to spend its limited resources on caring for veterans, not paying excessive fees to a government contractor" (Advisory Board 2018). While the VCP represented significant progress in improving access to care for veterans, it was far from a panacea. As Sen. John Boozman (R-AR) observed, the VCP "had its own share of troubles. Specifically, we heard repeated stories of difficulties navigating the complex and confusing bureaucratic process. Despite the new reforms, many veterans were still facing unacceptably long wait times at VA medical centers" (Boozman 2019).

In May 2018, Congress passed S. 2372, the VA Maintaining Internal Systems and Strengthening Integrated Outside Networks (MISSION) Act of 2018. The VA MISSION Act won endorsements from more than 30 veterans' groups and 7 former leaders of the VA (U.S. Senate Committee on Veterans' Affairs 2018a). The VA MISSION Act passed the House by a vote of 347–70 and the Senate by an overwhelming margin of 92–5. President Donald Trump signed the VA MISSION Act into law on the anniversary of D-Day, June 6, 2018. As the U.S. Senate Committee on Veterans' Affairs noted, the VA MISSION Act consolidated seven separate VA community care programs into one unified program, ended the "arbitrary 30-day/40-mile barriers to veterans' care in the community," improved veterans' ability to access care at walk-in community clinics, streamlined agreements with local providers to "remove bureaucratic red tape," and established new reimbursement standards for private providers (U.S. Senate Committee on Veterans' Affairs 2018b).

Many veterans' service organizations expressed concerns, however, that increased use of private providers would divert much-needed resources from the VA's own hospitals and clinics (Steinhauer and Phillips 2019). As one representative for VoteVets.org noted, "Each time you're taking resources out and putting them into the private sector, you're leaving [the] VA dying on the vine" (Shane

2019b). The Veterans of Foreign Wars (VFW) raised similar concerns: "Congress and the administration must fix what is wrong with the VA health care system—improve hiring authorities, expand and fix its aging infrastructure, improve access, customer service—and not just simply turn to the private sector when VA facilities are having problems" (Shane 2018a). The executive director of the Vietnam Veterans of America expressed reservations about the growing emphasis on private providers. He declared, "We don't like it. This thing was initially sold as to supplement the VA, and some people want to try and use it to supplant" (Steinhauer and Philipps 2019). However, some female veterans strongly supported proposals to expand access to community care. As a former Marine Corps captain wrote in an op-ed in the *New York Times*, "Far too many veterans who have experience gender-based discrimination or sexual violence in the military also suffer immeasurably by being forced to use VA facilities" (Bhagwati 2019).

The Trump administration issued new rules to implement the VA MISSION Act in 2019. The new community access standards allowed veterans to seek care from private-sector providers if they had to drive 30 minutes or more to a VA facility or if they needed to wait 20 or more days for primary care or mental health appointments. Veterans could seek care from outside specialists if they lived more than a 60-minute drive from a facility or faced a 28-day wait. VA Secretary Robert Wilkie described the new rules as "the most transformative piece of legislation since the passage of the GI Bill" (Steinhauer 2019). "These proposed access standards will ensure veterans have better access to health care and will give them more choices in how they receive their care," said Dan Caldwell, the executive director of Concerned Veterans for America. "These standards are simple and straightforward, eliminating much of the confusion created by the Veterans Choice Program and the VA's other community care programs" (Steinhauer 2019). Testifying before Congress in October 2019, a senior VHA executive declared "the MISSION Act is a success. We have improved how we do all aspects of our business, from scheduling of appointments to referring veterans to specialists, thus resulting in enhanced services for our enrolled veterans" (U.S. Department of Veterans Affairs 2019a).

The new access standards faced widespread criticism from Democrats and some veteran service organizations. Former VA Secretary David Shulkin warned, "The path now chosen, if allowed to continue, will leave veterans with fewer options, a severely weakened VA, and a private health care system not designed to meet the complex requirements of high-need veterans" (Arnsdorf 2019).

Democrats on Veterans' Health Care

Democrats argue that encouraging veterans to seek care outside of the VA system will lower the quality of services for all veterans, particularly for those who continue to use the VA as a principal source of care. Coordination of care and the availability of health care services tailored to the unique needs of veterans made the

VA the first, and best, choice for veterans. On the campaign trail in 2016, Hillary Clinton acknowledged that "many veterans have to wait an unacceptably long time to see a doctor or to process disability claims and appeals" and promised to "make the Veterans Health Administration (VHA) a seamless partner in health care." Nevertheless, she did "not believe that privatization will solve the problems that the VHA is facing" (Clinton 2019).

Democrats worry that expanding access to private-sector providers hinders the VA's efforts to modernize its facilities and improve the quality of care. A week after the signing of the VA MISSION Act in June 2018, Sen. Bernie Sanders (I-VT)—one of only two members of the Veterans' Affairs Committee who opposed the bill—warned about the dangers of privatization. According to Sanders, "This bill provides $5 billion for the Choice program. It provides nothing to fill the vacancies at the VA. That is wrong. My fear is that this bill will open the door to the draining, year after year, of much needed resources from the VA" (Gordon and Craven 2018). Rep. Mark Takano (D-CA), the most senior Democrat on the House Veterans' Affairs Committee, expressed similar concerns. He declared that "the Veterans Health Administration represents our promise to provide high-quality healthcare to our nation's veterans. We owe it to them to uphold that commitment and make sure their healthcare is never sold out to profiteers in the for-profit healthcare industry" (Takano 2018). At a Senate hearing on the implementation of the VA MISSION Act in December 2018, Sen. Jon Tester (D-MT) sounded a similar warning, claiming that "if you move further down this path—gutting the VA health care system for those veterans who want and need to use it—you'll end up bringing down the whole ship" (Tester 2018).

Democrats also describe proposals to increase the use of community-based providers as unnecessary, citing numerous peer-reviewed studies affirming that the VA provides high-quality care to most veterans. Furthermore, Democrats pointed out that most patients are highly satisfied with the health care services they receive through the VA health care system. Speaking in 2016, President Barack Obama observed that "even as more veterans are coming to VA for more care, nearly 97% of those appointments are completed within 30 days of the veteran's preferred date or the date that is clinically appropriate. And 90% of veterans surveyed are either 'satisfied' or 'completely satisfied' with the timeliness of their care" (Obama 2016). In addition, Democrats argued that VA providers are uniquely positioned to care for the special needs of veterans, many of whom are managing multiple health conditions and often struggle with PTSD, traumatic brain injury, or other mental health needs, in an integrated fashion. "If you listen to veterans all across this country as I do they will tell you sure there are problems with the VA but by and large once they get into the system they are proud of the quality care that the VA provides," added Sanders (Tillett 2018).

By referring patients outside of the VA for care, Democrats warned that veterans will be at greater risk for uncoordinated or duplicative care. After the publication of the Trump administration's new access standards in 2019, Democratic senators wrote a scathing letter to VA Secretary Robert Wilkie opposing "any diminishment of VA's internal capacity to provide health care, only for veterans to be sent into the private care sector that Dartmouth, RAND, and others have found is often of lower quality" (Tester et al. 2019). The Dartmouth study, which compared quality of care measures for both VA and private hospitals in 121 different local health care markets around the United States, found that VA hospitals often had the best health care outcomes. As William Weeks, a health policy researcher at Dartmouth Medical School observed, "Our findings suggest that, despite some recent negative reports, the VA generally provides truly excellent care. If that is the case, outsourcing VA care to non-VA settings solely for patient convenience should be reconsidered" (Dartmouth Institute 2018). Furthermore, the senators noted that "the Department's wait times in primary care and several specialty care services have improved since 2014 and are competitive, if not better as is the case with primary care, cardiology, and dermatology, than the private sector" (Tester et al. 2019).

Instead of sending more veterans outside of the VA to reduce waiting times, Democrats propose to strengthen the VA by giving it the resources it needs to reduce waiting times within its own facilities. While recognizing the need for veterans to access community-based care, Democrats warn that without additional funding, increased use of private providers will consume resources that could be used to fill existing staffing gaps within the VA. In 2018, Rep. Mark Takano (D-CA), the ranking Democrat on the House Veterans' Affair Committee, noted that "VA health care is on par with, if not better than, private sector care. The problem is access to that care. So let's work on access to that care, enhanced internal capacity" (Shane 2018). During the 2020 presidential campaign, Sanders pledged to add physicians, nurses, and allied health professionals to improve the accessibility of services within the VA health care system (Bernie 2020 2019). He promised to "fully fund the VA with the staff and infrastructure needed to ensure our country keeps its promise to our veterans. The overwhelming majority of veterans are happy with the care they receive from the VA and it's our job to make it easier—not harder—for them to get that high-quality care" (Bernie 2020 2019).

Other Democratic legislators expressed similar concerns about the impact of the MISSION Act on the financial stability of the VA. Sen. Jon Tester (D-MT), for example, worried that veterans "would ultimately bear the brunt of cuts to other services or benefits to cover the increased costs of community care. And that will be a bad deal for veterans" (Tester 2018). Without significant increases in overall funding for the VA, Democrats argued that expanded choice of private providers would create a fiscal day of reckoning. Congressman Takano warned that if the "VA fails to implement these access standards properly, or if VA makes them too broad, then the number of veterans receiving expensive private healthcare in the community will increase exponentially, undermining veterans' healthcare and creating an unsustainable strain on VA resources" (Takano 2018).

The publication of the Trump administration's proposed access standards for receiving care from community-based providers in January 2019 sparked a backlash among Democratic legislators. Twenty-eight Democratic senators wrote to VA Secretary Robert Wilkie to express their concerns about the implementation of the new Veterans Community Choice program: "Given that the administration opposes increasing overall federal spending, these increased costs for community care will likely come at the expense of VA's direct system of care. And that is something we cannot support" (Tester et al. 2019). Takano charged that "hastily rolling out new access standards places core VA services and vital research programs at risk by shifting money towards care outside VA without involving providers, VSOs and Congress." He argued that "rather than working to find an equilibrium within the system by building up VA's ability to deliver high quality care, fill the more than 40,000 vacancies within the department, continue working to reduce wait times, and raise the caliber of service we provide for our nation's veteran population, today's announcement places VA on a pathway to privatization" (Takano 2018.

Republicans on Veterans' Health Care

Republicans assert that encouraging veterans to seek care outside of the VA system will reduce waiting times and allow veterans to obtain the latest treatments and services offered by private-sector providers. According to Sen. John Boozman (R-AR), "Updating the VA distance requirement will ensure that more veterans qualify for improved access to timely, reliable and dependable health services they earned. Allowing additional veterans to meet the qualifications of the Veterans Choice Program will improve health care with my colleagues and Veterans Service Organizations to encourage enrollment in this program that improves access to health services for our veterans" (Boozman 2015).

Republicans in Congress point to long waiting times for patients seeking care within the VA as evidence that the system cannot accommodate all veterans' needs. In addition, in some states, veterans must travel hours to the nearest VA facility, creating significant burdens for veterans seeking care. Sen. Joni Ernst (R-IA) declared in 2016, "Our veterans shouldn't be forced to wait weeks on end for an appointment at the VA." On the eve of the vote for the VA MISSION Act, Sen. John Hoeven (R-ND) observed, "So we have veterans traveling hundreds of miles now, round trip, inconvenienced, making it very difficult for them and their families. No more. Under this legislation, that 40-mile requirement and the 30-day limit is taken away. If it is most convenient for a veteran to access care from a private provider in their community, they can do it" (U.S. Congress 2018).

Conservative health policy scholars such as Sally Pipes expressed support for the changes as well. "Empowering veterans to seek health care in the private sector would free them of the endless waiting, the poor quality and rank incompetence that plague our publicly run system," Pipes wrote. "The next VA secretary should strive to make sure that all veterans have the option of obtaining care from private health care providers" (Pipes 2018.

At the signing ceremony for the VA MISSION Act, President Donald Trump noted that "during the [2016 presidential] campaign I'd go out and say, 'Why can't they just go see a doctor instead of standing in line for weeks and weeks and weeks?' Now they can go see a doctor. It's going to be great" (Trump 2018). Republicans expressed frustration with the ongoing delays veterans experienced in seeking treatment outside of the VA. As Sen. Mike Enzi (R-WY) recalled, "Since the VA Choice Program was enacted in 2014, I have received hundreds of letters and calls from people across Wyoming who were so frustrated with the program that they felt they had no other choice but to call their Senator. I have been contacted by veterans who could not access timely follow-up care or critical screenings because of unpaid claims, leading to providers dropping patients" (U.S. Congress 2018).

Republicans dismiss Democratic accusations that they are seeking to privatize the VA. Rep. Phil Roe, the chair of the House Committee on Veterans Affairs, quipped in 2018, "If we're trying to privatize, we're not doing a very good job. . . . We've gone from 250,000 employees in the VA in 2009 to 370,000 employees, and we've gone from a $93.5 billion budget to what the president's asked this year is $198 billion. It sounds like we've been an utter failure if we're trying to privatize" (U.S. Department of Veterans Affairs 2018). Other congressional Republicans also disputed the notion that the VA MISSION Act would weaken the VA. As Sen. Johnny Isakson argued, "When healthcare in the private sector can be utilized for the convenience of the veteran—not as a competitor to the VA—we can use it as a force multiplier to lower the number of people we have to hire and, in addition, lower the number of hospitals we have to build and instead provide that money for services to our veterans. It is a win-win proposition for the VA and for all of us. It is no secret why every former VA Secretary who has served this country has endorsed the VA MISSION bill" (U.S. Congress 2018).

Republicans view improved access to private-sector providers as a necessary and appropriate response to chronic waiting times for needed care within the VA. After the publication of a scathing report by the VA inspector general on unauthorized wait lists in Phoenix and other VA medical centers in 2014, Rep. Jeff Miller (R-FL) argued that the investigation "confirmed beyond a shadow of a doubt what was becoming more obvious by the day: wait time schemes and data manipulation are systemic throughout the VA and are putting veterans at risk in Phoenix and across the country" (Oppel and Shear 2014). The waiting list scandal became a flashpoint for Republican concerns about other alleged performance issues within the VA. Sen. Jerry Moran (R-KS) expressed the growing frustration among many legislators about "instances of systemic dysfunction and lack of leadership at the VA. . . . We do not need more damage control—we need to eliminate the damage being done to our nation's veterans" (Moran 2014). Campaigning for Congress in 2018, Rep. Mike Coffman (R-CO) charged, "The Department of Veterans Affairs (VA) is mired in a culture of bureaucratic incompetence and corruption where no one responsible for wrongdoing is ever held accountable. The VA has failed to meet our nation's obligations to the men and women who have served our nation in uniform" (Ballotpedia 2019). With the passage of the VA MISSION Act, Sen. Johnny Isakson (R-GA) declared, "We have finally dealt with the accessibility of healthcare to our veterans. There will be no more headlines of veterans dying because they can't get an appointment because they are going to be able to get an appointment" (U.S. Congress 2018).

Finally, Republicans championed the virtues of choice itself. At the signing of the VA MISSION Act in June 2018, President Trump declared, "This is truly a historic moment, historic time for our country. I'll be signing landmark legislation to provide healthcare choice—what a beautiful word that is, 'choice'—and freedom to our amazing veterans" (Trump 2018). Republicans argue that more choice of providers will force the VA to improve the quality and accessibility of its services to keep veterans within the system. During the debate over the VA MISSION Act in May 2018, Sally Pipes, president and CEO of the Pacific Research Institute, a conservative policy think tank, argued that "giving vets vouchers, for example, would empower them to take control of their care. Doctors and hospitals would compete for vets' business, driving quality up and cost down in the process. Such competition would reward excellence and, equally important, weed out corruption and waste" (Pipes 2018).

Republicans argue that every veteran should be able to select the care (and setting) that best fits their individual needs, and Sen. Thom Tillis (R-NC) declared that "the VA MISSION Act will ensure that veterans have timely access to quality care, whether in a brick and mortar VA facility, or through one of the VA's community partners." House Majority Whip Steve Scalise (R-LA) described the new law as "great news for veterans who will now have more choice in the care they receive" (White House 2018). Choice also fits with Republicans' larger health care reform agenda, which they describe as one in which patients are empowered to shop for care in a free marketplace. "Most Americans can already choose the health care providers that they trust, and President Trump promised that Veterans would be able to do the same," said Robert Wilkie, the Trump administration's VA secretary. "With the VA's new access standards, the future of the VA health care system will lie in the hands of veterans—exactly where it should be" (Katz 2019). Sens. Phil Roe (R-TN) and Johnny Isakson (R-GA) summarized the prevailing mood of the GOP caucus when they expressed confidence that "these new standards will enable veterans to receive care that best fits their individual needs while making the VA healthcare system stronger" (Katz 2019).

Robert B. Hackey, Delaney Mayette, and Erin Walsh

Further Reading

Advisory Board. 2018. "Veterans Still Face Long Wait Times as Costs for Private Care Program Soar, Investigation Finds." December 20. Accessed November 6, 2019. https://www.advisory.com/daily-briefing/2018/12/20/veterans.

Arnsdorf, Isaac. 2019. "How Donald Trump Turned to a Comics Titan to Shape the VA." ProPublica, October 22. Accessed November 4, 2019. https://www.propublica.org/article/how-donald-trump-turned-to-a-comics-titan-to-shape-the-va.

Auerbach, David, William Weeks, and Ian Brantley. 2013. "Health Care Spending and Efficiency in the U.S. Department of Veterans Affairs." RAND Corporation. Accessed November 22, 2019. https://www.jstor.org/stable/10.7249/j.ctt5hhv36.1.

Ballotpedia. 2019. "Mike Coffman (Colorado)." Accessed September 3, 2019. https://ballotpedia.org/Mike_Coffman_(Colorado).

Bernie 2020. 2019. "Honoring Our Commitment to Veterans." Accessed November 13, 2019. https://berniesanders.com/issues/honoring-veterans/.

Bhagwati, Anuradha. 2019. "Donald Trump Is Getting It Right on Veterans Care." *New York Times*, February 3. Accessed September 3, 2019. https://www.nytimes.com/2019/02/03/opinion/trump-veterans-health-care.html.

Boozman, John. 2015. "Press Release: VA Updated Criteria Allows Better Access to Health Care for Veterans." March 24. Accessed September 23, 2019. www.boozman.senate.gov/public/index.cfm/2015/3/boozman-va-updated-criteria-allows-better-access-to-health-care-for-veterans.

Boozman, John. 2019. "Veterans' Affairs Oversight." *Congressional Record* (February 14): S1353–S1354. Accessed October 7, 2019. https://www.congress.gov/116/crec/2019/02/14/CREC-2019-02-14-pt1-PgS1353-2.pdf.

Clinton, Hillary. 2019. "Veterans, the Armed Forces, and Their Families" Office of Hillary Rodham Clinton. Accessed September 9, 2019. https://www.hillaryclinton.com/issues/veterans/.

Dartmouth Institute. 2018. "Veterans Health Administration Hospitals Outperform Non–VHA Hospitals in Most Healthcare Markets." December 10. Accessed October 17, 2020. https://tdi.dartmouth.edu/news-events/veterans-health-administration-hospitals-outperform-non-vha-hospitals-most-healthcare-markets.

Devine, Curt. 2015. "307,000 Vets May Have Died Awaiting VA Care, Report Says." CNN, September 3. Accessed September 9, 2019. https://www.cnn.com/2015/09/02/politics/va-inspector-general-report/index.html.

Elmendorf, Douglas. 2014. Letter to Sen. Bernie Sanders from Congressional Budget Office, June 11. Accessed November 5, 2019. https://www.cbo.gov/sites/default/files/113th-congress-2013-2014/costestimate/s24501.pdf.

Fandos, Nicholas. 2018. "Senate Sends Major Overhaul of Veterans Health Care to Trump." *New York Times*, May 23. Accessed December 4, 2019. https://www.nytimes.com/2018/05/23/us/politics/veterans-health-care.html.

Fonseca, Maria, Mary Smith, Robert Klein, and George Sheldon. 1996. "The Department of Veterans Affairs Medical Care System and the People It Serves." *Medical Care* 34, no. 3. Accessed November 22, 2019. https://www.jstor.org/stable/3766802.

Giroir, Brett P., and Gail R. Wilensky. 2015. "Reforming the Veterans Health Administration—Beyond Palliation of Symptoms." *New England Journal of Medicine* 373, no. 18: 1693–1695. Accessed December 4, 2019. https://www.nejm.org/doi/10.1056/NEJMp1511438.

Gordon, Suzanne, and Jasper Craven. 2018. "Trump Is Sabotaging a Veterans' Health Care Law He Just Signed." *Washington Monthly*, June 13. Accessed October 7, 2019. https://washingtonmonthly.com/2018/06/13/trump-is-sabotaging-a-veterans-health-care-law-he-just-signed/.

Heath, Sarah. 2018. "VA Patient Appointment Schedule Tool Receives GAO Approval." Accessed September 23, 2019. https://patientengagementhit.com/news/va-patient-appointment-schedule-tool-receives-gao-approval.

Katz, Eric. 2019. "Trump Administration Issues Guidelines to 'Revolutionize' Private Sector Role in Veterans Health Care." Government Executive, January 30. Accessed September 3, 2019. https://www.govexec.com/management/2019/01/trump-administration-issues-guidelines-revolutionize-private-sector-role-veterans-health-care/154536/.

Kesling, Ben. 2019. "An Influx of Women Tests the VA." *Wall Street Journal*, March 2–3: A3.

Kizer, Kenneth, John Demakis, and John Feussner. 2000. "Reinventing VA Health Care: Systematizing Quality Improvement and Quality Innovation." *Medical Care* 38, no. 6. Accessed November 22, 2019. https://www.jstor.org/stable/3767341.

Moran, Jerry. 2014. "Sen. Moran Takes Action on VA Scandal in Senate Appropriations Committee." May 22. Accessed November 10, 2019. https://www.moran.senate.gov/public/index.cfm/2014/5/sen-moran-takes-action-on-va-scandal-in-senate-appropriations-committee.

Moulton, Seth. 2016. "Moulton's Faster Care for Veterans Bill Signed into Law." December 16. Accessed September 11, 2019. https://moulton.house.gov/legislative-center/moultons-faster-care-for-veterans-bill-signed-into-law/.

Obama, Barack. 2014. "President Obama Signs Bill to Give the VA the Resources It Needs." August 7. Accessed November 6, 2019. https://obamawhitehouse.archives.gov/blog/2014/08/07/president-obama-signs-bill-give-va-resources-it-needs.

Obama, Barack. 2016. "Fact Sheet: A Recording of Serving Our Veterans." July 31. Accessed September 3, 2019. https://obamawhitehouse.archives.gov/the-press-office/2016/07/31/fact-sheet-record-serving-our-veterans.

Oliver, Adam. 2007. "The Veterans Health Administration: An American Success Story?" *Milbank Quarterly* 85, no. 1: 5–35.

Oppel, Richard, and Michael Shear. 2014. "Severe Report Finds V.A. Hid Waiting Lists at Hospitals." *New York Times*, May 28. Accessed November 13, 2019. https://www.nytimes.com/2014/05/29/us/va-report-confirms-improper-waiting-lists-at-phoenix-center.html.

Pew Research Center. 2019. "Public Expresses Favorable Views of a Number of Federal Agencies." October 1. Accessed November 13, 2019. https://www.people-press.org/2019/10/01/public-expresses-favorable-views-of-a-number-of-federal-agencies/.

Pipes, Sally. 2018. "Privatizing the VA." *Washington Times*, May 14. Accessed September 3, 2019. https://www.washingtontimes.com/news/2018/may/14/privatizing-the-va/.

Shane, Leo. 2018. "Incoming Chairman's Top Goal for 2019: Building Up VA, Not Outside Care Programs" *Military Times*, December 21. Accessed September 23, 2018. https://www.militarytimes.com/news/pentagon-congress/2018/12/31/incoming-chairmans-top-goal-for-2019-building-up-va-not-outside-care-programs/.

Shane, Leo. 2019a. "New VA Health Care Rules: Trump Overreach or More Choice for Vets?" *Military Times*, January 31. Accessed October 23, 2019. https://www.militarytimes.com/news/pentagon-congress/2019/01/31/new-va-health-care-rules-trump-overreach-or-more-choice-for-vets/.

Shane, Leo. 2019b. "Vets Groups and Lawmakers Say They're against It—But What Does "Privatization" of Veterans Affairs Really Mean?" *Military Times*, April 10. Accessed November 13, 2019. https://www.militarytimes.com/veterans/2018/04/11/vets-groups-and-lawmakers-say-theyre-against-it-but-what-does-privatization-of-veterans-affairs-really-mean/.

Sheetz, Kyle, and David Shulkin. 2018. "Why the VA Needs More Competition." *New England Journal of Medicine* 378, no. 25. Accessed November 22, 2019. https://www.nejm.org/doi/full/10.1056/NEJMp1803642.

Shulkin, David. 2016. "Beyond the VA Crisis—Becoming a High-Performance Network." *New England Journal of Medicine* 374, no. 11: 1003–1005. Accessed October 23, 2019. https://www.nejm.org/doi/full/10.1056/NEJMp1600307.

Shulkin, David. 2019. "I Ran the VA under President Trump until He Fired Me. Our First Trump Tower Meeting Was a Job Interview unlike Any Other" *Time*, October 16. Accessed November 13, 2019. https://time.com/5701364/david-shulkin-donald-trump/.

Steinhauer, Jennifer. 2019. "Veterans Will Have More Access to Private Health Care under New V.A. Rules." *New York Times*, January 30. Accessed October 7, 2019. https://www.nytimes.com/2019/01/30/us/politics/veterans-health-care.html.

Steinhauer, Jennifer, and Dave Philipps. 2019. "V.A. Seeks to Redirect Billions of Dollars into Private Care." *New York Times*, January 12. Accessed September 9, 2019. https://www.nytimes.com/2019/01/12/us/politics/veterans-administration-health-care-privatization.html?searchResultPosition=3.

Stires, David. 2006. "Technology Has Transformed the VA." *Fortune*, May 9. Accessed November 22, 2019. https://archive.fortune.com/2006/05/08/news/companies/va_3stocks_fortune_051506/index.htm.

Takano, Mark. 2018. "Takano Statement following Joint Hearing on VA MISSION Act Implementation." December 19. Accessed September 23, 2019. https://veterans.house.gov/news/press-releases/takano-statement-following-joint-hearing-va-mission-act-implementation.

Tester, Jon. 2018. "Tester Opening Statement on 'Implementation of the VA MISSION Act Hearing'" U.S. Senate, December 19. Accessed September 9, 2019. https://www.veterans.senate.gov/newsroom/minority-news/tester-opening-statement-on-implementation-of-the-va-mission-act-hearing.

Tester, Jon, et al. (with 27 other Democratic senators). 2019. Letter to Robert Wilkie, Secretary of Veterans Affairs, January 28. Accessed September 3, 2019. https://www.veterans.senate.gov/imo/media/doc/2019-01-28%20Letter%20to%20Wilkie%20re%20MISSION%20Act%20access%20standards.pdf.

Tillett, Emily. 2018. "Sen. Bernie Sanders Says Privatizing the VA Is a Very, Very, Very Bad Idea." CBS News, April 1. Accessed September 9, 2019. https://www.cbsnews.com/news/sen-bernie-sanders-face-the-nation-says-privatizing-department-of-veterans-affairs-va-a-very-very-bad-idea/.

Trump, Donald. 2018. "Remarks by President Trump at Signing of the VA MISSION Act of 2018." Accessed April 19, 2021. https://trumpwhitehouse.archives.gov/briefings-statements/remarks-president-trump-signing-va-mission-act-2018/.

U.S. Congress. Senate. 2018. "Executive Session." *Congressional Record*, no. 85 (May 23, 2018): S2846. Accessed November 4, 2019. https://www.congress.gov/115/crec/2018/05/23/CREC-2018-05-23-pt1-PgS2846-3.pdf.

U.S. Department of Veterans Affairs. 2017. "10 Things about the Veterans Choice Program." Veterans Health Administration, July 25, 2017. Accessed September 11, 2019. https://www.va.gov/health/newsfeatures/2017/july/things-to-know-about-the-veteran-choice-program.asp.

U.S. Department of Veterans Affairs. 2018. News Release—Debunking the VA Privatization Myth." April 5. Accessed December 4, 2019. https://www.va.gov/opa/pressrel/includes/viewPDF.cfm?id=4034.

U.S. Department of Veterans Affairs. 2019a. "Dr. Stone Testifies on Community Care Success, Recruitment Needs." *VAntage Point* (blog), October 4. Accessed November 4, 2019. https://www.blogs.va.gov/VAntage/66836/vhas-dr-stone-testifies-community-care-success-recruitment-needs/.

U.S. Department of Veteran Affairs. 2019b. "Veterans Health Administration—About VHA." Accessed October 28, 2019. https://www.va.gov/health/aboutvha.asp.

U.S. Senate Committee on Veterans' Affairs. 2018a. "Isakson, Tester Urge Senate to Pass Landmark VA Legislation." May 22. Accessed November 13, 2019. https://www.veterans.senate.gov/newsroom/majority-news/isakson-tester-urge-senate-to-pass-landmark-va-legislation-.

U.S. Senate Committee on Veterans' Affairs. 2018b. "The VA MISSION Act of 2018." Accessed February 28, 2021. https://www.veterans.senate.gov/imo/media/doc/One%20Pager_The%20VA%20MISSION%20Act%20of%202018.pdf.

Vespa, Jonathan. 2020. "Those Who Served: America's Veterans from World War II to the War on Terror—American Community Survey Report." U.S. Census Bureau. Accessed October 17, 2020. https://www.census.gov/content/dam/Census/library/publications/2020/demo/acs-43.pdf.

Weeks, William, and David Auerbach. 2014. "A VA Exit Strategy." *New England Journal of Medicine* 371, no. 9: 789–91. Accessed April 19, 2021. https://www.nejm.org/doi/full/10.1056/NEJMp1407535.

White House. 2018. "Support for President Donald J. Trump's Signing of the VA MISSION Act." June 8. Accessed April 19, 2021.https://trumpwhitehouse.archives.gov/briefings-statements/wtas-support-president-donald-j-trumps-signing-va-mission-act/.

Zezima, Katie. 2014. "Everything You Need to Know about the VA—and the Scandals Engulfing It." *Washington Post*, May 30. Accessed November 15, 2019. https://www.washingtonpost.com/news/the-fix/wp/2014/05/21/a-guide-to-the-va-and-the-scandals-engulfing-it/.

Women's Reproductive Health

At a Glance

Democrats and Republicans continue to debate the ethical, economic, and legal implications of women's reproductive health policy—namely, the regulation of abortion and birth control. The connection between party positions on abortion and birth control is rooted, in part, in landmark U.S. Supreme Court decisions, such as the 1973 *Roe v. Wade* decision that legalized abortion in the United States. Because *Roe v. Wade* concluded that the right to an abortion is only unrestricted in the first trimester—but allowed states to regulate the procedure to protect maternal health in the second trimester—the decision set in motion state-level efforts to regulate or proscribe the procedure and numerous court cases about what kinds of regulations are "reasonably related" to promoting maternal health.

During the 1980s and 1990s, the court gradually narrowed the circumstances under which abortion is allowed with momentous decisions in several cases: *Planned Parenthood v. Casey* (1992) applied an undue burden standard for subsequent abortion restrictions, and *Harris v. McRae* (1980) upheld the Hyde Amendment, a provision passed by Congress that prohibited federal funding of abortion services and curtailed access to abortion among Medicaid recipients.

The two political parties differ over both a woman's right to abortion and the state's authority to regulate it to protect the potentiality of human life and maternal health, whether through "heartbeat bills" that prohibit abortion after the detection of a fetal heartbeat or regulations that limit where or how physicians are allowed to perform the procedure.

The two parties interpret contraceptive policy along similar lines, often viewing government-mandated access to affordable birth control as either an endorsement of basic reproductive health rights or an affront to religious beliefs and moral standards. Over the past decade, though, Americans have agreed that birth control is a morally acceptable behavior. In 2019, for example, one public opinion survey found that 90 percent of Republicans and 93 percent of Democrats considered birth control to be "morally acceptable" (Brenan 2019). However, despite widespread agreement on this issue,

Democrats and Republicans differ on what role government should have in making contraceptives accessible and affordable. Since 2012, the Affordable Care Act's (ACA) contraceptive coverage mandate (added as a subsequent administration rule) became a touchpoint in a decades-long policy debate pitching reproductive freedom against religious liberty. The Obama administration issued regulations requiring commercial health plans to cover all FDA-approved contraceptive methods without cost sharing.

In response, employers with religious affiliations issued legal challenges that ultimately reached the U.S. Supreme Court in 2014. In *Burwell v. Hobby Lobby*, the court ruled that companies owned by Christian families could not be required to pay for contraceptive coverage as mandated by the ACA. The Trump administration expanded exemptions from the ACA contraceptive mandate for religious or moral reasons. These broader exemptions were derided by Democrats, who argued that many women stood to lose their health benefits, but were upheld by the Supreme Court in *Little Sisters of the Poor v. Pennsylvania* in 2020.

Democrats argue that women have a constitutional and moral right to reproductive freedom, which includes the right to abortion. Supporters of abortion rights argue that abortion access promotes economic freedom and quality of life for women and their families. Many Democrats also maintain that state and federal regulation of abortion should not prevent access to abortion and challenge Republican efforts to restrict abortion. Democrats consider birth control to be a basic reproductive health service that should be accessible and affordable to all women without any cost sharing. The party also strongly supports Planned Parenthood.

Republicans argue that a fetus is a person under the law and believe that abortion violates their religious beliefs. As such, they see restricting or ending abortion as imperative to protect the unborn. Current Republican efforts to restrict abortion trace back to state-level legislative efforts in the decade following *Roe*, and Republicans continue to maintain that the federal government should allow states to regulate and restrict abortion. Following the 2016 presidential election of Donald Trump, Republican-led states introduced increasingly strict state-level abortion restrictions, and GOP lawmakers at all levels of government have vowed to overturn *Roe*. Republicans also argue that the religious freedom should not be infringed upon by contraceptive mandates that require employers to subsidize birth control for employees. The party also opposes government funding for Planned Parenthood.

According to Many Democrats . . .

- Women have a right to control their own bodies and make their own reproductive health decisions.

- The Hyde Amendment, which prohibits federal funding for abortion, should be repealed.
- Federal funding should support Planned Parenthood and other family planning services.
- Contraception should be covered by Medicaid and private health plans, with no cost sharing.
- The *Roe v. Wade* Supreme Court decision that legalized abortion in the United States was decided correctly and should be strongly defended.

According to Many Republicans . . .

- The federal government should allow states to determine regulations that govern access to abortion and other reproductive health services.
- The fetus is a person under the law.
- The Hyde Amendment should be made permanent, and no public funding for abortion should be allowed.
- Religious freedom should not be infringed upon by contraceptive mandates.
- The *Roe v. Wade* decision that legalized abortion in the United States was wrongly decided and should be struck down.

Overview

Over the past 50 years, Democrats and Republicans have debated how to define and regulate women's reproductive health rights. In 1973, the U.S. Supreme Court recognized for the first time a woman's legal right to abortion under its landmark *Roe v. Wade* decision. The 7–2 majority opinion, written by Justice Harry Blackmun, set the precedent for future abortion cases in the United States by holding that any state law banning abortions outright was unconstitutional. The court affirmed a woman's right to abortion under the Fourteenth Amendment but stipulated that states had discretion regarding whether to allow abortion during the second and third trimesters of pregnancy.

As the court concluded, the government could not restrict a woman's ability to abort during the first trimester. Following the point of viability, however, "the State in promoting its interest in the potentiality of human life [410 U.S. 113, 165] may, if it chooses, regulate, and even proscribe, abortion except where it is necessary, in appropriate medical judgment, for the preservation of the life or health of the mother" (*Roe et al. v. Wade, District Attorney of Dallas County* 1973). In the decade that followed, pro-life legislators repeatedly sought to ban abortion via constitutional amendment, but all of the "Human Life Amendment" proposals during the 1970s and early 1980s failed (Westfall 1982).

Roe v. Wade accentuated an emerging chasm between Democrats and Republicans, as positions on abortion rights became increasingly tied to party identity. In particular, fetal personhood became an ongoing focal point highlighting the philosophical differences between Democrats and Republicans on abortion. *Roe v. Wade* spurred voter realignment within the political parties, bringing Catholics into the Republican tent in greater numbers, for example, after decades of Democratic alignment (Greenhouse and Siegel 2011).

During the 1980 presidential campaign, Republican candidate Ronald Reagan's antiabortion stance appealed to otherwise politically inactive evangelical Christians (Johnson 2019). Republicans received strong support from evangelical voters, who fostered a political push to restrict abortion. Since then, Republicans have advocated for the human rights of the unborn, emphasizing fetal personhood, and described abortion as "a fundamental assault on the sanctity of innocent human life" (Republican National Committee 2008). Meanwhile, the party's 2016 platform indicated that "the unborn child has a fundamental right to life which cannot be infringed" (Republican National Committee 2016). This perspective has driven many local and state efforts by conservative Republicans to make abortions harder to obtain. As Sen. Tom Cotton (R-AR) explained, "As long as we have unelected judges making the basic rules for abortion . . . we should try to find ways in which we can protect the most innocent lives that can survive" (Fearnow 2019).

Similarly, official Democratic party platforms released after *Roe* have consistently expressed support for a woman's right to abortion. Between 1992 and 2004, the platforms called for abortion to be safe yet rare, echoing Bill Clinton's famous phrase. During the 1992 presidential campaign, Clinton remarked that abortion should be "safe, legal, and rare," inspiring the succeeding generation of pro-choice Democrats to employ the phrase (Flanagan 2019). By 2008, the Democratic party platform affirmed that the party "strongly and unequivocally supports *Roe v. Wade* and a woman's right to choose a legal and safe abortion" (Democratic National Committee 2008). By 2019, only four Democrats in the U.S. House of Representatives identified as pro-life (Hellmann 2019). As Rep. Pramila Jayapal (D-WA) put it, "You can't say you're a Democrat . . . if you're against abortion" (Thebault 2019).

Not surprisingly, given the firm abortion stances adopted by the two major parties since the 1980s, public opinion polls suggest that abortion views vary dramatically depending on party affiliation and allegiance. For example, one 2019 Pew Research Center poll found 75 percent of Democrats support legal abortion and 65 percent of Republicans oppose legal abortion (Pew Research Center 2019).

Abortion policy continued to be hard fought for two decades after *Roe v. Wade* (Schoen 2015). The Hyde Amendment, introduced by Rep. Henry Hyde (R-IL) in 1976 and renewed annually thereafter, barred the use of federal funds to pay for abortions. In 1984, the Reagan administration introduced the Mexico City Policy, banning foreign nongovernmental agencies that receive U.S. global health

Defend Reproductive Justice

On the floor of the U.S. House of Representatives, in March 2020, Rep. Rosa DeLauro (D-CT) expressed her concern with recent nationwide efforts to restrict abortion rights.

Madam Speaker, we are at a critical juncture for abortion rights in America.

Abortion is health care and a fundamental right. But, across the street from the Capitol, the Supreme Court appears ready to overturn precedent to go after reproductive justice. June Medical Services v. Russo is the first abortion case to be heard by anti-abortion Justices Neil Gorsuch and Brett Kavanaugh. They could pave the way for states to ban abortion for 25 million people in the United States.

So, we are standing up. Because we will not be standing by.

Regardless of where they live or how much money they make, individuals deserve the right to control their own bodies and future, and to get the healthcare that they want and need. When women can make decisions about their own reproductive healthcare, including whether and when to have children, they have autonomy over their lives, and their economic security.

So, reproductive justice is about economic justice. That is what is under threat.

Source

Congressional Record, vol. 166, no. 44 (March 4, 2020): E268–E269. Accessed March 11, 2021. https://www.congress.gov/116/crec/2020/03/05/CREC-2020-03-05-pt1-PgE268-5.pdf.

assistance from performing or promoting abortion as a family planning option. Court decisions in the late 1980s focused on restrictions through various means: for example issuing spousal notifications, obtaining parental consent, or watching "educational" videos.

In 1992, the U.S. Supreme Court upheld *Roe v. Wade* in a 5–4 decision cowritten by Justices Sandra Day O'Connor, Anthony Kennedy, and David Souter. While *Planned Parenthood v. Casey* reaffirmed abortion as a constitutional right, the case also altered the standard by which subsequent restrictions upon that right would be measured. *Casey* set a new legal precedent by ruling that states cannot impose "a substantial obstacle in the path of a woman seeking an abortion before the fetus attains viability" (*Planned Parenthood of Southeastern Pennsylvania v. Casey* 1992). Following the *Casey* decision, public opinion shifted slightly toward antiabortion sentiment favored by Republicans. Gallup poll results indicate that the percentage of voters who identified as "pro-choice" fell from 56 percent to 48 percent between 1995 and 2000; during the same time span, those who identified as "pro-life" increased from 33 percent to 43 percent (Gallup 2019). As the court developed new legal tests to evaluate abortion cases—for example, asking whether a particular regulation is "reasonably related" to promoting maternal health or determining what constitutes a substantial obstacle—each decision fostered state experimentation to devise new ways to restrict abortion practices in ways that could pass legal muster.

Most Americans favor some regulation of abortion but still support keeping it legal; smaller percentages favor unrestricted access or complete prohibition. In a 1975 Gallup poll on abortion law, 22 percent of Americans indicated that abortion should be illegal. In 2018, 18 percent of Americans held the same opinion (Jones 2018). The slight majority of Americans who support legal abortion has hovered between 50 percent and 60 percent of the population across decades and different polling organizations (Gallup 2019). Polling indicates that the majority of Americans has opposed overturning *Roe* by a two-to-one margin since 1989 (Neufeld 2018).

Although the Supreme Court affirmed a woman's right to abortion and then later narrowed the circumstances under which abortion is allowed, it also established privacy rights related to contraception and reproductive health through a series of decisions in the 1960s and 1970s. The court's 1965 decision in *Griswold v. Connecticut* affirmed that married couples had a constitutional right to privacy, and, as such, married women had a right to contraception. Seven years later, the court's decision in *Eisenstadt v. Baird* extended the right to contraception to all single and unmarried citizens. In 1978, the court ruled in a third case, *Carey v. Population Services*, that minors have the same privacy rights as adults, and thus it is unconstitutional to prohibit advertising or distribution of nonprescription contraceptives.

Democrats and Republicans differ in how they view insurance coverage for contraceptives. During the 1990s, more than half of the states passed contraceptive coverage laws that required insurers that covered prescription drugs to also cover FDA-approved contraceptives. While these state laws improved accessibility to an extent, the mandates did not apply to self-funded plans, nor did they prohibit cost sharing (Sobel, Salganicoff, and Kurani 2015). In response to these state-level efforts, in 1997, Sens. Harry Reid (D-NV) and Olympia Snowe (R-ME) introduced the Equity in Prescription Insurance and Contraceptive Coverage Act (EPICC), which would have established contraceptive equity at the federal level. The bill received a 1998 hearing but no vote during the 105th Congress, and Democrats and moderate Republicans, including Snowe and Rep. James Greenwood (R-PA), reintroduced subsequent versions of the bill to no effect during each of the next six congressional terms.

The history of federal legislative failures led the Obama administration to expand on existing state laws by requiring private health plans to cover birth control as an essential preventive health benefit under the Affordable Care Act (ACA) with no cost sharing (Sobel, Salganicoff, and Kurani 2015). In February 2012, Sen. Roy Blunt (R-MO) introduced an amendment that would allow a "moral conviction" exemption from the contraceptive coverage mandate, but the amendment failed in the Senate (Blunt 2012). The Obama administration subsequently developed accommodations for houses of worship and other religious employers that oppose contraceptive services, allowing insurers to provide birth control coverage separately (Pear 2012).

In response, two privately held companies—Conestoga Wood Specialties and Hobby Lobby—alleged that the contraceptive coverage mandate in the ACA violated their First Amendment right to religious freedom. The case reached the U.S. Supreme Court in 2014, with the Court deciding in *Burwell v. Hobby Lobby* that some for-profit employers with religious objections to contraceptive use could refuse to cover contraception in their health insurance plans. Justice Samuel A. Alito Jr. delivered the majority opinion, which held that religiously affiliated institutions have the religious freedom to decline covering birth control under their employees' health insurance plans.

Democrats condemned the court's decision as deeply flawed and argued that the decision to strike down the provision would jeopardize the government's ability to close coverage and affordability gaps for low-income women. Sen. Patrick Leahy (D-VT) warned that "by ruling that the owners of corporations may impose their religious beliefs on their employees, women are no longer guaranteed the right to make their own health care decisions" (U.S. Congress 2014). Republicans, meanwhile, hailed the Hobby Lobby decision. Sen. Mike Lee (R-UT) declared that the decision "did not promulgate national health care policy nor did it render any opinion on the virtues of contraception and religious faith. No, the issue in Hobby Lobby involved not a dispute of competing rights but a straightforward application of plainly written law" (U.S. Congress 2014). Public opinion on the *Hobby Lobby* ruling was also highly partisan. In one Kaiser Family Foundation poll, 70 percent of Democrats disapproved of the decision, while 71 percent of Republicans expressed support (Hamel, Firth, and Brodie 2014).

Partisan differences carry over into disagreement with respect to government funding for abortion, family planning, and other reproductive health services. The ACA designated 10 "essential health benefits" for which all state plans must provide coverage. Although the ACA granted each state discretion with respect to covering abortion services, abortion was explicitly excluded from the list and from federal funding, with two exceptions: if pregnancy endangered a woman's life or was the result of rape or incest. Republicans voiced concern that the ACA established new routes for federal funding of abortion by allowing insurers to sell plans with abortion coverage on many state exchanges. During the final Senate debate on the bill, a compromise reached by Sens. Barbara Boxer (D-CA) and Ben Nelson (D-NE)—one an advocate of abortion rights, the other a staunch opponent—allowed state health insurance exchanges discretion to prohibit exchange plans from covering abortion. The compromise underscored the social significance of the abortion debate, fundamentally changing the ACA to secure Nelson's much-needed support for the politically charged bill. As Boxer observed, "You have both sides criticizing it, which means what we did [and] what we had to do, we compromised in a fair way" (Associated Press 2009). Republicans remained steadfastly opposed to the ACA, however, with Rep. Tom Coburn (R-OK) claiming that "the negotiations, whoever did them, threw unborn babies under the bus" (Bogardus 2009).

The ACA passed entirely along party lines, and President Obama issued a separate executive order that affirmed the prohibition of federal funding for abortion (Obama 2010). Although congressional Republicans were unable to secure language in the ACA that would have made the Hyde Amendment a permanent part of the reform plan, they made subsequent codification attempts. During a 2011 press conference introducing the No Taxpayer Funding for Abortion Act, House Speaker John Boehner (R-OH) argued that "a ban on taxpayer funding of abortion is the will of the people and ought to be the law of the land" (Smith and Boehner 2011). By June 2019, 16 state health insurance exchanges included at least one health insurance plan that offered abortion coverage, while 34 states did not.

According to Democrats, the taxing power granted to the federal government by the Constitution allows for the federal government to fund family planning centers that offer a full array of contraceptive options. The Title X Family Planning Program, first established under the Nixon administration in the 1970s, has allocated more than $250 million annually to Planned Parenthood and other family planning centers, enabling them to provide contraception, treatment for sexually transmitted infections, preventive screening services, and counseling on an income-based sliding fee scale.

Republican policy makers argue the opposite. In March 2019, the Trump administration proposed revoking funding for U.S. health clinics that perform abortions or refer patients to other clinics that do. Under the rule, health care providers may still offer nondirective abortion counseling so long as no procedure or referral is given; in the case of a medical emergency, the provider is permitted to give abortion referrals. Additionally, Title X recipients are required to refer pregnant women for prenatal care, even if a woman does not intend to keep her pregnancy (U.S. Department of Health and Human Services 2019). Although grant recipients have always been barred from using government funds for abortions, conservative think tanks such as the Heritage Foundation have argued for even greater separation. In 2017, the Heritage Foundation observed that "because money is fungible, any taxpayer funds given to abortion providers will free up other money to fund abortion" (Israel 2019). At the state level, similar policy proposals to tighten abortion restrictions have moved forward in several Republican-led states. In June 2019, Gov. Greg Abbott (R) of Texas signed SB 22, which prohibited local and state governments from partnering with organizations that perform abortions. While Texas state senator Donna Campbell (R) maintained that "this bill just prevents taxpayer dollars from being used to support or prop up abortion providers," Texas state representative Donna Howard (D) argued that "it's sacrificing women and their health to achieve a political agenda by shutting down Planned Parenthood" (Sundram 2019). In August 2019, Planned Parenthood announced that rather than comply with the Trump administration's "gag rule," the group would withdraw from the Title X program (Ollstein 2019a).

The Trump administration's Title X policy changes sparked discontent on both sides of the aisle. While 47 percent of Republican voters supported the changes, 48 percent opposed them (Kirzinger et al. 2019). Democrats such as Sen. Patty Murray (WA) argued that the rule changes reflected a Republican strategy to "use every vehicle they have, whether it's rulemaking or administrative executive action or budget, to take away women's rights" (Ollstein 2019b). Sen. Elizabeth Warren (D-MA) similarly accused the Trump administration of "deliberately obstructing low-income people's access to basic healthcare services" (Pilkington 2019). By early 2019, over 20 abortion-related lawsuits filed by Planned Parenthood and other family planning centers against state health departments were in the appeals process. Some lawsuits pertained to bans on dilation and evacuation abortions during the second trimester; others responded to state-imposed mandatory waiting periods between a woman's abortion consultation and the procedure.

Given advances in medical technology and neonatal intensive care units (NICUs), the point of viability continues to shift earlier over time. Although *Casey* set a standard that legalized abortion until a fetus reached viability, usually at 24–28 weeks into a woman's pregnancy, some traditionally conservative states—including Alabama, Georgia, Kentucky, and Louisiana—later limited legal abortion at 22 weeks. In 2013, Arkansas and North Dakota passed abortion restriction bills that were subsequently struck down by the courts. In Arkansas, the Republican-led state legislature overrode the veto of Gov. Mike Beebe (D), who argued that the bill did not adhere to the viability standard set by *Roe*. In March 2014, U.S. District Court Judge Susan Webber Wright struck down Arkansas's law that had restricted abortion beginning 12 weeks into a woman's pregnancy. Wright concluded that "the Supreme Court has . . . stressed that it is not the proper function of the legislature or the courts to place viability at a specific point in the gestation period" (Associated Press 2014). In January 2016, the North Dakota Supreme Court blocked the state's "fetal heartbeat" law, which had been one of three abortion restriction bills signed into law by Gov. Jack Dalrymple (R) in March 2013 (Ferris 2016).

Throughout 2019 and 2020, several Republican-led states began introducing increasingly rigorous abortion restriction laws in anticipation that one or more of them would eventually form the basis of a legal challenge to *Roe v. Wade* that would reach the U.S. Supreme Court, which had tilted conservative in the mid to late 2010s. These restrictions coincided with public polls that recorded the highest level of dissatisfaction with national abortion policy since 2001, including higher numbers of Democrats calling for less strict abortion laws (Saad 2020). As campaigning for the 2020 presidential election intensified during this time, presidential contenders offered statements that exemplified the increasingly partisan nature of abortion rights. In January 2020, Trump became the first U.S. president to speak in person at the annual March for Life rally in Washington, DC, where he claimed that "[the Democrats] are coming after me because I am fighting for you and we are fighting for those that have no voice" (Egan 2020). In February 2020, senator and Democratic presidential candidate Bernie Sanders (I-VT) declared that "being pro-choice is an absolutely essential part of being a Democrat" (Schor 2020).

The COVID-19 pandemic deepened partisan debates on reproductive health and abortion in particular. During March and April 2020, Republican-led states that already had restrictive abortion policies in place also classified abortion as a nonessential medical procedure and prohibited the procedure while pandemic-related emergency declarations remained in effect (Sobel et al. 2020). In Arkansas, the state health department prohibited surgical abortions. Following a series of court actions, the state revised its directive to allow elective surgeries, including abortion, but required patients to have a negative COVID-19 test result within 48 hours prior to the procedure. In Alabama, Ohio, and Tennessee, federal district courts issued preliminary injunctions that allowed abortions to continue.

In response to these efforts to categorize abortion as a nonessential procedure, the Democratic Attorneys General Association reaffirmed its support of abortion access. As New York Attorney General Letitia James remarked, "We will not allow any government agency or government official to use the coronavirus as an excuse to limit a woman's reproductive freedom" (McCammon 2020).

Democrats on Women's Reproductive Health

Democrats argue that preserving a woman's fundamental right to bodily autonomy also protects her reproductive freedom and economic well-being. For example, Democrats called the Supreme Court's 2014 *Hobby Lobby* decision an infringement on women's bodily autonomy. Sen. Patty Murray (D-WA) suggested that employer health plans in the years after the court decision could "threaten a worker's right to make their own autonomous decisions about everything from vaccinations to HIV treatment" (Leonard 2015). Public opinion polls also indicated that around 70 percent of Democrats opposed the decision (Lipka 2014).

According to Democrats, the contraceptive mandate made birth control affordable and accessible for all women. In 2014, Rep. Charlie Rangel (D-NY) explained, "The denial of contraception for women hampers progress towards creating a constitutional right to access various types of contraception and even threatens women's access to basic healthcare" (Goldberg 2014). Further, Democrats believe that removing a woman's ability to access and afford birth control threatens the security of other autonomous health-related decisions. Sen. Elizabeth Warren (D-MA) pronounced the *Hobby Lobby* decision as a "radical assault on women's health care and reproductive rights" (U.S. Congress 2015).

Democrats support abortion rights and oppose Republican efforts to restrict abortion access or reverse *Roe v. Wade*. Most recently, Democrats have called for the repeal of the Hyde Amendment, challenged "heartbeat bills," and opposed the Trump administration's Title X domestic gag rule. Democrats assert that state and federal regulation should protect, not prevent, access to abortion services. Support for abortion rights is now a litmus test for the Democratic party. In one 2019 poll, 85 percent of Democrats indicated that states should protect women's access to abortions (Kirzinger et al. 2020). In May 2019, Sen. Kirsten Gillibrand (D-NY) suggested that "as a party, we should be 100 percent pro-choice, and it should be nonnegotiable" (Greve and Alfaro 2019). In November 2019, the Democratic Attorneys General Association became the first Democratic entity to announce that it would only endorse candidates who support abortion rights (Lerer 2019).

The shift toward party near uniformity regarding abortion rights is relatively recent. The 2000 Democratic party platform acknowledged intraparty differences of opinion on abortion policy as "a source of strength" (Democratic National Committee 2000). In 2008, the party recruited a dozen antiabortion candidates to run in congressional districts won by President George W. Bush in 2004 (Hernandez 2008). Between 2007 and 2019, however, public opinion polls indicated that the proportion of Democrats favoring legal abortion increased from 63 percent to 82 percent (Pew Research Center 2019). In 2013, President Barack Obama became the first sitting president to speak at Planned Parenthood's national conference (Eilperin 2013). As Democrats emphasized reproductive justice for all women as a policy goal, public opinion polls indicated that by 2018, 61 percent of Americans trusted Democrats to do a better job ensuring women's access to reproductive health services than Republicans (Kirzinger, Muñana, and Brodie 2018). As of 2020, Democrats with pro-life or antiabortion positions are increasingly rare. As Kristen Day, the executive director of Democrats for Life of America, lamented, "We're politically homeless" (Smith 2020). Ahead of the 2020 Democratic National Convention, Democrats for Life encouraged the party to readopt the abortion language included in the 2000 party platform, but to no avail (Birenbaum 2020).

Opposition to the Hyde Amendment is representative of Democratic calls for reproductive justice. The Democratic party platform called for repealing the Hyde Amendment for the first time in 2016, and the 2020 platform affirmed that "every woman should have access to high-quality reproductive health care services, including safe and legal abortion" (Democratic National Committee 2020). During the 2020 Democratic presidential primary campaign, repealing the Hyde Amendment garnered support from all leading candidates. Former Vice President Joe Biden previously supported the Hyde Amendment but reversed his stance during the primaries. The president of NARAL Pro-Choice America announced, "We're pleased that Joe Biden has joined the rest of the 2020 Democratic field in coalescing around the Party's core values—support for abortion rights, and the basic truth that reproductive freedom is fundamental to the pursuit of equality and economic security in this country" (Glueck 2019). The campaign focus on the Hyde Amendment echoed earlier congressional calls for its repeal, notably through the Equal Access to Abortion Coverage in Health Insurance (EACH Woman) Act introduced by Sen. Tammy Duckworth (D-IL) and Rep. Barbara Lee (D-CA) in March 2019.

As of August 2020, the bill had 24 Democratic Senate cosponsors and 183 Democratic cosponsors in the House.

Democrats also voice strong support for Planned Parenthood. In one 2018 poll, 89 percent of Democrats held a favorable view of Planned Parenthood (Norman 2018). When the Trump administration announced its domestic gag rule in 2019, Democrats defended Planned Parenthood as an integral provider of basic reproductive health services for millions of women. In 2018, Planned Parenthood provided care to 2.4 million patients, and abortion procedures constituted only 4 percent of the organization's reproductive health services, which ranged from breast exams and HIV tests to emergency contraception kits (Planned Parenthood 2019). The Democratic National Committee issued a statement affirming that "Democrats support the right to quality, affordable health care, including abortion, and we stand with Planned Parenthood and our other partners today as they continue that important work, with or without Title X funding" (Democratic National Committee 2019). In return, Planned Parenthood endorsed Joe Biden's presidential candidacy in June 2020, emphasizing his commitment to "fighting for reproductive justice and rights for all" (Solender 2020).

As Republican-led state legislatures across the country introduced abortion restriction bills subsequently signed into law by Republican governors, Democrats argued that state governments were obligated to respect women's bodily autonomy and preserve their reproductive rights. Public opinion polling indicated that 65 percent of Democrats opposed the Republican-led abortion restriction measures (Kirzinger et al. 2019). When the Kentucky legislature was considering its abortion restriction measures in early 2019, Kentucky state representative Mary Lou Marzian (D) spoke for many in her party when she countered that "these choices must be kept sacred as a personal, private medical decision" (Ballentine 2019). Missouri State House Minority Leader Crystal Quade (D) responded to Missouri's abortion ban at eight weeks by arguing that the law stripped women of their personhood by regarding them as "little more than fetal incubators with no rights or role in the decision, even in cases of rape and incest" (Ballentine 2019).

Democrats have also sought to limit the impact of restrictive Republican measures by removing or easing those restrictions when they regain control of state legislatures and governorships. In May 2019, Gov. Steve Sisolak (D) of Nevada signed SB 179, the Trust Nevada Women Act, which removed abortion restrictions that had been incorporated into state law by Republicans, including a requirement that physicians discuss "emotional implications" of abortion with patients. As Sisolak explained upon signing the bill, "In light of increasing attacks at the federal level and in other states such as Georgia, Alabama, Missouri, and Louisiana, SB179 reaffirms Nevada's commitment to protecting reproductive freedom and access to reproductive health care" (Stracquarlursi and Boyette 2019). The following month, Gov. Janet Mills (D) of Maine signed one bill that allowed health care providers who are not physicians to perform abortions and another that required insurers that covered maternity care to also cover abortion services. Like Sisolak, Mills drew explicit attention to efforts to restrict abortion access elsewhere around the country: "While other states are seeking to undermine, rollback, or outright eliminate a woman's right to make her own personal medical decisions, Maine is defending the rights of women and taking a critical step towards equalizing access to their care" (Kelly 2019b).

In early 2020, Democrats undertook multiple legislative efforts to expand abortion access. In Virginia, Gov. Ralph Northam (D) signed bills passed by the Democratic-led state legislature that allowed nurse practitioners to perform abortions and removed ultrasound and counseling requirements that had been introduced by state Republicans over the preceding decade. As Virginia state senator Jennifer McClellan (D) remarked, "We have finally put an end to these medically unnecessary barriers to women's reproductive health care" (Kelly 2020). In Missouri, House Democrats sought to remove a requirement for abortion providers to perform pelvic examinations before abortions (Driscoll 2020). In Kentucky, Gov. Andy Beshear (D) vetoed Senate Bill 9, which would have granted immediate powers to the state's Republican attorney general to regulate abortion clinics in the state and also prohibited abortion procedures during the COVID-19 pandemic (Yetter 2020).

Democrats have also worked to codify and expand abortion rights through new state statutes or constitutional amendments. In January 2019, Gov. Andrew Cuomo (D) of New York signed the Reproductive Health Act, which decriminalized abortion within the state in the event that a conservative-led U.S. Supreme Court overturned *Roe*. As Cuomo emphasized, "We are sending a clear message that whatever happens in Washington, women in New York will always have the fundamental right to control their own body" (Russo 2019). In Illinois, the Democratic-led state legislature repealed the state's existing abortion statutes, removed criminal penalties for medical providers who perform abortions, and eliminated restrictions on late-term abortions virtually along party lines. As Gov. J. B. Pritzker (D) proclaimed, the legislative reform "ensures that women's rights do not hinge on *Roe v. Wade* or the whims of an increasingly conservative supreme court in Washington" (Kelly 2019a). In June 2019, Gov. Gina Raimondo (D) of Rhode Island signed the Reproductive Privacy Act, which prohibited the state government from interfering with a woman's decision to obtain an abortion before viability (North 2019). By early 2020, more than a dozen states and the District of Columbia had laws protecting the right to abortion, either prior to viability or throughout pregnancy. Although Vermont's Democratic-led legislature had already reaffirmed a woman's right to abortion in 2019, a separate proposal to amend the state's constitution to guarantee abortion rights moved forward pending another vote by the legislature in 2020 and a statewide referendum in 2022 (Rathe 2019).

Over the past decade, congressional Democrats have had nominal success challenging Republican efforts to restrict abortion at the national level. Republicans retook the U.S. House of Representatives following the 2010 midterm elections, and Democrats did not regain the chamber until the 2018 midterm elections. Although President Barack Obama won reelection in 2012, Democrats ceded control of the Senate following the 2014 midterm elections. In 2013, 2015, and then again in 2017, House Republicans advanced bills that proposed banning most abortions after either 20 or 22 weeks. While the bills passed along party lines in the Republican-led House, Senate Democrats blocked passage in all three cases (Thorp 2015). In February 2020, Senate Democrats blocked two abortion measures, virtually along party lines. One bill, sponsored by Sen. Lindsey Graham (R-SC), would have banned nearly all abortions after 20 weeks, while the other bill, sponsored by Sen. Ben Sasse (R-NE), would have required physicians to care for babies after failed abortion attempts (Stolberg 2020).

Some Democratic officeholders in red states express opposition to abortion, just as some moderate Republicans in blue states advocate in favor of preserving abortion rights. In Louisiana, Democratic state senator Katrina Jackson authored the 2014 law that required abortion providers in the state to have admitting privileges at a local hospital (Crisp 2020). The law spurred legal challenges that culminated in *June Medical Services, LLC v. Russo* reaching the U.S. Supreme Court in March 2020. In June 2020, the court voted 5–4 to strike down the law, with Chief Justice John Roberts siding with the court's liberal judges in ruling that the law placed an unconstitutional, undue burden on women seeking abortions (*June Medical Services L.L.C. et al. v. Russo* 2020). In 2019, Louisiana state legislators passed another bill modeled after Mississippi's "heartbeat" law (which had been under legal challenge) that they set to go into effect if Mississippi's law was upheld (De Vogue 2019). Louisiana state representative John Milkovich (D), who wrote and sponsored the bill, proclaimed, "We believe this is an important step in dismantling the attack of the abortion cartel on our next generation" (Blinder 2019). Gov. John Bel Edwards (D) of Louisiana justified signing SB 184 into law as the embodiment of being "pro-life for the whole life" (Kantor and Thebault 2019).

During the first months of 2020, several Democratic-led states included specific abortion protections in their COVID-19 health emergency declarations, while Republican-led states effectively banned abortion (albeit temporarily) by classifying abortion as a nonessential medical procedure. For example, Gov. Phil Murphy (D) of New Jersey and Gov. Ralph Northam (D) of Virginia excluded all family planning services and procedures from their respective emergency declaration orders. In Pennsylvania, Gov. Tom Wolf (D) vetoed a bill that would have mandated insurers to pay for telemedical visits, in part because a provision excluded remote prescribing of abortion-inducing drugs (Caruso 2020). As the 2020 presidential election campaign moved into the summer months of 2020, former Vice President Joe Biden reiterated the Democratic party's commitment to preserving *Roe v. Wade*. After the Supreme Court's ruling in *June Medical Services v. Russo*, Biden pledged, "As President, I will codify *Roe v. Wade* and my Justice Department will do everything in its power to stop the rash of state laws that so blatantly violate a woman's protected, constitutional right to choose" (Biden 2020).

Republicans on Women's Reproductive Health

Republicans insist that reproductive health rights should not trump religious freedom, and they generally oppose contraceptive coverage mandates and government funding of certain reproductive health services. Notably, the Supreme Court's 2014 *Hobby Lobby* decision deepened the Republican position on religious freedom and reproductive health. Following the decision, one public opinion poll indicated that 71 percent of Republicans approved of the court's ruling (Lipka 2014). Speaker of the House Paul Ryan (R-WI) declared the decision a "landmark day for religious liberty" (Pear, Ruiz, and Goodstein 2017). Rep. Diane Black (R-TN) celebrated the decision as well, declaring that it would end the "persecution of ordinary Americans who for years have been seeking only the freedom to live in accordance with their faith, free from government interference" (Pear, Ruiz, and Goodstein 2017).

When the Trump administration expanded exemptions to the Affordable Care Act's (ACA) contraceptive mandate, Attorney General Jeff Sessions (R) argued that the federal government must consider religious freedom a fundamental part of American culture and law. Sessions pointed out that "the protections for this right, enshrined in our Constitution and laws, serve to declare and protect this important part of our heritage" (Levy and Neuhauser 2017). Republicans have used this framing to maintain that employers with religious objections should not have to pay for employees' contraception under their health plans. As President Donald Trump put it in 2019, employers should not be "bullied by the federal government because of their religious beliefs" (Pear 2019).

The Republican party's long-standing opposition to abortion, at least from the 1970s onward, is grounded in the belief that the state has a compelling interest in the "potentiality of human life" as referenced in the *Roe v. Wade* decision. Republicans reject the notion of public funding for abortion and argue that states should be able to determine how to restrict access to abortion and other reproductive health services. President Ronald Reagan, a profound abortion opponent, remains a celebrated figure within the pro-life movement and the party. The Republican party's commitment to overturning *Roe* shapes judicial nominations to district and appellate courts as well as the U.S. Supreme Court. Most recently, the Trump administration continued to rely on endorsements from the Federalist Society, a conservative legal advocacy organization committed to identifying pro-life judicial candidates, to remake the federal judiciary (Montgomery 2019). In 2018, President Donald Trump's appointment of Brett Kavanaugh to the Supreme Court reaffirmed a conservative majority on the court. Nomination hearings for Kavanaugh in 2018 and Neil Gorsuch the year before were controversial, in part, due to the pro-life inclinations of both candidates. Republicans voted almost unanimously for both candidates: all 51 Republicans present voted to confirm Gorsuch (with one Republican absent for health reasons), while 49 of 50 Republicans present voted to confirm Kavanaugh (with one Republican absent for family reasons and another, Lisa Murkowski from Alaska, voting "present").

Republican efforts to populate the federal judiciary with pro-life judges coincide with ongoing state-level legislative efforts to restrict abortion. Following Trump's inauguration, pro-life legislators across the country introduced various measures to restrict abortion: banning medical abortion via telehealth appointment, requiring waiting periods, mandating the burial of fetal remains, or requiring physicians at abortion clinics to have admitting privileges at local hospitals. For example, Kentucky legislators instituted abortion restriction measures in 2017 and 2018 that had previously been struck down as unconstitutional. In 2017, U.S. District Judge David Hale ruled that Kentucky's HB 2, which had required physicians to perform ultrasounds and show and describe the fetus and fetal heartbeat to women seeking abortions, violated physicians' freedom of speech (Costello and Yetter 2017). In 2018, U.S. District Judge Greg Stivers overturned another Kentucky state law that required abortion clinics to have written agreements with hospitals and ambulance services. In his opinion, Stivers concluded that "scant medical benefits from transfer and transport agreements are far outweighed by the burden on Kentucky women seeking abortions" (Yetter 2018). In March 2019, though, Gov. Matt Bevin (R) of Kentucky signed into law another series of abortion restrictions. The signature bill, SB 9, banned abortions after the detection of a fetal heartbeat, while the others required physicians to inform patients about the reversibility of medication abortions and called for an absolute abortion ban in the event that *Roe* were overturned. Soon thereafter, Judge Hale instituted and subsequently extended a court injunction (Associated Press 2019a).

The Supreme Court's new conservative majority under the Trump administration spurred a new wave of "heartbeat bills" and other antiabortion measures introduced by Republican legislators and signed into law by Republican governors with the ultimate aim of challenging *Roe v. Wade*. Republican lawmakers such as Ohio state senator Kristina Roegner explained that although the primary purpose of pro-life bills "is to save human life," Republicans are "not going to shy away from it going to the Supreme Court with the intention of overturning *Roe v. Wade*" (Mindock 2019). Similarly, Iowa state senator Rick Bertrand (R) declared that an Iowa bill continuing new abortion restrictions could be "the vehicle that will ultimately provide change and provide the opportunity to overturn *Roe v. Wade*" (Levenson and Baldacci 2019).

Legislators who introduce and vote for "heartbeat bills" argue that they are protecting the human rights of the unborn fetus. Georgia state representative Ed Setzler (R), who sponsored the Living Infants Fairness and Equality Act, argued in March 2019 that "a child in the womb should be worthy of full legal protection" (Williams and Blinder 2019b). Similarly, after Polk County District Judge Michael

Huppert struck down Iowa's fetal heartbeat law in January 2019, Gov. Kim Reynolds (R) declared, "I am incredibly disappointed in today's court ruling, because I believe that if death is determined when a heart stops beating, then a beating heart indicates life" (Leys 2019). When Gov. Phil Bryant (R) of Mississippi signed a fetal heartbeat bill that also revoked state medical licenses for medical professionals who violated the statute, he claimed, "We think that this is showing the profound respect and desire of Mississippians to protect the sanctity of that very unborn life whenever possible" (Pettus 2019). In May 2019, U.S. District Judge Carlton Reeves, who had previously struck down a 2018 Mississippi law banning abortion at 15 weeks, blocked the 2019 abortion law banning abortions after the detection of fetal heartbeat at 6 weeks. As Reeves remarked, "Mississippi has passed another law banning abortions prior to viability" (Pettus 2019).

In April 2019, Gov. Mike DeWine (R) of Ohio signed SB 23, a bill that banned abortion after the detection of a fetal heartbeat. DeWine's predecessor, John Kasich (R), had twice vetoed the same measure, which he deemed unconstitutional. When Kasich issued one of those vetoes in 2016, he stated that his intent was to dissuade "additional challenges to Ohio's strong legal protections for unborn life" (Kasich 2016). DeWine, however, described his signing of the same measure that Kasich had vetoed as part of "our duty, I believe, and an essential form of government, to protect those who cannot protect themselves" (Associated Press 2019b). Similar to the challenge lodged against the Mississippi abortion restriction, a federal judge temporarily blocked SB 23 in July 2019, arguing that the law "places an 'undue burden' on a woman's right to choose a pre-viability abortion" (Balmert and Borchardt 2019).

The most stringent pro-life measures proposed by Republicans include no exceptions when restricting or criminalizing abortion. In May 2019, Gov. Kay Ivey (R) signed HB 314, the Alabama Human Life Protection Act. The act criminalized all abortion in the state, rendered performing an abortion a felony, and included no exception for rape or incest. When she signed the bill into law, Ivey proclaimed, "This legislation stands as a powerful testament to Alabamians' deeply held belief that every life is precious and that every life is a sacred gift from God" (Ivey 2019). Ivey's signing was presaged by the November 2018 midterm elections, during which 59 percent of state voters supported adding antiabortion language to the Alabama State Constitution (Chandler and Paterson 2019). In October 2019, a federal judge blocked the measure, arguing that "Alabama's abortion ban contravenes clear Supreme Court precedent" (Brown and Lyman 2019).

Further north, in May 2019, Gov. Mike Parson (R) of Missouri signed HB 126, which criminalized abortion beyond eight weeks except in cases of medical emergency. Republican legislators voiced strong support for the Missouri Stands for the Unborn Act. As Missouri state representative Holly Rehder (R) asked abortion opponents who "stand on this floor and say, 'How could someone look at a child of rape or incest and care for them?' I can say how we can do that. We can do that with the love of God" (Tavernise and Hassan 2019). In August 2019, a federal

Protect the Unborn

On the floor of the U.S. Senate, in February 2020, Sen. Joni Ernst (R-IA) spoke in favor of the Pain-Capable Unborn Child Protection Act and the Born-Alive Abortion Survivors Protection Act.

> Women I talk to will often comment on the amazing feeling and bond they will have with that child who is growing in their womb. They experience that heartbeat in the womb. And even to the effects that maybe we don't like to reflect on—I remember the swollen ankles I had in the last month of pregnancy. No offense to Fred Flintstone, but I had Fred Flintstone feet. Even things like that we can reflect on. But the impact of having that child stays with me. It changed me forever.
>
> I know that other mothers know that whether it is from the beginning of a pregnancy with a healthy, full-term child or whether it is a scary premature birth or, for some, the difficult and life-ending decision to abort, the fact remains that the tiny human being carried within us has forever left a mark on their mother. This truth spurs me on to fight even harder to protect the undeniable value that every human life has. Every human life has value.
>
> So today I stand with my pro-life colleagues in asking our pro-choice friends—many of whom are mothers and fathers themselves—to meet us in the middle. We may not be able to get on the same page when it comes to recognizing the inherent value each of these lives holds, but surely we can agree that protecting our most vulnerable from painful death is a unifying and humanitarian cause.

Source

Congressional Record, vol. 166, no. 36 (February 24, 2020): S1110. Accessed March 11, 2021. https://www.congress.gov/116/crec/2020/02/24/CREC-2020-02-24-pt1-PgS1105.pdf.

judge issued a temporary injunction that was subsequently appealed by the state attorney general.

Even as judges struck down "heartbeat bills" throughout 2019, Republicans maintained that the federal government should allow states to determine how to govern access to abortion and other methods of family planning. For example, one public opinion poll found that 77 percent of Republican women and 64 percent of Republican men supported these restriction measures (Kirzinger et al. 2019).

While Republicans continued to mobilize legal challenges in hopes of overturning *Roe*, in July 2020, the Supreme Court issued a 7–2 decision in two consolidated cases—*The Little Sisters of the Poor Saints Peter and Paul Home v. Pennsylvania* and *Trump v. Pennsylvania*—that upheld Trump administration rules that expanded exemptions to the ACA's contraceptive mandate for religious and moral reasons. White House Press Secretary Kayleigh McEnany framed the decision as "a big win for religious freedom and freedom of conscience" (Barnes 2020).

A clear majority of Republicans view Planned Parenthood unfavorably. In one 2018 poll, for example, 63 percent of Republicans held an unfavorable view of the organization (Norman 2018). Republican opposition to Planned Parenthood is explicitly tied to the organization's status as an abortion provider. In 2018, Sen. Rand Paul (R-KY) introduced a measure to defund Planned Parenthood that failed to pass when two moderate Republican senators, Susan Collins (R-ME) and Lisa Murkowski (R-AK), joined with Democrats to vote no (Werner 2018). In January 2019, Rep. Vicki Hartzler (R-MO) introduced the Defund Planned Parenthood Act, which she described as motivated by her conviction that "taxpayers should not have to pay for Planned Parenthood's abortion industry" (Hartzler 2019). Days later, Sen. Joni Ernst (R-IA) and 31 Republican colleagues cosponsored S. 141, the Protect Funding for Women's Health Care Act, which was another bill prohibiting federal funding of Planned Parenthood. That same month, newly elected Sen. Marsha Blackburn (R-TN) introduced S. 105, the Title X Abortion Provider Prohibition Act, as her first legislative action. As of October 2020, none of the bills had received a vote in committee in the 116th Congress.

Even as Republican politicians seek to defund Planned Parenthood, public opinion polls indicate that Republican voters are less likely to support defunding Planned Parenthood if government funding would only be used for non-abortion-related health services (Quinnipiac University Poll 2017). Similarly, in the wake of the Trump administration's announcement that it would revoke Title X funding for health clinics that perform abortions or refer patients to other clinics that do, some Republicans—and Republican women in particular—broke with the party. In 2019, for example, 62 percent of Republican women considered it important for the federal government to fund reproductive health services for lower-income women (Kirzinger et al. 2019).

Although Republicans have tied opposition to abortion to their party identity since the 1980s, a small contingent of moderate Republicans, typically those holding elective office in blue states, have voiced support for abortion rights. Most notably, Sens. Susan Collins (R-ME) and Lisa Murkowski (R-AK) have publicly supported *Roe v. Wade* during their respective political careers. Following the June 2018 announcement of Supreme Court Justice Anthony Kennedy's retirement, Collins acknowledged that "from my perspective, *Roe v. Wade* is an important precedent and it is settled law" (Kim 2018). Collins subsequently drew sharp criticism from Democrats when she voted in favor of Brett Kavanaugh's Supreme Court nomination several months later.

Moderate Republican governors also issued abortion policy decisions out of sync with the party's conservative wing. In May 2019, Gov. Phil Scott (R) of Vermont signed H 57, which reaffirmed a woman's right to abortion in the state. As the legislation outlined, Vermont would "recognize as a fundamental right the freedom of reproductive choice" and also "prohibit public entities from interfering with or restricting the right of an individual to terminate the individual's pregnancy" (Vermont General Assembly 2019). Although a Republican governor presiding over a state with a liberal congressional delegation, Scott remarked when signing the bill that "this legislation affirms what is already allowable in Vermont—protecting reproductive rights and ensuring those decisions remain between a woman and her health care provider" (Folley 2019). Nonetheless, national public opinion polling heading into the 2020 presidential election indicated that 50 percent of Republican voters supported overturning *Roe v. Wade* (Holzberg and Kamisar 2020). On the eve of Amy Coney Barrett's October 2020 confirmation to replace Justice Ruth Bader Ginsburg and establish a 6–3 conservative majority on the Supreme Court, 57 percent of Republicans identifying as "very conservative" supported overturning *Roe v. Wade* (Clement and Guskin 2020).

Todd M. Olszewski and Olivia Braga

Further Reading

Associated Press. 2009. "Abortion Compromise Was Carefully Crafted." NBC News, December 21. Accessed August 27, 2020. http://www.nbcnews.com/id/34514852/ns/politics/t/abortion-compromise-was-carefully-crafted/.

Associated Press. 2014. "U.S. Judge Strikes Arkansas' 12-Week Abortion Ban." *USA Today*, March 15. Accessed September 22, 2019. https://www.usatoday.com/story/news/nation/2014/03/15/arkansas-abortion-ban/6453807/.

Associated Press. 2019a. "Judge Extends Temporary Ban on 2 New Kentucky Abortion Laws." March 27. Accessed September 22, 2019. https://www.apnews.com/04b6cd071a844a93bc5cd1f84b6df979.

Associated Press. 2019b. "Ohio Governor Sign Ban on Abortion after 1st Heartbeat." April 12. Accessed September 22, 2019. https://www.apnews.com/0b1deb8c1f5d41d8ab4c9e32446a55ce.

Ballentine, Summer. 2019. "Missouri Governor Signs Bill Banning Abortions at 8 Weeks." Associated Press, May 24. Accessed September 22, 2019. https://www.apnews.com/80bfa84a31cb449cb5a60e1a24d7f8a7.

Balmert, Jessie, and Jackie Borchardt. 2019. "Federal Judge Blocks Ohio's 'Heartbeat Bill' Abortion Ban." *Cincinnati Enquirer*, July 3. Accessed September 22, 2019. https://www.cincinnati.com/story/news/politics/2019/07/03/federal-judge-blocks-ohios-heartbeat-bill-abortion-ban/1559819001/.

Barnes, Robert. 2020. "Supreme Court Says Employers May Opt Out of Affordable Care Act's Birth Control Mandate over Religious, Moral Objections." *Washington Post*, July 8. Accessed September 10, 2020. https://www.washingtonpost.com/politics/courts_law/supreme-court-obamacare-birth-control-mandate/2020/07/08/0b38a352-c123-11ea-b4f6-cb39cd8940fb_story.html.

Biden, Joe. 2020. "My Statement on *June Medical Services vs. Russo*." Medium, June 29. Accessed August 25, 2020. https://medium.com/@JoeBiden/my-statement-on-june-medical-services-vs-russo-6e903c5b1e7e.

Birenbaum, Gabby. 2020. "Democrats for Life Urge DNC to Change Party Platform on Abortion." The Hill, August 14. Accessed August 25, 2020. https://thehill.com/policy/healthcare/abortion/511967-democrats-for-life-dnc-change-party-platform-abortion.

Blinder, Alan. 2019. "Louisiana Moves to Ban Abortions after a Heartbeat Is Detected." *New York Times*, May 29. Accessed September 22, 2019. https://www.nytimes.com/2019/05/29/us/louisiana-abortion-heartbeat-bill.html.

Blunt, Roy. 2012. "Senator Blunt's Response to President Obama's Remarks on HHS Mandate." February 10. Accessed September 9, 2020. https://www.blunt.senate.gov/news/press-releases/senator-blunts-response-to-president-obamas-remarks-on-hhs-mandate.

Bogardus, Kevin. 2009. "Coburn: Nelson Agreement with Leaders 'Threw Unborn Babies under the Bus.'" The Hill, December 19. Accessed August 26, 2020. https://thehill.com/homenews/senate/73081-coburn-nelson-agreement-with-leaders-threw-unborn-babies-under-the-bus.

Brenan, Megan. 2019. "Birth Control Still Tops List of Morally Acceptable Issues." Gallup, May 29. Accessed September 9, 2020. https://news.gallup.com/poll/257858/birth-control-tops-list-morally-acceptable-issues.aspx.

Brown, Melissa, and Brian Lyman. 2019. "Alabama's Tough Abortion Ban Blocked by Federal Judge: Law Would've Made Most Abortions a Felony." *USA Today*, October 29. Accessed August 25, 2020. https://www.usatoday.com/story/news/2019/10/29/alabama-abortion-ban-blocked-tough-law-nixed-judge-myron-thompson/2495753001/.

Bush, George W. 2003. "President Bush Signs Partial Birth Abortion Act of 2003." White House, November 5. Accessed September 22, 2019. https://georgewbush-whitehouse.archives.gov/news/releases/2003/11/20031105-1.html.

Caruso, Stephen. 2020. "Amid COVID-19, Wolf Vetoes Telemedicine Bill over Abortion Concerns." *Pennsylvania Capital-Star*, April 29. Accessed June 1, 2020. https://www.penncapital-star.com/blog/amid-covid-19-wolf-vetoes-telemedicine-bill-over-abortion-concerns/.

Chandler, Kim, and Blake Paterson. 2019. "Alabama Governor Invokes God in Banning Nearly All Abortions." Associated Press, May 16. Accessed September 22, 2019. https://www.apnews.com/7a47ddc761dc4b72a017b0836da3a87b.

Clement, Scott, and Emily Guskin. 2020. "A Slim Majority of Voters Oppose Barrett Hearings, though a Consistent Majority Support High Court Upholding *Roe v. Wade*, Post-ABC Poll Finds." *Washington Post*, October 12. Accessed October 31, 2020. https://www.washingtonpost.com/politics/poll-trump-court-abortion/2020/10/12/ec11a880-0bd1-11eb-8a35-237ef1eb2ef7_story.html.

Costello, Darcy, and Deborah Yetter. 2017. "Judge's Order Ends 'Invasive, Demeaning, and Humiliating' Kentucky Abortion Law, Lawyer Says." *Louisville Courier-Journal*, September 27. Accessed September 22, 2019. https://www.courier-journal.com/story/news/2017/09/27/judge-strikes-down-kentucky-abortion-law-saying-violates-physicians-free-speech/711049001/.

Crisp, Elizabeth. 2020. "Meet the Anti-Abortion Louisiana Democrat at the Heart of the Supreme Court's Abortion Debate." *The Advocate*, February 29. Accessed June 1, 2020. https://www.theadvocate.com/baton_rouge/news/politics/article_0ee860ec-59a3-11ea-a903-bb38c5a9d9f4.html.

De Vogue, Ariane. 2019. "Louisiana Asks Supreme Court to Allow State Abortion Law to Go into Effect." CNN, July 19. Accessed September 22, 2019. https://www.cnn.com/2019/07/19/politics/louisiana-abortion-law-supreme-court/index.html.

Democratic National Committee. 2000. "2000 Democratic Party Platform Online." Online by Gerhard Peters and John T. Woolley, the American Presidency Project. Accessed August 25, 2020. https://www.presidency.ucsb.edu/documents/2000-democratic-party-platform.

Democratic National Committee. 2008. "2008 Democratic Party Platform Online." Online by Gerhard Peters and John T. Woolley, the American Presidency Project. Accessed August 25, 2020. https://www.presidency.ucsb.edu/documents/2008-democratic-party-platform.

Democratic National Committee. 2019. "DNC Statement of Support for Planned Parenthood." August 19. Accessed September 10, 2020. https://democrats.org/news/dnc-statement-of-support-for-planned-parenthood/.

Democratic National Committee. 2020. "2020 Democratic Party Platform." Democratic National Convention. Accessed August 25, 2020. https://www.demconvention.com/wp-content/uploads/2020/08/2020-07-31-Democratic-Party-Platform-For-Distribution.pdf.

Driscoll, Jaclyn. 2020. "Missouri House Democrats Push Measure to Stop Requiring Pelvic Exams before Abortions." St. Louis Public Radio, March 3. Accessed June 1, 2020. https://news.stlpublicradio.org/post/missouri-house-democrats-push-measure-stop-requiring-pelvic-exams-abortions#stream/0

Egan, Lauren. 2020. "Trump 'Truly Proud' to be First President to Attend March for Life." NBC News, January 24. Accessed June 1, 2020. https://www.nbcnews.com/politics/donald-trump/trump-becomes-first-sitting-president-attend-march-life-rally-n1122246.

Eilperin, Juliet. 2013. "Why Obama Decided to Be the First Sitting President to Address Planned Parenthood." *Washington Post*, April 25. Accessed August 20, 2020. https://www.washingtonpost.com/news/the-fix/wp/2013/04/25/why-obama-decided-to-be-the-first-sitting-president-to-address-planned-parenthood/.

Fearnow, Benjamin. 2019. "Republican Sen. Tom Cotton Says Life Begins at Conception, Fetus Has Constitutional Rights Protecting from Abortion." *Newsweek*, May 19. Accessed September 22, 2019. https://www.newsweek.com/tom-cotton-abortion-life-begins-conception-rape-incest-constitutional-right-1429858.

Ferris, Sarah. 2016. "Supreme Court Won't Let North Dakota Enforce 'Fetal Heartbeat' Law." The Hill, January 25. Accessed September 22, 2019. https://thehill.com/policy/healthcare/266871-scotus-north-dakota-cannot-enforce-fetal-heartbeat-law.

Flanagan, Caitlin. 2019. "Losing the *Rare* in 'Safe, Legal, and Rare.'" *The Atlantic*, December 6. Accessed August 25, 2020. https://www.theatlantic.com/ideas/archive/2019/12/the-brilliance-of-safe-legal-and-rare/603151/

Folley, Aris. 2019. "GOP Vermont Governor Signs Sweeping Abortion Rights Bill into Law." The Hill, June 11. Accessed September 22, 2019. https://thehill.com/homenews/state-watch/448006-gop-vermont-governor-signs-sweeping-abortion-rights-bill-into-law.

Gallup. 2019. "Abortion." Accessed August 4, 2019. https://news.gallup.com/poll/1576/abortion.aspx.

Glueck, Katie. 2019. "Joe Biden Denounces Hyde Amendment, Reversing His Position." *New York Times*, June 6. Accessed August 20, 2020. https://www.nytimes.com/2019/06/06/us/politics/joe-biden-hyde-amendment.html.

Goldberg, Dan. 2014. "Local Pols React to Supreme Court's Contraception Ruling." Politico, June 30. Accessed September 10, 2020. https://www.politico.com/states/new-york/city-hall/story/2014/06/local-pols-react-to-supreme-courts-contraception-ruling-000000.

Greenhouse, Linda, and Reva Siegel. 2011. "Before (and after) *Roe v. Wade*: New Questions about Backlash." *Yale Law Journal* 120: 2028–2087. Accessed August 26, 2020. https://law.yale.edu/sites/default/files/documents/pdf/Faculty/Siegel_BeforeAndAfterRoeVWadeNewQuestionsAboutBacklash.pdf.

Greve, Joanie, and Mariana Alfaro. 2019. "The Daily 202: Kirsten Gillibrand's Trip to Georgia Showcases the Changing Politics of Abortion for Democrats in 2020." *Washington Post*, May 16. Accessed August 26, 2020. https://www.washingtonpost.com/news/powerpost/paloma/daily-202/2019/05/16/daily-202-kirsten-gillibrand-s-trip-to-georgia-showcases-the-changing-politics-of-abortion-for-democrats-in-2020/5cdc4c581ad2e5092403d1d9/.

Hamel, Liz, Jamie Firth, and Mollyann Brodie. 2014. "Kaiser Health Tracking Poll: July 2014." Kaiser Family Foundation, August 1. Accessed October 4, 2020. https://www.kff.org/health-reform/poll-finding/kaiser-health-tracking-poll-july-2014/.

Hartzler, Vicky. 2019. "Hartzler Introduces the Defund Planned Parenthood Act of 2019." January 9. Accessed September 10, 2020. https://hartzler.house.gov/media-center/press-releases/hartzler-introduces-defund-planned-parenthood-act-2019.

Hellmann, Jessie. 2019. "Anti-Abortion Democrats Take Heat from Party." The Hill, June 2. Accessed August 4, 2019. https://thehill.com/policy/healthcare/446438-anti-abortion-democrats-take-heat-from-party.

Hernandez, Raymond. 2008. "Democrats Carrying Anti-Abortion Banner Put More Congressional Races in Play." *New York Times*, October 25. Accessed August 26, 2020. https://www.nytimes.com/2008/10/26/us/politics/26abortion.html.

Holzberg, Melissa, and Ben Kamisar. 2020. "Poll: Majority of Adults Don't Support Overturning *Roe v. Wade*." NBC News, September 29. Accessed October 4, 2020. https://www.nbcnews.com/politics/2020-election/poll-majority-adults-don-t-support-overturning-roe-v-wade-n1241269.

Israel, Melanie. 2019. "Defending Life: Recommendations for the 116th Congress." Heritage Foundation, July 24. Accessed August 4, 2019. https://www.heritage.org/node/14726055/print-display.

Ivey, Kay. 2019. "Governor Ivey Issues Statement after Signing the Alabama Human Life Protection Act." Office of the Governor, State of Alabama, May 15. Accessed September 22, 2019. https://governor.alabama.gov/statements/governor-ivey-issues-statement-after-signing-the-alabama-human-life-protection-act/.

Johnson, Emily. 2019. *This Is Our Message: Women's Leadership in the New Christian Right*. Oxford, UK: Oxford University Press.

Jones, Jeffrey. 2018. "U.S. Abortion Attitudes Remain Closely Divided." Gallup, June 11. Accessed August 4, 2019. https://news.gallup.com/poll/235445/abortion-attitudes-remain-closely-divided.aspx.

June Medical Services L.L.C. et al. v. Russo, syllabus, 591 U.S. __ (2020). Accessed July 10, 2020. https://www.supremecourt.gov/opinions/19pdf/18-1323_c07d.pdf.

Kantor, Jacqueline, and Reis Thebault. 2019. "Louisiana's Democratic Governor Just Defied His Party and Signed an Abortion Ban into Law." *Washington Post*, May 30. Accessed September 22, 2019. https://www.washingtonpost.com/nation/2019/05/29/louisiana-passed-an-abortion-ban-its-democratic-governor-plans-defy-his-party-sign-it/.

Kasich, John. 2016. "Veto Messages. Statement of the Reasons for the Veto of Items in Amended Substitute House Bill 493." State of Ohio Executive Department, Office of the Governor, December 13. Accessed September 22, 2019. http://cdn.cnn.com/cnn/2019/images/01/25/veto_message.pdf.

Kelly, Caroline. 2019a. "Illinois Governor Signs Sweeping Abortion Protection Bill into Law." CNN, June 12. Accessed September 22, 2019. https://www.cnn.com/2019/06/12/politics/illinois-governor-signs-abortion-protection-law/index.html.

Kelly, Caroline. 2019b. "Maine Laws Expanding Abortion Access Go into Effect." CNN, September 19. Accessed September 22, 2019. https://www.cnn.com/2019/09/19/politics/maine-abortion-access-expansion-laws-trnd/index.html.

Kelly, Caroline. 2020. "Virginia Governor Signs Abortion Protections into Law." CNN, April 10. Accessed June 1, 2020. https://www.cnn.com/2020/04/10/politics/virginia-abortion-protections/index.html.

Kim, Seung Min. 2018. "'Everyone Is Focused on Lisa and Susan': The Two Most Powerful Senators in the Fight to Replace Kennedy." *Washington Post*, June 28. Accessed August 25, 2020. https://www.washingtonpost.com/politics/everyone-is-focused-on-lisa-and-susan-the-two-most-powerful-senators-in-the-fight-to-replace-kennedy/2018/06/28/d7f7f72e-7ae6-11e8-93cc-6d3beccdd7a3_story.html.

Kirzinger, Ashley, Lunna Lopes, Alina Salganicoff, Brittni Frederiksen, Cailey Muñana, Usha Ranji, and Mollyann Brodie. 2019. "KFF Poll: Public Opinion and Knowledge on Reproductive Health Policy." Kaiser Family Foundation, May 3. Accessed September 3, 2019. https://www.kff.org/womens-health-policy/poll-finding/kff-poll-public-opinion-and-knowledge-on-reproductive-health-policy/.

Kirzinger, Ashley, Cailey Muñana, and Mollyann Brodie. 2018. "Public More Likely to Trust Democratic Party to Do a Better Job Dealing with Most Health Care Issues." Kaiser Family Foundation, October 19. Accessed August 20, 2020. https://www.kff.org/health-reform/issue-brief/public-more-likely-to-trust-democratic-party-to-do-a-better-job-dealing-with-most-health-care-issues/.

Kirzinger, Ashley, Cailey Muñana, Audrey Kearney, Mollyann Brodie, Gabriela Weigel, Brittni Fredericksen, Usha Ranji, and Alina Salganicoff. 2020. "Abortion Knowledge and Attitudes: KFF Polling and Policy Insights." Kaiser Family Foundation, January 22. Accessed August 27, 2020. https://www.kff.org/coronavirus-covid-19/issue-brief/state-action-to-limit-abortion-access-during-the-covid-19-pandemic/.

Leonard, Kimberly. 2015. "After Hobby Lobby, a Way to Cover Birth Control." *U.S. News & World Report*, July 10. Accessed September 10, 2020. https://www.usnews.com/news/articles/2015/07/10/after-hobby-lobby-ruling-hhs-announces-birth-control-workaround.

Lerer, Lisa. 2019. "Abortion Is New Litmus Test for Democratic Attorneys General Group." *New York Times*, November 18. Accessed August 25, 2020. https://www.nytimes.com/2019/11/18/us/politics/democratic-attorneys-general-abortion.html.

Levenson, Eric, and Marlena Baldacci. 2019. "Iowa's 'Fetal Heartbeat' Abortion Restriction Declared Unconstitutional." CNN, January 23. Accessed September 22, 2019. https://www.cnn.com/2019/01/23/us/iowa-fetal-heartbeat-abortion-unconstitutional/index.html.

Levy, Gabrielle, and Alan Neuhauser. 2017. "Birth Control Mandate Narrowed, Religious Freedom Rules Expanded." *U.S. News & World Report*, October 6. Accessed September 10, 2020. https://www.usnews.com/news/national-news/articles/2017-10-06/trump-administration-narrows-birth-control-mandate-expand-religious-freedom-rules.

Leys, Tony. 2019. "Iowa's 'Fetal Heartbeat' Abortion Restriction Declared Unconstitutional." *USA Today*, January 23. Accessed September 22, 2019. https://www.usatoday.com/story/news/nation/2019/01/23/iowa-fetal-heartbeat-abortion-law-ruling/2655252002/.

Lipka, Michael. 2014. "Kaiser: Americans' Views of Hobby Lobby Ruling Are Evenly Divided." Pew Research Center, August 1. Accessed September 10, 2020. https://www.pewresearch.org/fact-tank/2014/08/01/kaiser-americans-views-of-hobby-lobby-ruling-are-evenly-divided/.

McCammon, Sarah. 2020. "State Officials Battle over Abortion during Medical Supply Shortage." NPR, March 27. Accessed June 1, 2020. https://www.npr.org/sections/coronavirus-live-updates/2020/03/27/822656455/state-officials-battle-over-abortion-during-medical-supply-shortage.

Mindock, Clark. 2019. "'The Point Is to Overturn *Roe v. Wade*': How a Quiet Republican Effort to Limit Abortion Rights Has Blown Up into a Full Scale Attack on Women's Rights." *Independent*, May 18. Accessed September 3, 2019. https://www.independent.co.uk/news/world/americas/us-politics/abortion-ban-republican-roe-v-wade-bill-law-gop-alabama-heartbeat-ohio-trump-kavanaugh-a8919431.html.

Montgomery, David. 2019. "Conquerers of the Courts." *Washington Post*, January 2. Accessed August 20, 2020. https://www.washingtonpost.com/news/magazine/wp/2019/01/02/feature/conquerors-of-the-courts/.

Neufeld, Jennie. 2018. "What the Polls Say about Americans, Abortion, and the Supreme Court." Vox, July 9. Accessed September 3, 2019. https://www.vox.com/2018/7/9/17525410/polls-abortion-roe-v-wade-supreme-court.

Norman, Jim. 2018. "Sixty-Two Percent View Planned Parenthood Favorably." Gallup, June 27. Accessed September 10, 2020. https://news.gallup.com/poll/236126/sixty-two-percent-view-planned-parenthood-favorably.aspx.

North, Anna. 2019. "While Some States Try to Ban Abortion, These States Are Expanding Access." Vox, June 20. Accessed September 22, 2019. https://www.vox.com/identities/2019/6/12/18662738/abortion-bill-illinois-maine-laws-new-york.

Obama, Barack. 2010. "Executive Order 13535—Ensuring Enforcement and Implementation of Abortion Restrictions in the Patient Protection and Affordable Care Act." American Presidency Project, March 24. Accessed September 22, 2019. https://www.presidency.ucsb.edu/documents/executive-order-13535-ensuring-enforcement-and-implementation-abortion-restrictions-the.

Ollstein, Alice Miranda. 2019a. "Planned Parenthood Pulls Out of Family Planning Program over Trump Abortion Rule." Politico, August 19. Accessed August 26, 2020. https://www.politico.com/story/2019/08/19/planned-parenthood-trump-administration-1468561.

Ollstein, Alice Miranda. 2019b. "Trump Abortion Rule Has Both Sides Digging In." Politico, February 22. Accessed August 4, 2019. https://www.politico.com/story/2019/02/22/trump-planned-parenthood-abortion-title-x-1204937.

Pear, Robert. 2012. "U.S. Clarifies Policy on Birth Control for Religious Groups." *New York Times*, March 16. Accessed September 10, 2020. https://www.nytimes.com/2012/03/17/health/policy/obama-administration-says-birth-control-mandate-applies-to-religious-groups-that-insure-themselves.html.

Pear, Robert. 2019. "Court Blocks Trump Administration Restrictions on Birth Control." *New York Times*, January 14. Accessed September 10, 2020. https://www.nytimes.com/2019/01/14/us/politics/court-trump-birth-control.html.

Pear, Robert, Rebecca Ruiz, and Laurie Goodstein. 2017. "Trump Administration Rolls Back Birth Control Mandate." *New York Times*, October 6. Accessed September 9, 2020. https://www.nytimes.com/2017/10/06/us/politics/trump-contraception-birth-control.html.

Pettus, Emily Wagster. 2019. "'Here We Go Again': Judge Blocks Mississippi Abortion Ban." Associated Press, May 24. Accessed September 22, 2019. https://www.apnews.com/9a5b239465744bde92ff0fdcfad4ef88.

Pew Research Center. 2019. "U.S. Public Continues to Favor Legal Abortion, Oppose Overturning *Roe v. Wade*." August 29. Accessed August 25, 2020. https://www.pewresearch.org/politics/2019/08/29/u-s-public-continues-to-favor-legal-abortion-oppose-overturning-roe-v-wade/#partisan-gap-in-views-of-legal-abortion-has-widened-in-recent-years.

Pilkington, Ed. 2019. "Female Democrats Rally around Planned Parenthood amid Abortion Rule Dispute." *The Guardian*, August 20. Accessed September 3, 2019. https://www.theguardian.com/us-news/2019/aug/19/planned-parenthood-title-x-withdraws-trump-rule.

Planned Parenthood. 2019. "Annual Report 2018–2019." Accessed October 30, 2020. https://www.plannedparenthood.org/uploads/filer_public/2e/da/2eda3f50-82aa-4ddb-acce-c2854c4ea80b/2018-2019_annual_report.pdf.

Planned Parenthood of Southeastern Pennsylvania v. Casey. 1992. 505 U.S. 833. June 29. Accessed September 22, 2019. https://www.law.cornell.edu/supremecourt/text/505/833.

Quinnipiac University Poll. 2017. "Use a Scalpel, Don't Amputate Obamacare, U.S. Voters Tell Quinnipiac University National Poll; Voters Oppose Fund Cut for Planned Parenthood 7-1." January 27. Accessed September 10, 2020. https://poll.qu.edu/connecticut/release-detail?ReleaseID=3660.

Rathke, Lisa. 2019. "Vermont Governor Signs Bill Protecting Abortion Rights." *The Columbian*, June 11. Accessed September 22, 2019. https://www.columbian.com/news/2019/jun/11/vermont-governor-signs-bill-protecting-abortion-rights/.

Republican National Committee. 2008. "2008 Republican Party Platform Online." Online by Gerhard Peters and John T. Woolley, the American Presidency Project. Accessed August 25, 2020. https://www.presidency.ucsb.edu/documents/2008-republican-party-platform.

Republican National Committee. 2016. "2016 Republican Party Platform Online." Online by Gerhard Peters and John T. Woolley, the American Presidency Project. Accessed August 25, 2020. https://www.presidency.ucsb.edu/documents/2016-republican-party-platform.

Roe et al. v. Wade, District Attorney of Dallas County. 410 US 113 (1973). Accessed August 26, 2020. https://cdn.loc.gov/service/ll/usrep/usrep410/usrep410113/usrep410113.pdf.

Russo, Amy. 2019. "Andrew Cuomo Signs Abortion Bill into Law, Codifying *Roe v. Wade*." HuffPost, January 23. Accessed September 22, 2019. https://www.huffpost.com/entry/andrew-cuomo-abortion-bill_n_5c480bebe4b0b66936751a47.

Saad, Lydia. 2020. "Dissatisfaction with U.S. Abortion Laws at New High." Gallup, January 22. Accessed June 30, 2020. https://news.gallup.com/poll/283916/dissatisfaction-abortion-laws-new-high.aspx.

Schoen, Johanna. 2015. *Abortion after* Roe. Chapel Hill: University of North Carolina Press.

Schor, Elana. 2020. "Democrats Diverge on Outreach to Anti-Abortion Swing Voters." Associated Press, February 18. Accessed June 30, 2020. https://apnews.com/f1bcf5ca695fdbb9214980727ebb22ca.

Smith, Chris, and John Boehner. 2011. "Cong. Smith, Speaker Boehner Hold Press Conference on New Pro-Life Legislation." January 21. Accessed September 22, 2019. https://chrissmith.house.gov/news/documentsingle.aspx?DocumentID=220960.

Smith, Kate. 2020. "Anti-Abortion Democrats Head into Super Tuesday without a Candidate to Support." CBS News, February 28. Accessed August 20, 2020. https://www.cbsnews.com/news/anti-abortion-democrats-head-into-super-tuesday-without-a-candidate-to-support/.

Sobel, Laurie, Amrutha Ramaswamy, Brittni Frederiksen, and Alina Salganicoff. 2020. "State Action to Limit Abortion Access during the COVID-19 Pandemic." Kaiser Family Foundation, August 10. Accessed August 25, 2020. https://www.kff.org/coronavirus-covid-19/issue-brief/state-action-to-limit-abortion-access-during-the-covid-19-pandemic/.

Sobel, Laurie, Alina Salganicoff, and Nisha Kurani. 2015. "Coverage of Contraceptive Services: A Review of Health Insurance Plans in Five States." Kaiser Family Foundation. Accessed September 9, 2020. https://www.kff.org/report-section/coverage-of-contraceptive-services-introduction/.

Solender, Andrew. 2020. "Planned Parenthood Endorses Biden after Pledging to Triple Election Spending in 2020 over 2016." *Forbes*, June 15. Accessed September 9, 2020. https://www.forbes.com/sites/andrewsolender/2020/06/15/planned-parenthood-endorses-biden-after-pledging-to-triple-election-spending-in-2020-over-2016/#77f73e23385f.

Stolberg, Sheryl Gay. 2020. "Democrats Block Abortion-Related Bills as Republicans Seek Election Advantage." *New York Times*, February 25. Accessed June 1, 2020. https://www.nytimes.com/2020/02/25/us/politics/democrats-abortion-bills-republicans.html.

Stracquarlursi, Veronica, and Chris Boyette. 2019. "Illinois and Nevada Approve Abortion Rights Bills That Remove Long-Standing Criminal Penalties." CNN, June 1. Accessed September 22, 2019. https://www.cnn.com/2019/06/01/politics/illinois-nevada-abortion-protections-bill/index.html.

Sundram, Arya. 2019. "Texas Passes Bill Banning Cities from Partnering with Planned Parenthood on Any Services." *Texas Tribune*, May 24. Accessed September 22, 2019. https://www.texastribune.org/2019/05/24/texas-abortion-bill-called-biggest-threat-planned-parenthood-passes/.

Tavernise, Sabrina, and Adeel Hassan. 2019. "Missouri Lawmakers Pass Bill Criminalizing Abortion at about 8 Weeks of Pregnancy." *New York Times*, May 17. Accessed September 22, 2019. https://www.nytimes.com/2019/05/17/us/missouri-abortion-law.html.

Thebault, Reis. 2019. "Another Red State Could Soon Pass an Abortion Ban. Only This Time a Democrat Will Sign It into Law." *Washington Post*, May 25. Accessed September 22, 2019. https://www.washingtonpost.com/nation/2019/05/25/another-red-state-could-soon-pass-an-abortion-ban-only-this-time-democrat-will-sign-it-into-law/.

Thorp, Frank, V. 2015. "Senate Democrats Block 20-Week Abortion Ban Bill." NBC News, September 22. Accessed August 26, 2020. https://www.nbcnews.com/news/us-news/senate-democrats-block-20-week-abortion-ban-bill-n431641.

U.S. Congress. Senate. 2014. "Protect Women's Health from Corporate Interference Act of 2014—Motion to Proceed." 113rd Cong., 2nd sess. *Congressional Record* 160, no. 111: S4528–S4534. Accessed September 10, 2020. https://www.congress.gov/113/crec/2014/07/16/modified/CREC-2014-07-16-pt1-PgS4528.htm.

U.S. Congress. Senate. 2015. "Restoring Americans' Healthcare Freedom Reconciliation Act of 2015." 114th Cong., 1st sess. *Congressional Record* 161, no. 175: S8326–S8357. Accessed September 10, 2020. https://www.congress.gov/114/crec/2015/12/03/modified/CREC-2015-12-03-pt1-PgS8326-2.htm.

U.S. Department of Health and Human Services. 2019. "Compliance with Statutory Program Integrity Requirements." 84 FR 7714 (March 4): 7714–7791. Accessed September 22, 2019. https://www.federalregister.gov/documents/2019/03/04/2019-03461/compliance-with-statutory-program-integrity-requirements.

Vermont General Assembly. 2019. "H.57. Bill as Introduced." Accessed September 22, 2019. https://legislature.vermont.gov/Documents/2020/Docs/BILLS/H-0057/H-0057%20As%20Introduced.pdf.

Wallace, Danielle. 2019. "Bernie Sanders Says He'd Back US Funding for Third World Abortions, Birth Control as Part of Climate Plan." Fox News, September 5. Accessed September 10, 2020. https://www.foxnews.com/politics/bernie-sanders-climate-change-abortion-birth-control-julian-castro-aoc-family-cycle.

Werner, Erica. 2018. "Senate Easily Defeats Measure to Defund Planned Parenthood." *Washington Post*, August 23. Accessed September 10, 2020. https://www.washingtonpost.com/politics/senate-easily-defeats-measure-to-defund-planned-parenthood/2018/08/23/7103b168-a726-11e8-97ce-cc9042272f07_story.html.

Westfall, David. 1982. "Beyond Abortion: The Potential Reach of a Human Life Amendment." *American Journal of Law and Medicine* 8, no. 2: 97–135. Accessed August 26, 2020. https://pubmed.ncbi.nlm.nih.gov/7148834/.

Williams, Timothy and Alan Blinder. 2019a. "Lawmakers Vote to Effectively Ban Abortion in Alabama." *New York Times*, May 14. Accessed September 22, 2019. https://www.nytimes.com/2019/05/14/us/abortion-law-alabama.html.

Williams, Timothy, and Alan Blinder. 2019b. "Mississippi Bans Abortions if Heartbeat Can Be Heard. Expect a Legal Fight." *New York Times*, March 21. Accessed September 22, 2019. https://www.nytimes.com/2019/03/21/us/abortion-laws-states.html.

Yetter, Deborah. 2018. "Federal Judge Strikes Down Kentucky Restriction on Abortion Clinics." *Louisville Courier-Journal*, September 28. Accessed September 22, 2019. https://www.courier-journal.com/story/news/2018/09/28/federal-judge-rules-challenge-regulations-ky-using-try-close-abortion-clinics/1069036001/.

Yetter, Deborah. 2020. "Gov. Beshear Vetoes Abortion Bill That Gives More Power over Clinics to Attorney General." *Louisville Courier-Journal*, April 24. Accessed June 1, 2020. https://www.courier-journal.com/story/news/politics/ky-legislature/2020/04/24/beshear-vetoes-abortion-bill-expands-power-attorney-general/5165325002/.

Index

About the Authors and Contributors

Authors

Robert B. Hackey, PhD, is a professor of health policy and management at Providence College. He is the author of *Cries of Crisis: Rethinking the Health Care Debate*, *The New Politics of State Health Policy*, and *Rethinking Health Policy: The New Politics of State Regulation*.

Todd M. Olszewski, PhD, is an associate professor of health policy and management at Providence College, where he also serves as associate director of the Center for Teaching Excellence. He was previously a Stetten Fellow in the History of the Biomedical Sciences at the National Institutes of Health.

Contributors

Morgan Bjarno, a 2019 graduate of the Department of Health Policy and Management at Providence College, is a health and benefits analyst at Willis Towers Watson.

Olivia Braga has a double major in biology and health policy and management from Providence College.

Anne Capozzoli earned a BS in health policy and management from Providence College in 2020. She is a systems analyst for UPMC in Pittsburgh, Pennsylvania, and is pursuing MS in health informatics at Chatham University.

Theresa Durkee earned a BS in health policy and management from Providence College in 2020. She is a benefits analyst at Boston Benefit Partners, LLC.

Bethany Evans earned a BS in health policy and management from Providence College in 2020. She is a research assistant at Brigham and Women's Hospital.

Anxhela Hoti graduated from Providence College in 2021 with a BS in health policy and management. She is a member service guide at Devoted Health.

Delaney Mayette, a 2020 graduate of the Health Policy and Management Program at Providence College, is pursuing an MHA degree at Virginia Commonwealth University.

Shannon McGonagle earned a BS in health policy and management from Providence College in 2019. She is a benefits analyst at Boston Benefit Partners, LLC.

Amanda McGrath, a 2019 graduate in health policy and management from Providence College, is a clinical data manager at ECOG-ACRIN Cancer Research Group.

Maureen Murphy is a student majoring in health science at Northeastern University.

Shannon Rowe graduated from Providence College in 2020 with a BS in health policy and management. She is a patient experience representative at Boston Children's Hospital.

Rose Shelley graduated from Providence College in 2019 with a BS in health policy and management. She is a reputation and risk management strategist for Syneos Health.

Keith Vieira Jr., earned a BA in mathematics and a BS in health policy and management from Providence College in 2021.

Erin Walsh, a 2020 graduate of the Health Policy and Management Program at Providence College, is a clinical data associate at ECOG-ACRIN Cancer Research Group.